Third Edition

RESEARCH DESIGN AND EVALUATION IN SPEECH-LANGUAGE PATHOLOGY AND AUDIOLOGY

Asking and Answering Questions

FRANKLIN H. SILVERMAN
Marquette University
Medical College of Wisconsin

Prentice Hall, Englewood Cliffs, New Jersey 07632

Library of Congress Cataloging-in-Publication Data

SILVERMAN, FRANKLIN H., [date]
  Research design and evaluation in speech-language pathology and
  audiology : Asking and answering questions / Franklin H. Silverman.
  —3rd ed.
    p. cm.
  Includes bibliographical references and index.
  ISBN 0-13-755448-6
  1. Speech disorders—Research—Methodology. 2. Language
  disorders—Research—Methodology. 3. Audiology—Research—
  Methodology. I. Title.
    [DNLM: 1. Hearing Disorders. 2. Language Disorders. 3. Research—
  methods. 4. Speech Disorders. WM 475 S587r]
  RC423.S519 1993
  616.85'5'0072—dc20
  DNLM/DLC
  for Library of Congress   91-40158

Acquisitions editor: *Carol Wada*
Editorial/production supervision and interior design: *Edie Riker*
Cover design: *Carol Ceraldi*
Prepress buyer: *Kelly Behr*
Manufacturing buyer: *Mary Ann Gloriande*

To Professor Dean E. Williams of the University of Iowa
for facilitating my development
as both a researcher and a research methodologist

Printed in the United States of America

10 9 8 7 6 5 4 3 2

ISBN   0-13-755448-6

Prentice-Hall International (UK) Limited, *London*
Prentice-Hall of Australia Pty. Limited, *Sydney*
Prentice-Hall Canada Inc., *Toronto*
Prentice-Hall Hispanoamericana, S.A., *Mexico*
Prentice-Hall of India Private Limited, *New Delhi*
Prentice-Hall of Japan, Inc., *Tokyo*
Simon & Schuster Asia Pte. Ltd., *Singapore*
Editora Prentice-Hall do Brasil, Ltda., *Rio de Janeiro*

Contents

Preface

In this Third Edition of *Research Design and Evaluation in Speech-Language Pathology and Audiology*, I have sought not only to bring the text up to date but to strengthen it in several ways.

There are two new chapters. The first, Chapter 4, provides information needed for doing literature searches with abstracts journals and online, interactive computer-based information retrieval systems (such as Medline). The second, Chapter 14, deals with legal and ethical restrictions and obligations when doing clinical research.

The material on single subject research has been expanded considerably (see Chapter 6). Also, new material has been added to Chapter 8 on strategies for generating qualitative and quantitative data. In addition, there is greater emphasis on the use of computers for data analysis in Chapter 9 and 10 and in Appendix A. With regard to the latter, the commands required for doing some of the exercises with the MINITAB Statistical Software are presented. This program, which was developed in 1972 at Pennsylvania State University to help teach introductory courses in statistics, is utilized in such courses at more than 1500 colleges and universities and is available for almost all mainframes and minicomputers as well as Macintosh and IBM-compatible microcomputers. These exercises, of course, can be done with other statistical software packages.

It is impossible to give credit to all of the sources from which the concepts presented in this book have been drawn. The book is the result of years of reading and thousands of hours of conversation with students and colleagues in the areas of communicative disorders and research methodology. Thus, I often cannot credit this or that concept to a specific person, but I can say thank you to all who have helped, particularly my graduate students at Marquette University whose questions and criticisms through the years have helped me to clarify my own ideas. Some special thanks are due to Wendy Wolfgram for keyboarding the entire Second Edition (with practically no typos) to enable me to use it as a starting point for this revision.

I am pleased by reports that the first two editions of the text have helped to break down the dichotomy in the minds of many speech-language pathologists and audiologists between clinical work and clinical research. I am also pleased by reports that it has provided many with information needed to become informed consumers and producers of research. Hopefully, the information they gain from functioning as a clinician-investigator will help them fulfill the ASHA ethical injunction "to hold paramount the welfare of persons served professionally."

Franklin H. Silverman

1

Need for Research in Speech-Language Pathology and Audiology

This chapter demonstrates the relevance of pure (or basic) and applied research to evaluation and therapy (clinical process) in speech-language pathology and audiology. *Pure research* is intended to increase our understanding of the etiology (that is, the predisposing, precipitating, and maintaining causes) of communicative disorders. *Applied research* is intended to increase our understanding of how to prevent the development of, or modify behaviors contributing to, communicative disorders. Some research serves both functions: it provides data relevant to the etiology of communicative disorders as well as to their diagnosis, prevention, or treatment.

The term *research* in this book refers to the processes underlying the *asking and answering* of questions as well as to the "answers" that can be abstracted from the observations provided by such processes. In a sense, the overall objective of this book is to clarify and elaborate upon this definition of research as it applies to clinical process in speech-language pathology and audiology.

You, the reader of this book, have to make some assumption(s) about the relevance of research to your activities before deciding how much to invest in acquiring a knowledge of research methodology. The amount you are willing to invest to attain a goal is at least partially a function of the return you anticipate. If you expect a substantial return, you usually will be willing to invest more than if you anticipate little, if any, return. The stronger your belief that learning certain material will directly benefit you, the more time and energy you are likely to invest in doing so. Also, the stronger your belief that learning certain material will benefit you, the more willing you are likely to be to tackle material you expect to be difficult, such as statistical and research design concepts. And the more willing you are to tackle such material and the more time and energy you devote to doing so, the more likely you are to master it. Some persons who have difficulty understanding statistical and research design concepts do *not* appear to experience it because of a lack of ability, but because they are not convinced that learning such concepts will be helpful to them in the "real world" and, hence, they do not invest the time and energy necessary to grasp them. One of my goals in this chapter and the one that follows is to strengthen your belief in the relevance of research and research design concepts to your functioning as a clinician.

QUESTIONING AND CLINICAL EFFECTIVENESS

We will begin our discussion of the relevance of research to clinical process in speech-language pathology and audiology with the following premise: To be even minimally effective, a clinician must be able to at least partially answer certain questions. These questions include:

1. Is the communicative behavior of the child or adult whom I am evaluating "within normal limits"?
2. If his or her communicative behavior is not "within normal limits," what is the reason?
3. How can his or her communicative behavior be modified to bring it "within normal limits," or as close as possible to this goal?

If we are not aware of "normal limits" for the various attributes of speech, language, and hearing, we will be unable to determine with an acceptable degree of accuracy whether a child or adult (particularly a child) has a communicative disorder. We will tend to make one or both of the following errors more often than we should: (1) classifying a person whose communicative behavior is "within normal limits" as having a communicative disorder, or (2) classifying a person who has a communicative disorder as having communicative behavior "within normal limits." We may, for example, classify a three-year-old who has an IQ of approximately 100 and consistently substitutes /w/ for /r/ as not being "within normal limits." Also, we might classify a three-year-old who is "effortlessly" repeating some syllables as beginning to stutter. To answer questions concerning the normality of a three-year-old's communicative behavior, we must have information concerning the communicative behavior of "normal" three-year-olds. That is, we must have access to relevant normative data.

If the answer to the first question is no (that is, if we do not judge the person's communicative behavior to be "within normal limits"), we then attempt to answer the second, or "why," question. To answer this question, we have to be able to specify the possible causes for the deviation or deviations we have observed. We need this information to perform a differential diagnosis—to rule in and rule out possible causes systematically. We also need this information to plan therapy. For a therapy strategy to have maximum probability of success, it should be based upon, or derived from, our assumption or assumptions about why a client's communicative behavior is not "within normal limits" (Williams, 1968).

Once we have at least partially established the reason or reasons for a client's communicative behavior not being "within normal limits," we then develop an intervention strategy that will hopefully either bring it "within normal limits" or as close as possible to the goal. To develop such a strategy, or to answer the "how" question, we need information concerning the relative effectiveness of the various strategies that could be used. For each possible strategy, we also need related information, including negative side effects and susceptibility to relapse. Such information provides guidelines for answering the "how" question and thereby helps to maximize the probability of achieving the therapy goal or goals.

NEED FOR SYSTEMATIC OBSERVATION IN ANSWERING QUESTIONS

How do we go about answering questions such as the three previously discussed so that the probability of a correct answer is maximized? Answering questions in this manner requires the type of data that results from systematic observation. The term *data* as used here refers to numerical and verbal descriptions of attributes of events. Attributes of the event "speech," for example, would include "voice quality" and "amount of syllable repetition." And attributes of the event "listening" would include "sound discrimination ability" and "level of comprehension." Numerical descriptions of attributes of events are referred to as *quantitative* and verbal as *qualitative.*

Systematic observation is a process that permits us to describe individual attributes of events. We decide in advance which attributes of which events we wish to describe and then for each attribute devise a "filter" that will permit us to make the desired observations. The filter makes each target attribute—each attribute we seek to describe—stand out sufficiently from the others so that it can be described reliably. The filter, then, enhances the figure-background relationship (the target attribute being the figure and the other attributes the background). The filter may include instrumentation to enhance our ability to restrict our observational processes, or it may consist solely of a "set" we give ourselves to do so. Speech-language pathologists usually give themselves such a set during the administration of a picture articulation test, since they pay most attention to the particular speech sound each picture was included to elicit. This sound would be the figure (i.e., the target attribute); the other sounds in the word would be the background. Instrumentation used by speech-language pathologists and audiologists for this purpose is described in Chapter 8.

Systematic observation maximizes the probability that the data used to answer questions will yield correct answers by maximizing the probability that they will possess adequate validity and reliability for the purpose. By adequate *validity* in this context, we mean that the filter used to observe and describe a particular attribute of a particular event actually permits us to observe and describe that attribute of that event. If we wished, for example, to determine how frequently a child produced a lateral /s/ (attribute) during conversational speech (event), having observers listen to tape recordings of the child's conversational speech and identifying instances of lateral /s/ on typescripts of the recordings should yield data which possess adequate validity for this purpose.

By maximizing the probability that the data used to answer a question will possess adequate *reliability*, we mean that the filter used to observe and describe an attribute of an event permits this to be done with a *sufficient level of accuracy*—that is, a level that permits the minimum desired degree of confidence in the correctness of the answer. The less distortion (or error) introduced by the filter, the more reliable will be the resulting data. As indicated in the previous paragraph, a valid method for estimating how frequently a child produced a lateral /s/ probably would be to tape record his conversational speech and have trained listeners indicate instances of lateral /s/ on a typescript of the recording. For this methodology to be adequately reliable as well as valid, the tape recordings would have to be of sufficiently high quality that instances of lateral /s/ could be identified from them with minimal error.

Systematic observation, in addition to maximizing the probability that the data used to answer a question will possess adequate levels of validity and reliability for the purpose, also provides a methodology for determining whether this goal has been achieved. In fact, this methodology permits us to estimate the validity and reliability levels of a set of data. These constructs will be discussed further in Chapter 11.

SATISFYING THE NEED FOR SYSTEMATIC OBSERVATION

The preceding section discussed why systematic observation could be expected to yield the type of data that maximizes the probability of correct answers to questions. We will now consider how pure and applied research can satisfy, at least partially, the need for systematic observation.

Systematic observation is used in both pure and applied research. It is, in fact, a component (as will be shown in Chapter 3) of the scientific method that underlies almost all research. For this reason, data yielded by both types of research can be used by speech-language pathologists and audiologists to answer questions of professional interest, including those on clinical process.

The previous section discussed three questions that a clinician needs to be able to answer to function effectively. *How can data from pure and applied research help to maximize the probability of a correct answer to each question?*

The first of these questions was: Is the communicative behavior of the child or adult whom I am evaluating "within normal limits"? To maximize the probability of a correct answer, a clinician needs *normative data*—data that help to define "normal limits" for each attribute of communicative behavior being evaluated. Such data have been reported for a number of attributes of communicative behavior in research papers appearing in such journals as the *American Journal of Audiology: A Journal of Clinical Practice*, the *American Journal of Speech-Language Pathology: A Journal of Clinical Practice*, the *Journal of Speech and Hearing Disorders*, the *Journal of Speech and Hearing Research*, and *Language, Speech, and Hearing Services in Schools*.

The second question was: If the client's communicative behavior is not "within normal limits," what is the reason? To answer this question, we need to know the possible causes for each deviation from "normal limits" a client exhibits. Considerable relevant research-based information has appeared in the *American Journal of Audiology: A Journal of Clinical Practice*, the *American Journal of Speech-Language Pathology: A Journal of Clinical Practice*, the *Journal of Speech and Hearing Disorders*, the *Journal of Speech and Hearing Research*, and *Language, Speech, and Hearing Services in Schools*. Such research-based information, incidentally, is the source of lists of possible causes of articulation disorders, voice disorders, fluency disorders, children's language disorders, hearing loss, and other communicative disorders that appear in speech-language pathology and audiology textbooks.

The final question was: How can the client's communicative behavior be modified to bring it "within normal limits," or as close as possible to this goal? To answer this question, we need information concerning the possible impacts of each intervention strategy we are considering, on the client in general and his or her communicative behavior in particular. We are not only interested in information about the possible positive effects of an intervention strategy on a client's communicative disorder, but also in information about possible negative side effects and the permanence of changes in a client's communicative behavior resulting from its use. Relevant data for some therapy approaches used to treat communicative disorders have been reported in such journals as the *American Journal of Audiology: A Journal of Clinical Practice*, the *American Journal of Speech-Language Pathology: A Journal of Clinical Practice*, the *Journal of Speech and Hearing Disorders*, and *Language, Speech, and Hearing Services in Schools*. There is a need for considerably more therapy outcome research. This need is explored further in Chapters 2 and 13.

QUESTIONS AND ANSWERS

To demonstrate the relevance of research to clinical decision making in speech-language pathology and audiology, we have argued that a clinician has to be able to answer certain questions to be even minimally effective. In this section we will indicate more specifically how research can provide the data needed to maximize the probability of correct answers to questions concerning evaluation and therapy. We will pose five questions a clinician might need to answer and indicate how data published in several *randomly* selected issues of the *Journal of Speech and Hearing Research* could provide at least a partial answer to each question. The format used for each question will be: (1) a statement of the question, (2) a reference for the data, (3) a description of the observational procedures, (4) a summary of the observations made (i.e., data) that are relevant to answering the question, and (5) a tentative answer to the question. In addition to demonstrating the relevance of research to clinical decision making, this presentation is also intended as an informal introduction to the structure of a research report.

1. ARE THE EARPHONES I USE FOR MY CLINICAL AUDIOLOGICAL EVALUATION LIKELY ENOUGH TO BECOME CONTAMINATED TO WARRANT THE EXPENSE OF ROUTINE DECONTAMINATION?

    Data Source. Talbott, R. E. (1969). Bacteriology of earphone contamination. *Journal of Speech and Hearing Research,* 12, 326–329.

    Observational Procedure. Bacterial samples of earphone earcushions used for clinical audiological evaluations in a hospital setting were examined for the presence of three pathogenic microorganisms that have been associated with otitis media and otitis externa.

    Observations Made. Staphylococcus aureus, a pathogenic microorganism, was recovered "in great quantities" from all earcushions sampled.

    Tentative Answer to Question. Earphones used for clinical audiological evaluations appear likely enough to become contaminated by pathogenic microorganisms to warrant the expense of routine decontamination.

    Remarks. A clinician also could obtain data to answer this question through systematic observations of his or her own earphones.

2. CAN SAMPLES OF CONVERSATIONAL SPEECH THAT ARE SUFFICIENTLY REPRESENTATIVE TO BE USEFUL FOR ASSESSING A FOUR-YEAR-OLD CHILD'S PRAGMATIC ABILITY BE ELICITED IN A PRESCHOOL PLAYROOM ENVIRONMENT?

    Data Source. Schober-Peterson, D., and Johnson, C. J. (1989). Conversational topics of four-year-olds. *Journal of Speech and Hearing Research,* 32, 857–870.

    Observational Procedure. Ten dyads (pairs) of four-year-old children were videotaped during play in a typical preschool playroom environment. Ten-minute samples were analyzed according to a number of topic-dependent measures.

    Observations Made. All dyads evidenced some lengthy topics (13–91 utterances). Longer topics were characterized by three text-level functions: enacting scenarios, describing, and problem solving.

Tentative Answer to Question. Samples of conversation that are likely to have adequate generality for revealing a four-year-old's pragmatic ability can be obtained by recording him or her during play in a preschool playroom setting.

3. SHOULD I ROUTINELY EVALUATE CHILDREN WHO HAVE RELATIVELY SEVERE ARTICULATION PROBLEMS FOR THE POSSIBILITY THAT THEY ARE AVOIDING TALKING?

Data Source. Shriner, T. H., Holloway, M. S., and Daniloff, R. G. (1969). The relationship between articulation defects and syntax in speech defective children. *Journal of Speech and Hearing Research, 12,* 319–325.

Observational Procedure. Each of 30 first- through third-grade children diagnosed by a speech clinician as having "severe problems with articulation" and 30 matched controls who had no speech problems told a story about a picture. Average sentence length (i.e., total number of words per response) was computed for each child.

Observations Made. The mean number of words per response was lower for the speech defective children.

Tentative Answer to Question. Since these data suggest that at least some children who have relatively severe articulation problems are apt to talk less than their peers, such children should be routinely evaluated for the possibility that they are avoiding talking.

4. WHAT FACTORS SHOULD I CONSIDER WHEN MAKING A PROGNOSIS FOR LANGUAGE RECOVERY FOLLOWING A STROKE?

Data Source. Holland, A. L., Greenhouse, J. B., Fromm, D., and Swingell, C. S. (1989). Predictors of language restitution following stroke: A multivariate analysis. *Journal of Speech and Hearing Research, 32,* 332–338.

Observational Procedure. A consecutive sample of 50 language impaired patients was evaluated prospectively during the first three to four months following a unilateral left- or right-hemisphere stroke with regard to the relative importance of eight variables on the likelihood of language recovery.

Observations Made. The variables that were found to be most strongly associated with language recovery were age (favoring younger patients) and length of hospital stay (favoring shorter stays). Gender (favoring males), type of stroke (favoring hemorrhages), and site of lesion (favoring right) also appeared to influence language recovery, but not as strongly as age and length of hospital stay. Neither race nor history of previous stroke appeared to influence language recovery.

Tentative Answer to Question. These data suggest that the age of the patient is probably the best single predictor of language recovery following stroke. If the length of the patient's hospital stay was not influenced by financial (insurance) considerations, this also could be a good predictor.

5. CAN A COCHLEAR IMPLANT INTERFACED WITH A WEARABLE SPEECH PROCESSING DEVICE ASSIST A DEAF PERSON IN UNDERSTANDING SPEECH?

Data Source. Dowell, R. C., Martin, L. F. A., Tong, Y. C., Clark, G. M., Seligman, P. M., and Patrick, J. F. (1982). A 12-consonant confusion study of a multiple-channel cochlear implant patient. *Journal of Speech and Hearing Research, 25,* 509–516.

Observation Procedure. A 49-year-old man with total bilateral deafness who had been fitted with a cochlear implant and a wearable speech processing device was asked to identify 12 consonant sounds (in a VCV context) spoken by a male and a female speaker. He could not see the speakers' faces. The percentage of the consonants that were correctly identified was determined.

Observations Made. The subject correctly identified 48 percent of the consonants.

Tentative Answer to Question. Judging by the fact that this subject was able to understand almost half of the consonant sounds, it would appear that a cochlear implant interfaced with a wearable speech processing device can significantly assist *some* deaf persons in understanding speech. More subjects, of course, would have to be tested before a reliable estimate could be made of the percentage of deaf persons who would be likely to benefit significantly from such an approach.

If you would like an additional demonstration of how research can provide the data needed to answer questions concerning clinical process, I would recommend that you read two papers (Jerger and Speaks, 1967; Lilly, Sherman, Compton, Fisher, and Carney, 1968) in which the authors attempted to indicate the clinical relevance of the data reported in two volumes of the *Journal of Speech and Hearing Research.* Though relatively old, they illustrate this well.

HAS THE NEED BEEN MET?

This chapter stressed the fact that existing research can provide data helpful in answering questions concerning clinical process. This was not meant to imply that the need for such data has been met. To the contrary, more such data are needed (The Task Force on Research, 1989). This need is, incidentally, one of the main reasons for my arguing in the next chapter that clinicians should be producers as well as consumers of research.

EXERCISES AND DISCUSSION TOPICS

1. Select any single issue of the *Journal of Speech and Hearing Research.* Formulate three questions a clinician might want to answer that could be at least partially answered using data reported in this issue. For each indicate the data source (i.e., the title of the paper) and summarize the observational procedures used and the observations made. Then indicate the tentative answer to each question. Five examples of this type of analysis are included in the chapter.

2. The need for systematic observation in answering research questions is explored in this chapter. Discuss why systematic observation also is needed for answering *clinical* questions, particularly those that clinicians attempt to answer when evaluating clients.

3. Suppose that there would be no further research on communicative disorders. What impacts would this have on clinical practice in speech-language pathology and audiology?

4. Select a paper from the *Journal of Speech and Hearing Research* or *Language, Speech, and Hearing Services in Schools* in which a therapy approach is described. Show how pure and applied research contributed to the development of the approach, using the studies cited in the paper.

5. You are a research audiologist working for a hearing aid manufacturer. Your employer has developed a new type of hearing aid and wants you to do research to evaluate its impacts on hard-of-hearing persons. What research questions might you attempt to answer to accomplish this objective?

2

Research
and the
Clinician

The previous chapter dealt with the need for research in speech-language pathology and audiology to answer questions relating to clinical practice. This chapter will present the need for clinicians to be able *both* to evaluate answers to such questions and to answer them through research. Specifically, we will argue that it is important for clinicians to function as both consumers and producers of research. Both roles require a knowledge of research methodology. It is used in the first for *evaluating* research and in the second for both *evaluating and designing* research.

THE CONSUMER ROLE

All speech-language pathologists and audiologists are consumers of research. They read research reports in professional journals and utilize information presented in them in their clinical practice. They need to understand research methodology (particularly that aspect dealing with descriptive and inferential statistics) to *evaluate* the information presented in them. Specifically, they need it to determine whether the data reported possess levels of validity, reliability, and generality that are adequate for them to be utilized clinically. Data reported in professional journals may not possess levels of one or more of these that would be adequate for this purpose. The reasons are discussed in Chapter 11.

THE PRODUCER, OR CLINICIAN-INVESTIGATOR, ROLE

The term *clinician-investigator* will be used in this book to designate a speech-language pathologist or audiologist who functions both as a clinician and a clinical investigator, or researcher. A hyphen was inserted between "clinician" and "investigator" to indicate that the two roles are not independent but interdependent. Thus, being a clinician would probably influence the kinds of research questions an investigator would ask, and being an investigator would probably influence a clinician's approach to problem solving in diagnosis and therapy. Also, a speech-language pathologist or audiologist might perform both functions simultaneously. That is, he or she might gather clinical research data while performing clinical functions (diagnosis and therapy). The individual clinical case study that utilizes data gathered as part of diagnosis or therapy, or both, illustrates this combined function (Bromley, 1986). The term *clinician-investigator*, incidentally, was derived from *teacher-investigator*, a term used in some colleges and universities to designate the dual interrelated roles of a professor—teaching and research.

Why should a clinician be a clinician-investigator? One of the most compelling reasons is to function in a manner that is consistent with the Code of Ethics of the American Speech-Language-Hearing Association. The current (1991) revision of the Code states that "individuals shall evaluate services rendered to determine effectiveness." Thus, for clinicians to function ethically they *must* systematically evaluate the impacts of the services they render. And to be able to do so they *must* acquire a knowledge of clinical research methodology.

There are a number of benefits in addition to satisfying the requirements of the ASHA Ethical Code that a clinician can derive from functioning as a clinician-investigator. The following discussion suggests several of them. The order in which they are discussed is not intended to reflect their relative importance.

First of all, functioning as a clinician-investigator would probably make one's job more stimulating, less routine, and would probably increase the possibilities for positive reinforcement. In addition to feeling successful at clinical activities, the clinician-investigator would have a second potential source of reinforcement—his or her research activities. This reinforcement could arise from any of the following factors: the feeling of accomplishment that comes from formulating a research question (or questions) and making the necessary observations to answer it (or them) at least partially; reporting the results of research to professional colleagues on the program of a professional meeting (that of a state speech and hearing association or the American Speech-Language-Hearing Association) or in a professional journal; and knowing that your professional efforts can help not only your own clients but also those of other speech-language pathologists and audiologists. Thus, communicating your clinical knowledge and experience with the communicatively handicapped can spread the benefits to others.

Functioning as a clinician-investigator also would help you to satisfy your employer's requirements for *accountability* (Olswang, 1990). Almost all speech-language pathologists and audiologists are required by their employers to document the impacts of their therapy programs on their clients. Incidentally, for speech-language pathologists employed in the public schools such documentation is mandated by Public Law 94–142.

Next, functioning as a clinician-investigator could probably help you become a more effective clinician, for several reasons. First, the dual role could provide answers to questions relevant to managing your own caseload. For example, it could help you to determine whether a therapy approach you are using is effective and whether, therefore, you should continue to use it. Or it could help you to determine whether a newer therapy approach is more effective than one you are currently using and, therefore, whether you should adopt the newer approach. It could also help you to establish whether your diagnostic procedures are adequately reliable and to provide normative data for diagnostic procedures you use that are not standardized on the specific populations in your caseload. Finally, it could provide information about the effectiveness of new clinical programs that could be useful when you are deciding whether to continue them.

Functioning as a clinician-investigator could improve effectiveness by helping to develop a more "scientific" approach to clinical decision making. The problem-solving approach based on the scientific method that is essential for functioning as an investigator is also desirable for functioning as a clinician. This approach has several aspects, including; (1) stating goals, or objectives, clearly; (2) asking questions that are "answerable" and stating hypotheses that are "testable"; (3) being systematic in making observations to answer questions and test hypotheses; and (4) being aware of the *tentative* nature of answers and hypotheses.

The need for clinical goals and objectives to be stated clearly has been discussed by a number of authors (e.g., Johnson, 1946; Silverman, 1984; Williams, 1968). Obviously, if a clinical objective or goal were not clearly stated, a clinician could never be reasonably certain whether or not it had been achieved. This situation probably would not be positively reinforcing for either client or clinician.

Another clinically relevant aspect of this approach is asking questions that are "answerable" and stating hypotheses that are "testable." Rather than asking, for example, whether a given therapy approach has been effective, you would ask whether it resulted in certain behavioral changes. (The reason why the second question would be more "answerable" than the first will be discussed in Chapter 5). Also, rather than hypothesizing that a child is slow in learning to talk because he is "emotionally disturbed," you would define operationally what you meant by being emotionally disturbed. This definition would suggest the diagnostic procedures you would need to test your hypothesis.

A third aspect is being systematic in making observations to answer questions and test hypotheses. The considerations described in Chapter 13 for designing research to evaluate the effects of therapies, for example, are relevant *clinically* for making observations to evaluate the effects of therapies you are using with clients. That is, the approaches used to answer systematically clinical questions for both clinical and research purposes are identical. The approaches used for both for making observations to "test" clinically relevant hypotheses are also identical. There should be no difference, therefore, in the way you would go about answering clinically relevant questions or testing clinically relevant hypotheses for clinical and research purposes. This similarity in approach is not surprising since no sharp line of demarcation exists between clinical work and clinical research. Overlap is particularly evident with regard to the individual case study and other clinical research that utilizes a single subject design (e.g., Barlow and Hersen, 1984; Connell and Thompson, 1986; Kazdin, 1982; Kearns, 1986; McReynolds and Kearns, 1983; McReynolds and Thompson, 1986; Tawney and Gast, 1984).

The final aspect of the scientific approach, being aware of the *tentative* nature of answers and hypotheses, is one of the most important, because it indicates that no answer to a question or test of a hypothesis is *final*. As new information becomes available, hypotheses that appeared viable may no longer appear so. The answer to every question and the viability of every hypothesis must therefore be regarded as tentative. Both have implicit qualifiers attached. For answers to questions, the implicit qualifier would be: "With the information I currently have available, the answer to the question is . . ." And for statements concerning the viability of hypotheses, the implicit qualifier would be: "Judging by the information I currently have available, the hypothesis seems viable."

The tentative nature of answers and hypotheses is due at least partially to the fact that observations are never complete. In other words, "the data are never all in." It is more appropriate to conclude, therefore, that available research *suggest* a therapy is effective, rather than available data *prove* a therapy is effective. This concept is discussed further in Chapter 3.

If clinicians functioned as clinician-investigators, furthermore, they would provide data needed for answering questions on diagnosis and therapy. The answers to many questions sought by clinicians require observations that can be made at least as validly and efficiently in the clinic as in the laboratory. If you wished to evaluate, for example, a therapy approach intended for use in a school setting, it probably would make most sense for you to evaluate it in a school setting. One reason is that the setting in which therapy is done may place constraints upon what can be done. Thus, a therapy approach that is effective but requires a child to be seen five days a week for an hour a day would not be practical in a typical school setting. Also, data on the long-term effects of therapies probably can be gathered as validly, and more efficiently, in a clinical setting as it can in a laboratory setting. Additionally, the populations that must be observed to answer certain clinical questions may be more available to an investigator who works in a setting where such cases are seen for therapy than to one who is not employed in such a setting.

Finally, the data necessary to answer many clinically relevant questions can be gathered over a period of time as a part of diagnosis and therapy. Some of the best data we have on the symptomatology, etiology, diagnosis, and treatment of communicative disorders have come from this source. One example is the data on psychogenic stuttering of adult onset reported by Roth, Aronson, and Davis, Jr. (1989).

A clinician often is in a better position to make the observation needed to answer questions of clinical interest than is an investigator not actively engaged in clinical work. As previously mentioned, a clinician sometimes can make and record such observations within the context of his or her clinical work. In fact, the observations a clinician makes and records during diagnosis and therapy may be used to answer clinically relevant questions. It is necessary, though, that these observations be made in such a way that they possess relatively high levels of validity and reliability. This, incidentally, would also be a requirement for making such observations for clinical purposes. Observations that are not adequately reliable and valid would not be particularly useful for these purposes, either.

A clinician may also be able to make the observations needed to answer certain questions more reliably than an investigator not actively engaged in clinical work because of his or her clinical background and experience. This would be especially likely, for example, if the observations were of performance on clinical diagnostic tests. An experienced administrator's and interpreter's observations of performance on a diagnostic test probably would be more reliable than those of an investigator who is not experienced with the test, particularly one who did not administer or interpret it prior to doing so for a research project.

A clinician-investigator would also probably be better able both to evaluate therapies and to design research for this purpose than would an investigator not actively engaged in clinical work. This is especially likely to be true if the research involves experimental therapy and the design calls for the investigator to serve as clinician. An experienced clinician probably would do a better job administering an experimental therapy than an inexperienced one would. Additionally, an experienced clinician would probably be more aware of the "reality" factors which have to be considered when designing clinical research, particularly those introduced by the environment in which the data are being gathered. It may not be realistic, for example, to expect a classroom teacher to consistently reinforce "target" behaviors in a specified manner.

Thus far we have argued that: (1) many questions to which clinicians seek answers require observations that are at least as validly made in the clinic as in the laboratory, and (2) a clinician may be in a better position to make the observations necessary to answer such questions than an investigator not actively engaged in clinical work. Hopefully, we have demonstrated why a speech-language pathologist or audiologist would have the *possibility* of functioning as a clinician-investigator. Is there a *need*, however, for speech-language pathologists and audiologists to function in this manner? We believe such a need exists for several reasons, including the following:

1. He or she may be in the best position to make the observations necessary to answer clinically relevant questions, particularly those related to diagnosis and therapy. There are several reasons why the clinician-investigator might be in an advantageous position to answer such questions, including: (a) the setting in which he or she works, (b) the populations in his or her caseload, (c) his or her background and experience, (d) the availability of equipment and facilities for making the necessary observations, (e) the availability of collaborators from other disciplines, (f) the availability of an existing research program as a part of which the desired observations could be made, and (g) the availability of consultants and other supportive research personnel. The first three reasons were discussed earlier in the chapter; let us briefly examine the others here.

A speech-language pathologist or audiologist may be in an excellent position to make the observations necessary to answer certain questions of clinical interest because of available facilities that are unique or not generally available. An audiologist, for example, may have testing instrumentation or facilities that are unavailable in most audiological settings because of their cost or relatively limited usefulness. A speech-language pathologist may have one or more instruments for behavior modification, augmentative communication, or diagnostic testing that are not available in most clinics. If a speech-language pathologist or audiologist is able to exploit such facilities or instrumentation, he or she may be in a unique position to gather data necessary to answer questions of clinical importance.

A speech-language pathologist or audiologist may also have the opportunity to collaborate with investigators in other disciplines. A speech-language pathologist might collaborate with an otolaryngologist to assess the effects of a therapy on vocal nodules, or with a reading specialist to determine the effect of articulation errors on reading ability. An audiologist might collaborate with a microbiologist to determine if audiometer earphones are likely to contain pathogenic microorganisms. Again, if a speech-language pathologist or audiologist "exploits" opportunities for interdisciplinary research, he or she may be able to make observations necessary for answering questions that are significant clinically.

Another opportunity for a speech-language pathologist or audiologist to gather clinically relevant data is to become involved with an ongoing research program, especially an interdisciplinary one. If a clinician is working in a setting where research is being conducted in a related area such as psychology, learning disabilities, physical therapy, occupational therapy, rehabilitation counseling, social work, medicine, or dentistry, he or she may be able to gather clinically relevant data on communicative disorders by participating in the research program. In fact, by becoming involved when such a program is being planned, the clinician may be able to arrange for relevant data on communicative disorders to be gathered at the same time subjects are being seen by the other discipline or disciplines involved. To illustrate how this combining of interests can be accomplished, in the late 1950s a group of audiologists at a Veteran's Administration Outpatient Center was able to gather data on the hearing of men well past the age of 70 by arranging to do an audiometric evaluation on each of a group of Spanish-American War veterans being seen at the Center for other reasons. In this way speech pathologists and audiologists can take advantage of available opportunities to gather the data they need to answer clinically relevant questions.

The final factor to consider is the availability of consultants and supportive research personnel. Included here would be persons with expertise in statistics and electronics. When such persons are available, a clinician with clinically relevant questions that require expertise in these areas can utilize the opportunity.

2. Much of the needed clinical research probably will not be done unless more clinicians are willing to function as clinician-investigators. In the first place, investigators who are not actively involved in clinical work are unlikely to be as *aware* as those who are of at least some clinically relevant questions that need to be answered. This is particularly true for practical questions concerning clinical program procedure. Such questions might deal with the effectiveness of paraprofessionals in various roles in speech, language, and hearing habilitation and rehabilitation, or with the efficacy of pediatrician referral for identifying children younger than three years who have or are "at risk" of developing a communicative disorder.

Second, investigators who are not clinicians are unlikely to be as *interested* as those who are in answering some questions of clinical interest, particularly those on clinical program procedure and therapy outcome. Such investigators may view questions on clinical program procedure as having limited theoretical significance. They may also be less interested in questions on therapy outcome for one or more of the following reasons: (a) the effects of extraneous variables are more difficult to control than in much laboratory research; (b) the time it takes to collect data may be longer than for many types of laboratory research; and (c) the likehood of a publishable result may not be as high in outcome research as in many types of laboratory research.

Third, investigators who are not clinicians might lack the *opportunity* to make the observations needed to answer many clinically relevant questions even if they were interested in doing so. Possible reasons for this lack of opportunity have already been discussed.

3. More clinicians functioning as clinician-investigators would probably help break down the clinician-researcher dichotomy that exists to some extent in speech-language pathology and audiology (Attanasio, 1986; Costello, 1979; Goldstein, 1972; Hamre, 1972; Jerger, 1963a, 1963b, 1964a; Powers, 1955; Ringel, 1972; Schultz, Roberts, and Yairi, 1972; Siegel and Spradlin, 1985). While this is certainly not the primary reason speech-language pathologists and audiologists should function as clinician-investigators, it nevertheless is an important one, since (for reasons previously discussed) it seems reasonable to conclude that clinical research and clinical practice are interdependent activities.

WHO CAN BE A CLINICIAN-INVESTIGATOR?

The previous section attempted partially to answer the question, "What benefits would a clinician derive from functioning as a clinician-investigator?" The word *partially* was inserted here to indicate that the reasons discussed are not the only possible ones. As general semanticists (e.g., Johnson, 1946) and others have pointed out, it is quite doubtful that any question can be completely answered or, for that matter, that everything can be said about anything.

This section will attempt partially to answer the question: "What attributes and competencies are necessary for a clinician to function successfully as a clinician-investigator, and how do these differ from those necessary to function solely as a clinician?" It will also attempt to answer the related question: "What attitudes and competencies are not essential for a clinician to function successfully as a clinician-investigator that might be regarded as necessary for him or her to function successfully in this role?" Its objective is to help the reader develop a more objective attitude toward research.

Why is it necessary for you to be concerned about developing a more objective attitude toward research? The term *objective attitude* is used here to indicate that your attitude toward research and your ability to function as a researcher should be as rational, or reality-oriented, as possible. If you were to view research as an activity possible for Ph.D.'s in universities but not for clinicians who have master's degrees, your attitude would not be objective. Speech-language pathologists and audiologists employed in clinical setting who are not Ph.D.'s both have done and continue to do research. Viewing research as an activity that requires extensive training in statistics and research methodology or a considerable expenditure of time is likewise not an objective attitude, because neither is absolutely essential for at least some clinical research.

The more objective your attitude toward research, the higher the probability you will consider functioning as a clinician-investigator. That is, the more certain you are that this is a possibility, the more likely you are to attempt to function in this role. Some clinicians do not function as clinician-investigators because their attitudes toward research are not objective, not because their interest is lacking. They may assume, for example, that to do clinical research, a speech-language pathologist or audiologist must have a doctoral degree, or advanced training in statistics or research design, or considerable time available, or certain personal attributes that are not generally regarded as essential for clinicians. While these are not the only such assumptions made by clinicians, they appear to be among the most frequent, judging by both the results of a survey of speech clinicians in Wisconsin (Silverman, Halbach, and Palmer, unpublished data) and a national survey of ASHA members certified in speech-language pathology (Kelly and McReynolds, 1987). For this reason, the validity of each assumption will be considered here.

Neither a Ph.D. degree nor extensive training in statistics is essential for a speech-language pathologist or audiologist to make many (but not necessarily all) of the observations needed to answer clinical questions and report the answers in oral convention presentations or journal articles. While training on a doctoral level is desirable for an investigator because it is usually in large part research training, it is not a prerequisite. The investigator responsible for the scientific exhibit that won First Prize for Scientific Excellence at the 1972 Annual Convention of the American Speech-Language-Hearing Association was a high school student. His competition consisted of 19 exhibits by speech-language pathologists, audiologists, and speech and hearing scientists with doctoral degrees (including the author). Perhaps the strongest evidence that a Ph.D. is not a prerequisite for at least some clinical research is the fact that clinical research done by speech-language pathologists and audiologists with master's degrees has been reported at annual conventions of the American Speech-Language-Hearing Association, those of state speech and hearing associations, as well as in clinical journals including those that are (or were) published by the American Speech-Language-Hearing Association (the *American Journal of Audiology: A Journal of Clinical Practice*, the *American Journal of Speech-Language Pathology: A Journal of Clinical Practice*, the *Journal of Speech and Hearing Disorders*, the *Journal of Speech and Hearing Research*, and *Language, Speech, and Hearing Services in the Schools*).

Extensive knowledge of statistics and research methodology, like doctoral-level training, though desirable for a speech-language pathologist or audiologist who wishes to function as a clinician-investigator, is not essential. The information presented in this book will suffice to formulate a plan for making the observations necessary to answer some questions. To answer others, the clinician-investigator may have to consult with persons who are knowledgeable in statistics and research design. Such consultants are available in many school systems, hospitals, rehabilitation centers, and other clinical settings. In addition, there may be faculty members at nearby colleges and universities who would be willing to consult with you about research design problems.

Another potentially unobjective attitude is that doing clinical research requires more time than a speech-language pathologist or audiologist would have available for the purpose. This reason was one of the most frequently mentioned for not doing research in the survey of Wisconsin speech clinicians cited previously. The objectivity of this attitude is a function of the question, or questions, the clinician seeks to answer. If these questions require observations that *the clinician has to make as part of his or her routine clinical responsibilities* (or observations he or she would not routinely make but could make within the context of his or her clinical responsibilities), this attitude would probably not be objective. Such questions might deal with the effectiveness of therapies being used with clients in the clinician's caseload. It seems reasonable to assume that the clinician would make some observations to evaluate the effectiveness of the therapies being used, if for no other reason than to satisfy his or her employers' demands for accountability. If these observations were reasonably reliable and valid (which also would be necessary for them to be useful clinically), they could be used for answering clinical research questions concerning therapy outcome. Gathering research data in this manner should not be particularly time-consuming.

Other research likely to place minimal demands upon a clinician's time is that which utilizes client folder data—i.e., the diagnostic and therapy data recorded in clients' folders or in computer database equivalents. For such data to be usable for this purpose, they must be easily retrievable: that is, the files must be organized so that the folders of clients in the "population" to be studied can be located fairly easily. A variety of clinically relevant questions can be answered, at least partially, through the use of such data. These would include those pertaining to: (1) factors influencing the prognosis for various communicative disorders, (2) interrelationships between test results (e.g., audiometric test results) for specific clinical "populations," (3) negative side effects of specific therapies, (4) positive effects of specific therapies upon specific communicative disorders, and (5) factors that influence the probability a client will terminate therapy before the clinician feels he or she is ready.

A final misconceived attitude is that clinicians, to do research, need to have more of certain personal attributes than are strictly necessary in their present role. The attribute most frequently mentioned by speech clinicians in the Wisconsin survey was "intelligence." More than a third of the clinicians surveyed indicated that they did not consider themselves sufficiently intelligent to do clinical research. Several assumptions appear to underlie this attitude. One is that clinical research is relatively homogeneous in the demands it places on an investigator's intelligence, that is, that the level of intelligence required to answer most questions of clinical interest is approximately the same. A second, related assumption implicit here is that the level of intelligence required to answer clinically relevant questions for research purposes exceeds that required to answer such questions for clinical purposes. (We are assuming here that a clinician would regard his or her level of intelligence as adequate for answering clinically relevant questions for clinical purposes.)

While clinical research may possibly be relatively homogeneous in the demands it places on an investigator's intelligence, this still seems quite unlikely, for several reasons. First, this assumption would violate the principle posited by general semanticists (e.g., Johnson, 1946) and others that the members of a "class of events" (clinical research studies would constitute such a class) are not identical in any attribute. In other words, events do not replicate themselves. Second, it would be necessary to assume that the observations required to answer clinically relevant questions place approximately equal demands on an investigator's intelligence. Such an assumption would be counterintuitive, since some observational procedures appear to place greater demands on an investigator's intelligence and ingenuity than others do. Questions that, to be answered, required an observational procedure that was well developed and standardized (such as a standardized test) would not intuitively appear to place as great a demand on an investigator as would those requiring an observational procedure the investigator has to devise and standardize.

The second assumption (probably the more important of the two with reference to the ability of a clinician to function as an investigator) is that the level of intelligence required to answer clinically relevant questions for research purposes exceeds that required to answer such questions for clinical purposes. If a clinician feels sufficiently intelligent to answer certain clinically relevant questions for clinical purposes, he or she should rationally also feel sufficiently intelligent to answer the same questions for research purposes.

Thus far, this section has dealt with attributes and competencies that do *not* appear to be essential for a speech-language pathologist or audiologist to function successfully as a clinician-investigator. What attributes and competencies *do* appear to be necessary for him or her to have a reasonable chance for success as a clinician-investigator? Since few relevant research data have been reported, the answers here should be regarded as speculative.

The personal attributes that appear necessary for a speech-language pathologist or audiologist to have a reasonable chance of functioning successfully as a clinician-investigator also appear, for the most part, necessary for him or her to have a reasonable chance of functioning successfully as a clinician. Partial support for this conclusion is provided by the findings of a study (Silverman, Halbach, and Palmer, unpublished data) in which a national random sample of speech-language pathologists ascribed essentially the same attributes to "a speech-language pathologist who does clinical work" as a second such random sample ascribed to "a speech-language pathologist who does clinical work and clinical research." While these data generally support the conclusion that the attributes of a successful clinician-investigator are essentially the same as those of a successful clinician, they obviously do not constitute a direct test of this hypothesis. A direct test would require comparing a number of personal attributes of a group of clinician-investigators with those of a group of clinicians who do not function as investigators.

What competencies are essential for speech-language pathologists or audiologists to function successfully as clinician-investigators? A general answer to this question would be that they must know how to: (1) formulate "answerable" questions and make the observations necessary to answer them with adequate levels of validity and reliability, (2) relate their answers to existing theories and knowledge, and (3) communicate questions, answers, and relations. The information in this book, hopefully, will assist in developing these competencies.

EXERCISES AND DISCUSSION TOPICS

1. Why might you as a clinician resist functioning as a clinician-investigator? How could such resistance be dealt with?

2. Indicate for each of the following statements whether you agree or disagree and why:

   a. "Diagnosis, therapy, and clinical research are interrelated activities."

   b. "I can visualize myself doing a research project and reporting the results in a professional journal."

   c. "I can visualize one or more of my classmates doing a research project and reporting the results in a professional journal."

   d. "Having a knowledge of clinical research methodology tends to make one a better clinician."

   e. "It is unethical for clinicians to use their clients for clinical research."

   f. "Male clinicians tend to be better suited for doing research than female ones."

   g. "I feel that I am smart enough to be a good clinician, but I do not feel that I am smart enough to do clinical research."

   h. "Clinicians usually do not have time available for doing therapy outcome research."

3

Research as a Process of Asking and Answering Questions

The first two chapters attempted to demonstrate that clinical research in speech-language pathology and audiology is needed and that speech-language pathologists and audiologists can help to satisfy this need by functioning as clinician-investigators. This chapter discusses the *scientific method* that underlies research. The primary objective will be to demonstrate that the scientific method, as applied to research, can be viewed as a set of rules for asking and answering questions and for evaluating answers to questions.

It is desirable for speech-language pathologists and audiologists to have an intuitive understanding of the scientific method. This is true regardless of whether they function as clinicians or clinician-investigators; they are obviously consumers of research in both roles. As such, they have to be able to assess the validity, reliability, and generality of research findings—that is, "answers" to research questions. To do this, they need an intuitive understanding of the method used to generate research findings from the frame of reference both of the philosophy of science (how it is supposed to function) and the history of science (how it has functioned). The methods used by investigators to answer questions (and to arrive, apparently, at "correct" answers) are not always those that philosophers of science regard as consistent with the scientific method (Bush, 1974; Kuhn, 1962). What the philosopher of science regards as the method of science is not always what the historian of science has found to be the case. For this reason, the scientific method will be considered in this chapter from both points of view. Several examples relevant to speech-language pathology and audiology will be presented to illustrate the difference between the two ways of regarding the scientific method, including Franz Joseph Gall's discovery of the importance of the anterior portion of the brain for motor speech.

In addition to understanding intuitively the set of rules used to answer questions based on the scientific method, speech-language pathologists and audiologists should also preferably understand the assumptions (or presuppositions) on which the scientific method and hence these rules are based. They should understand what they are required to accept on "faith" when they interpret research findings. This knowledge can enhance their ability to evaluate research reports critically as well as to help them develop an objective attitude toward research.

First, the intuitive understanding. To play a game successfully, you must understand the rules, and the scientific method can easily be viewed as a game. Like any game, it has both objectives and strategies for maximizing the probability of achieving these objectives. In fact, as Agnew and Pyke (1975) pointed out in their provocative and entertaining description of "the science game,"

> The ingredients of any great game can be found in science—massive effort, goals, great plays, mediocre plays, lousy plays; umpires making clear calls, judgment calls, biased calls, and of course, mistaken calls. There are prizes and penalties. You will find integrity, dignity, and deals, along with good luck and bad luck—but above all you will find commitment. (Agnew and Pyke, 1975, pp. vii–viii)

To learn the rules of the "game," the clinician-investigator should study them from the frame of reference of both the philosophy of science and the history of science. The philosophy of science provides information on strategies that, theoretically, should lead to success at the game; the history of science provides information on strategies that have led to success at the game in the past. Together, they provide a set of guidelines.

Speech-language pathologists and audiologists need an intuitive understanding of the scientific method just as much in their role as clinician. All else being equal, a speech-language pathologist or audiologist probably will be a more effective diagnostician and behavior modifier if he or she has at least some grounding in the scientific method. Diagnosis, particularly differential diagnosis, consists in large part of asking "answerable" questions (or forming "testable" hypotheses) and making the observations necessary to answer (or test) them. The scientific method offers a set of rules for maximizing the probability of "correct" answers to such questions (or of reliable and valid tests of such hypotheses). As such, it is relevant for the speech-language pathologist or audiologist who functions as a diagnostician. It is also relevant for the speech-language pathologist or audiologist who functions as a behavior modifier. Rules associated with the scientific method are applicable both to the administration of therapies (or behavior modification procedures) and to the evaluation of the effects produced by them. In fact, most approaches to behavior modification based on learning theory, including Skinnerian Operant Conditioning, are applied and their results evaluated by means of "rules" derived from the scientific method.

There is not universal agreement about the amount of impact that "rules" derived from the scientific method both do and should have on research and clinical practice in speech-language pathology and audiology. For lively discussions of this issue, see Bench (1989), Bloodstein (1988), Ingham and Siegel (1989), Panush (1989), Perkins (1986), Prutting, Mentis, and Nelson (1989), Ringel, Tachtman, and Prutting (1984), Siegel (1988), and Siegel and Ingham (1987).

WHAT IS THE SCIENTIFIC METHOD?

Now that we have briefly considered the "why" question (Why is knowledge of the scientific method relevant for speech-language pathologists or audiologists?), we are ready to deal with the "what" question: What is the scientific method? As a partial answer, some of its objectives, characteristics, and underlying assumptions will be delineated. These objectives, characteristics, and underlying assumptions are not the only ones that have been attributed to the scientific method, nor is there universal agreement that they are a necessary part of the scientific method. However, they are among those that tend to be most frequently mentioned by philosophers and historians of science.

Objectives

We will begin our discussion of the scientific method with its objectives. We will consider the functions it can serve, specifically the question: What can the scientific method do for a speech-language pathologist or audiologist? How and when might he or she use it?

The scientific method is a set of rules that can be used for *describing* events, *explaining* events, and *predicting* events. The term *event*, as used here, includes anything observable that occurs in time and thus includes phenomena usually classified as objects.

Description.   Describing events means partially answering questions beginning with "who," "what," "when," "where," "how," and "which," questions concerning events. The following are examples:

1. *Who* should be examined by an otolaryngologist before being scheduled for voice therapy?
2. *Who* can benefit from a particular type of hearing aid?

3. *What* factors cause a child to begin to stutter?
4. *What* factors influence speechreading ability?
5. *When* is a speech deviation a speech defect?
6. *When* is a hearing loss educationally significant?
7. *Where* do esophageal speakers have most difficulty communicating?
8. *Where* should ear protectors be worn?
9. *How* can a child who "lateralizes" /s/ be taught to produce a "frontal" /s/?
10. *How* can hearing loss be identified most reliably in neonates?
11. *Which* of two aphasia tests yields the most reliable and valid information concerning a stroke patient's ability to communicate?
12. *Which* approach to teaching the deaf is most likely to result in the highest level of ability to communicate with normal-hearing persons, the "oral" method or "total communication"?

The structures of these questions, of course, should be regarded as illustrative rather than exhaustive. Questions that result in answers that describe events can begin with various words. The process of structuring questions is further discussed in Chapter 5.

Speech-language pathologists and audiologists can use the scientific method whenever they have to describe something. It offers an approach for describing events (e.g., behavior) that both maximizes the reliability and validity of a description and permits its reliability and validity to be estimated. Since the meaningfulness of descriptive data is a direct function of their reliability and validity, the scientific method can perform a useful function for speech-language pathologists and audiologists in this regard.

Explanation. Explaining events means dealing with the "why" question—i.e., specifying the reason or reasons for events. Once an event has been described, we may be interested in explaining why it occurred. If a therapy approach employed by a speech-language pathologist or audiologist resulted in a reduction in the severity of a client's communicative disorder, the clinician probably would have some interest in being able to specify the reason or reasons why. If, for example, you could identify the aspect, or aspects, of the therapy that were responsible for the observed change, you might be able to "simplify" the therapy and thereby make it more efficient. Or if you could identify and isolate the active ingredient in the therapy, you might be able to incorporate it into a new therapy approach that would be more effective than the one you originally used. Also, if you could determine why the frequency, duration, and complexity of behaviors that contribute to communicative disorders vary in predictable ways under specified laboratory conditions, you might be able to incorporate the active components of such conditions into programs of therapy for communicative disorders. If, for example, you could explain why the frequency of stuttering decreases under certain laboratory conditions (e.g., reading in chorus), you might be able to incorporate the active components of such conditions into programs of therapy for stuttering. Or if you could explain the reasons for spontaneous recovery following damage to the central nervous system, you might be better able to devise therapy strategies to maximize it.

The scientific method is helpful in establishing the degree of certainty a speech-language pathologist or audiologist can have in answers to "why" questions—questions of causality. These questions are particularly difficult to answer with a high degree of certainty in the biological and behavioral sciences which, of course, are the areas to which most questions in speech-language pathology and audiology relate (Perkins and Curlee, 1969). Philosophers of science have pointed out several reasons why questions of causality are difficult to answer with a high degree of certainty, including the following:

First, *more than one explanation for an event may be possible from descriptions of it*. The existing data may support more than one explanation for an event. Even if the existing data support only one of the explanations posited for an event, they could conceivably support as well, or possibly even better, an explanation for the event that has not yet been posited. Also, while existing data may support one explanation of an event more than others, new data may become available that would make one of the other explanations appear more viable. Under these circumstances, no explanation of an event can be accepted as absolutely certain. All we can conclude based on the scientific method is that judging by what we know about an event, the most plausible explanation for it appears to be. . . . As the amount of information we have about an event increases, our judgment on the most plausible explanation for it may change. One of the most important rules, or principles, of the scientific method is that explanations for events *must be* regarded as tentative and subject to change when new information becomes available.

Second, *because two events are highly correlated does not necessarily mean that one is causally related to the other*. Even though auditory memory span is fairly highly related to articulation proficiency, for example, this does not necessarily mean that poor auditory memory span is a cause of articulation disorders. The two may be correlated because they are both related to a *third variable* such as mental age. If a child were developing mentally at a slower-than-normal rate, both auditory memory span and articulation proficiency would also be developing slowly. The possibility that two variables that appear closely related are actually both causally related to a third variable is another reason why explanations for events must be regarded as tentative and thus subject to change.

Third, *all events in a system are interrelated*. Causation, therefore, is apt to be complex. A system, for example, could be "centered" around a client and could include all events in both his internal and external environments that affect him. Because of the existence of such systems, if a client improves following a period of therapy, we can never be certain that the improvement was due solely to the therapy he or she received. Even if we isolate one aspect of therapy (event associated with therapy) that always seems to be present when improvement occurs, we cannot conclude this is the only event that has to be present for it to occur. In fact, we could not even be certain that the aspect isolated was related to the observed improvement. There could be other common aspects we have not abstracted, or identified, that were wholly or partially responsible for it.

Another possibility that needs to be considered here is that an aspect of therapy might be more likely to result in improvement if it is combined with a particular value of another variable, or variables. Organismic and therapist variables (Edwards and Cronbach, 1966) would be relevant here. A given therapy, for example, might be more effective with clients who have above-average intelligence than with those who have below-average intelligence. Also, this same therapy might be more effective if it were administered by a clinician who expected it to be effective (positive placebo effect) than if it were administered by one who did not expect it to be effective (negative placebo effect).

For a discussion both of problems that are likely to be encountered when attempting to establish causal relationships in communication disorders and of a strategy (path analysis) that can be helpful for doing so, see Duffy, Watt, and Duffy (1981).

We can conclude our discussion of the role of the scientific method in explanation with this generalization: Answers to "why" questions should be regarded as tentative and subject to change when new information becomes available.

Prediction. Predicting events means making probability statements about the likelihood of their future occurrence—that is, estimating the odds that a specific event will occur during a specific period of time. Once an event has been described and information becomes available concerning the conditions under which it occurs, its future occurrence may be predicted with "greater than chance" accuracy. The degree of accuracy with which such predictions can be made is at least partially a function of the amount of information available about the conditions under which the event occurs. The greater the available information about these conditions, the more accurately an event usually can be predicted.

Weather forecasting illustrates the application of the scientific method to predicting events. Weather forecasters estimate the odds a specific event (rain) will occur during a specific time period (next 24 hours). They base their predictions on available information about: (1) the conditions under which specific weather events occur, and (2) the conditions that are likely to be present during the period for which they are making their prediction. For each event they predict, they usually make a probability statement (20 percent chance of rain) about the likelihood of its occurrence.

What kinds of events do speech-language pathologists and audiologists attempt to predict? One is the probable outcome of therapy. This prediction is incorporated into the statement of prognosis. In this statement a speech-language pathologist or audiologist attempts to predict the probable impact of a specific program of therapy on a specific client's communicative disorder (possibly within a specific period of time). To make this statement, he or she consciously or unconsciously uses: (1) information about the conditions that have to be present for improvement to occur in persons who have a given communicative disorder and (2) his or her judgment concerning the likelihood that these conditions will be operative for the client. The statement of prognosis could have a statement of either verbal (little chance for further improvement) or numerical (less than a 10 percent chance for further improvement) probability attached to it.

Speech-language pathologists and audiologists also may have to make predictions relevant to program planning. A speech-language pathologist, for example, may be called upon to predict which young children who have sound substitutions are likely to correct them on their own and which most likely will require some form of therapy. These predictions usually are based on information about: (1) the conditions under which a child is likely to correct sound substitutions on his or her own ("error" phonemes are stimulable), and (2) whether these conditions appear to be present for a given group of children. A probability statement probably will be attached to such predictions (kindergarten-age children are quite likely to correct sound substitutions on their own if their "error" sounds are stimulable in both isolation and words).

The scientific method can assist the speech-language pathologist or audiologist in predicting events in a manner that permits him or her (at least roughly) to estimate accuracy of prediction. A number of statistical procedures have been developed that can be used for this purpose, including regression analysis and discriminant function analysis (both are discussed in Chapter 10).

Characteristics

We will now delineate some of the characteristics of the scientific method as they relate to speech-language pathology and audiology. Our primary goal is to help the reader develop an intuitive understanding of the method as an approach to describing, explaining, and predicting events. This discussion can be viewed as an *operational definition* (Bridgman, 1927) of the scientific method, because it describes how one would have to behave to function in a manner consistent with it. The terminology used is that of Feigl (1953).

Intersubjective Testability.   This term refers to "the requirement that the knowledge claims of science be in principle capable of test (confirmation or disconfirmation, at least indirectly and to some degree) on the part of any person properly equipped with intelligence and the technical devices of observation or experimentation" (Feigl, 1953, p. 11). If speech-language pathologists or audiologists devise therapeutic procedures which purport to reduce the severity of a communicative disorder, or diagnostic procedures which purport to be effective in determining the etiology of a communicative disorder, these claims should be capable of test by another person. Their procedure should be described in sufficient detail so that it can be tested by someone else. Before any claims can be accepted, they must be confirmed by others. They cannot be accepted on the basis of "authority" or appearance in print. A claim is not credible simply because a person regarded as an authority claims a procedure is effective and his or her claim appears in print. Claims have appeared in speech-language pathology and audiology literature that could not be confirmed by those who tested them.

That a claim should not be regarded as valid unless it has been adequately tested and reasonably well confirmed has relevance for speech-language pathologists and audiologists when they are deciding whether to adopt an intervention strategy. Before making such a decision, they should attempt to determine whether the claims made for it have been adequately tested and, if they have, whether the data appear to confirm or disconfirm them. Obviously, it would probably be safer to adopt an intervention strategy that has been tested and its claims confirmed than one that has not been tested. It is probably reasonable to assume that the claims made for some diagnostic and therapy procedures currently used by speech-language pathologists or audiologists have not been adequately tested. As indicated in Chapter 2, one of the reasons there is a need for speech-language pathologists and audiologists to function as clinician-investigators is simply to test such claims.

Reliability. The "knowledge-claims" of science are required to have "a sufficient degree of confirmation. This second criterion of scientific knowledge enables us to distinguish what is generally called 'mere opinion' (or worse still, 'superstition') from knowledge (well-sustained belief)" (Feigl, 1953, p. 12). Degree of confirmation can vary from none to considerable. Obviously, the weight given to a claim in decision making is partially a function of a degree to which it has been confirmed. The greater the degree to which a claim has been confirmed (and hence the greater its reliability), the more confidence one can place in it and the more weight it can be given in decision making.

The claims, or observations, that speech-language pathologists and audiologists utilize in clinical decision making have been confirmed to varying degrees. Some have been confirmed beyond reasonable doubt while others are no more than hunches. Examples of claims relevant to speech-language pathology and audiology that appear to have received enough degree of confirmation to be regarded as well-substantiated belief include:

1. Anticipation of stuttering is somehow involved in precipitating the moment of stuttering.
2. Damage to the anterior portion of the left cerebral cortex in right-handed persons is more likely to result in expressive aphasia than damage to the corresponding portion of the right cerebral cortex.
3. Vocal abuse in a cause of vocal nodules.
4. A characteristic of at least some types of noise-induced hearing loss is a greater degree of loss by air conduction at 4000 Hz than at 2000 Hz and 8000 Hz.

Definiteness and Precision.   It is necessary that "the concepts used in the formulation of scientific knowledge-claims be as definitely delimited as possible. On the level of the qualitative-classificatory sciences this amounts to the attempt to reduce all border-zone vagueness to a minimum. On the level of quantitative science the exactitude of the concepts is enormously enhanced through the application of the techniques of measurement" (Feigl, 1953, p. 12). Speech-language pathologists and audiologists are concerned with both qualitative-classificatory and quantitative concepts.

Why is it necessary that the concepts dealt with by science be as definitely delimited (and hence as precise) as possible? An event, or phenomenon, referred to by a concept cannot be investigated unless it can be defined with enough precision that it is likely to be identified both when it does and does not occur. Before we can determine the effect of a therapy on the "lateralized" /s/ (concept) we have to be able to detect with precision both when /s/ is and is not being lateralized. The meaning of precision in this context is illustrated by Figure 3.1. If precision is high, /s/ will be identified as lateralized when it is lateralized and will not be identified when it is not lateralized. Judgments will fall into one of the two cells marked with Xs. The

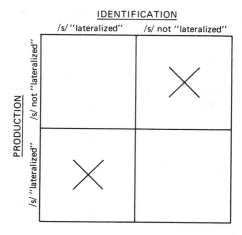

FIGURE 3.1   A four-cell bivariate table for assessing accuracy of judgments of /s/ lateralization. If accuracy is perfect, all judgments will fall into one of the two cells marked with Xs.

more frequently /s/ is judged to be lateralized when it is not lateralized and judged not to be lateralized when it is lateralized, the lower the precision of the judgments (and the lower the percentage of judgments that will fall into one of the two cells marked with Xs). To maximize the precision of such judgments, it would be necessary to define as precisely as possible what is meant by a lateralized /s/ and thereby reduce all border-zone vagueness between what is meant by a lateralized and nonlateralized /s/ to a minimum. Increased definiteness would be expected to lead to increased precision.

The borderline vagueness between categories sometimes can be reduced by supplementing verbal definitions with extensional ones. A category, or term, can be *defined extensionally* "by pointing to or exhibiting somehow the actual objects, phenomena, etc., to which the term refers" (Johnson, 1946, p. 507). Thus, the borderline vagueness between the categories "lateralized" and "nonlateralized" /s/ probably could be reduced by preparing an audiotape recording on which are both labeled examples of /s/ that the definer considers lateralized and labeled examples of /s/ he or she does not consider lateralized.

Thus far, we have considered why it is necessary for qualitative-classificatory concepts to be defined as precisely as possible. Speech-language pathologists and audiologists also deal with quantitative concepts. The events, or phenomena, referred to by such concepts are designated by numerals (rather than words) and hence constitute measurement. (Measurement, which can be defined as the assignment of numerals to events according to rules, is discussed in depth in Chapter 8). Quantitative concepts of interest to speech-language pathologists and audiologists include degree of hearing loss (in decibels), language age (in years), and frequency of stuttering (in percentage of words stuttered). Obviously, it is important that quantitative concepts be defined with precision.

How precisely do concepts have to be defined? How definitely delimited do they have to be? How much borderline vagueness can be tolerated? The answers to these questions are dependent upon the purpose for which a conceptual scheme is being used. For some purposes—i.e., to answer some questions—the conceptual scheme must be highly precise (have little borderline vagueness). To answer other questions, a conceptual scheme could have considerable borderline vagueness and still be adequate for the purpose. As Feigl has indicated "there is no point in sharpening precision to a higher degree than the problem in hand requires. (You need no razor to cut butter.)" (Feigl, 1953, p. 12).

Coherence of Systematic Structure.   In science we seek "not a mere collection of miscellaneous items of information, but a well-connected account of the facts" (Feigl, 1953, p. 12). This is true on both descriptive and explanatory levels.

On the *descriptive level,* the need for coherence or systematic structure "results, for example, in systems of classification of division, in diagrams, statistical charts and the like" (Feigl, 1953, pp. 12–13). An articulation test response form is a way of organizing information concerning the types of articulatory errors (i.e., substitutions, omissions, distortions, additions) a child produces. An audiogram is a diagram for organizing certain information concerning a person's hearing.

Items of information concerning a phenomenon can be viewed as pieces of a puzzle. As such items become available and are fitted together into a coherent whole, our ability to describe the phenomenon increases. When information concerning a person's hearing acuity at various frequencies is plotted on a pure-tone audiogram form and thus is made more coherent, our ability to describe his or her hearing problem (if one is present) increases. Similarly, when a child's articulation errors are recorded on an articulation test response form, patterns of misarticulations emerge that can be useful in clinical decision making.

To satisfy the need for coherence or systematic structure on the *explanatory level*, "sets of laws, or theoretical assumptions, are utilized. Explanation in science consists in the hypothetico-deductive procedure. The laws, theories, or hypotheses form the premises from which we derive logically, or logico-mathematically, the observed, or observable facts" (Feigl, 1953, p. 13). Thus, after we had plotted a person's hearing acuity in the left ear at various frequencies by air conduction and bone conduction on an audiogram form and connected the points for the air conduction curve (see Figure 3.2), we would attempt to explain the mechanisms responsible for the configurations

FIGURE 3.2   Pure-tone audiogram indicating degree of hearing in left ear by air conduction (x) and bone conduction (<).

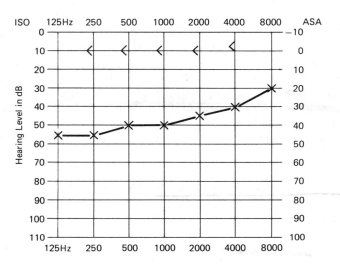

of the curves. We could hypothesize one or more mechanisms that could account for the observed configurations and then attempt to determine how well each hypothesized mechanism could explain it. Two hypotheses that might be offered to explain the configurations of the air and bone conduction pure-tone audiogram curves would be: (1) outer or middle ear pathology, and (2) inner ear pathology. We would state by *reasoning deductively* from each hypothesis what we would expect the configuration of the curves to be if it were the mechanism responsible. If this mechanism were pathology in the outer or middle ear, we would expect the air conduction curve to be relatively flat and the bone conduction curve to indicate essentially normal hearing. On the other hand, if the mechanism responsible were pathology in the inner ear, we would expect the configuration of the air conduction curve to indicate greater loss in the high frequencies than in the low frequencies; we would also expect the bone conduction curve to indicate approximately the same amount of loss as the air conduction curve. Since the configurations of the curves in Figure 3.2 more closely approximate what we would expect if the mechanism responsible were outer or middle ear pathology than inner ear pathology, we would conclude that outer or middle ear pathology appears to be the more viable explanation. In other words, we would conclude that the data plotted in Figure 3.2 are *consistent with the hypothesis* that the person has outer or middle ear pathology in his left ear.

Simply because a hypothesis is consistent with the data concerning a phenomenon, this does not necessarily mean it explains the phenomenon. There could be other hypotheses as consistent or even more consistent with the data. This dilemma was aptly described by Einstein and Infeld in *The Evolution of Physics*:

> In our endeavor to understand reality we are somewhat like a man trying to understand the mechanism of a closed watch. He sees the face and the moving hands, even hears it ticking, but he has no way of opening the case. If he is ingenious he may form some picture of a mechanism that could be responsible for all the things he observes, but he may never be quite sure his picture is the only one which could explain his observations. He will never be able to compare his picture with the real mechanism and he cannot even imagine the possibility or the meaning of such a comparison. But he certainly believes that, as his knowledge increases, his picture of reality will become simpler and simpler and will explain a wider and wider range of his sensuous impressions. (Einstein and Infeld, 1938)

This statement reinforces the conclusion we reached earlier in this chapter that explanations for phenomena must be regarded as tentative.

Comprehensiveness or Scope of Knowledge.

Instead of presenting a finished account of the world, the genuine scientist keeps his unifying hypotheses open to revision and is always ready to modify or abandon them if evidence should render them doubtful. This *self- corrective aspect* [italics added] of science has rightly been stressed as its most important characteristic. . . . It is a sign of one's maturity to be able to live with an unfinished world view. (Feigl, 1953, p. 13)

Speech-language pathologists and audiologists, whether they function as clinicians or clinician-investigators, have to be able to tolerate living professionally with an "unfinished world view." The "facts" they use concerning communicative disorders are not really facts but hypotheses subject to revision. Such facts (or beliefs) include those relevant to the symptomatology, incidence, etiology, prognosis, evaluation, prevention, and treatment of communicative disorders. Their beliefs about the etiology of communicative disorders may have to be modified or abandoned if new evidence renders these beliefs doubtful. Many speech-language pathologists who believed that stuttering resulted from lack of unilateral cerebral dominance, for example, abandoned this view when evidence appeared to render it doubtful (Bloodstein, 1987). Likewise, speech-language pathologists and audiologists have had to modify or abandon some of their beliefs concerning the symptomatology, incidence, prognosis, evaluation, prevention, and treatment of other communicative disorders.

How do we know when the evidence is sufficiently compelling to require us to modify or abandon a belief? There is no simple answer to this question. Several factors will influence the decision, including: (1) the internal standard of the person on what constitutes compelling evidence, (2) the evidence itself, and (3) the person's ego-involvement with the belief.

People differ in their internal standards of what constitutes compelling evidence. Evidence that one person would regard as compelling another may not. In part, this is a function of how critically you evaluate evidence. A person who did not evaluate the evidence relevant to a hypothesis critically might regard it as more compelling than one who did. (Considerations involved in evaluating evidence critically are discussed in Chapter 11.) One of the reasons, incidentally, why it is important for clinicians to develop an intuitive understanding of research methodology and the scientific method is to maximize their ability to evaluate evidence critically and thereby modify their internal standard of what constitutes compelling evidence.

Another relevant factor is the evidence itself. Some pieces of evidence will be judged stronger and more compelling than others, regardless of individual differences in internal standards among clinicians. Improved performance on a speech discrimination task would probably be considered more compelling evidence that a hearing aid has improved a hard-of-hearing person's ability to understand speech than would the person's own subjective report.

The third, and final, factor influencing the probability that evidence will be judged compelling is the person's ego-involvement with the belief. The greater the person's ego-involvement, the stronger the evidence would have to be before he or she would regard it as sufficiently compelling to modify or abandon his or her belief. Some persons become quite ego-involved with their beliefs and for this reason have difficulty evaluating them objectively. They tend to filter out evidence that might require them to modify or abandon their beliefs. In extreme cases, the filtering is so complete they communicate (verbally, nonverbally, or both) to anyone they feel might challenge their beliefs that *their minds are already made up and they don't wish to be confused by the facts.* Whether we function as clinicians, clinician-investigators, or investigators, we have to be constantly on guard against this consequence of ego-involvement. We should regard our beliefs as tentative and thus subject to modification and abandonment.

Underlying Assumptions

Thus far in our discussion of the scientific method we have dealt with its objectives and characteristics. We now will consider its underlying assumptions, or presuppositions. These must be accepted *on faith* by users of the method since they have not been, and presumably cannot be, either proven or disproven. They are being discussed here not only to help you develop an intuitive understanding of the method, but also to help you develop an objective attitude toward it. That is, you must realize that while the method is extremely useful because it provides a "set of rules" for asking and answering questions that maximizes the probability of correct answers, it is not completely objective, since it rests upon assumptions that are not empirically verifiable. Three such assumptions will be discussed here: (1) the principle of causality, (2) the principle of uniformity, and (3) the principle of the finitude of relevant factors.

Principle of Causality. One assumption, or presupposition, of the scientific method is that "every event has a cause" (Pap, 1949, p. 403). Without this assumption, two objectives of the scientific method—explanation and prediction—could not be achieved. To explain an event, we must assume it has a cause; otherwise, it would make no sense to try to explain it. Also, predicting an event requires a knowledge of its cause or causes. If events cannot be assumed to have causes, then attempting to predict their future occurrence with greater than chance accuracy makes no sense.

This assumption is implicitly or explicitly made every day by speech-language pathologists and audiologists, regardless of whether they function as clinicians or clinician-investigators. It underlies, for example, such statements as: "The cause of your speech disorder is . . ." or "The cause of your child's hearing problem is . . ."

Is it reasonable to assume that all events have causes? The success of the scientific method in explaining and predicting events during the past 300 years offers some support for the reasonableness of this assumption. If events did not have causes, then predicting their occurrence with greater-than-chance accuracy would be impossible. Whether *every* event has a cause, however, cannot be established until every event has been studied. This is, of course, an impossible condition to satisfy since new events are constantly occurring. The assumption is worth being made, nevertheless, since it has *heuristic value*. That is, by making it we are more likely to be able to explain and predict particular events than we are by not making it.

Principle of Uniformity. Another presupposition of the scientific method related to causality is the so-called principle of uniformity—i.e., "*'same cause, same effect'* [italics added]: it has been remarked that if an experiment, designed to prove a generalization 'if A, B, C, then D' is repeated several times under varied conditions, it is in order to make sure that A, B, C really are the essential conditions on which the effect D depends, and that the appearance of such a dependence was not due to some 'accidental' circumstance" (Pap, 1949, p. 405–406).

This assumption has relevance for speech-language pathologists and audiologists since without it they would have difficulty generalizing from their observations about causation. If they observed, for example, that a particular response-contingent reinforcer was likely to have a particular effect on a particular behavior exhibited by a particular subgroup of individuals with communicative disorders, they could not conclude without making this assumption that it would probably be as likely to have the same effect on the behavior in other members of the subgroup. Also, therapy outcome research would have limited generality and usefulness if this assumption were not made since whether the therapy evaluated would have the same effect on other clients who were similar to those studied in all relevant variables would be uncertain.

Principle of the Finitude of Relevant Factors. The third and final presupposition of the scientific method we will discuss—the principle of the finitude of relevant factors—states that "only a small, and in fact enumerable, set of circumstances is causally related to the observed effect" (Pap, 1953, p. 27). If we did not make this assumption implicitly or explicitly, we would be restricted in our ability to specify the reason or reasons for, or explain, events. We could not conclude with confidence, for example, that a person's communicative disorder probably was due to one or at most a small set of circumstances. We could not deal with causation as if it were relatively simple and employ relatively simple research designs when we wished to establish causation.

Is this assumption viable? Some relatively recent work historically in several disciplines, including general semantics (Korzybski, 1958), general systems theory (Buckley, 1968), and chaos theory (Briggs and Peat, 1989), suggests it might be more reasonable to assume the set of circumstances that are causally related to an observed effect is relatively complex. That is, it might be reasonable to assume that all parts of a system are interrelated—that all events within a system are, to some extent, causally related to all other events in that system. The value of such an assumption has been demonstrated in several fields including ecology and economics. The causes of such events as "environmental pollution" and "inflation" apparently are quite complex.

How crucial is this assumption to the scientific method? If causation could not be assumed to be relatively simple, would this invalidate the method? The assumption does not appear crucial to the validity of the method. However, substituting the opposite assumption would probably necessitate some revision in the methodology used to answer "why" questions and make predictions. Greater emphasis would be placed, for example, on the use of multivariate statistical techniques—techniques that permit us to assess the combined, or composite, effects of a number of variables—particularly nonlinear ones (Briggs and Peat, 1989). (The rationale for, and application of, such techniques is discussed in Chapter 10.)

Historical Perspective

Thus far, we have discussed the scientific method primarily from the frame of reference of the philosophy of science. There is a second frame of reference through which it may be viewed—that of the history of science. The first is concerned with how the scientific method is *supposed* to function; the second, with how it *has* functioned. The two may not, in fact, be synonymous (Bush, 1974; Kuhn, 1962). Scientists have made the observations necessary to answer questions accurately and to develop and test hypotheses by methods that deviated to some extent from the scientific method as defined by philosophers of science. For example, Gall in 1818 was apparently the first to hypothesize that the "faculty of speech" is located in the anterior portion of the brain. His hypothesis appears to have arisen from the following observations:

> . . . he was sent in his ninth year to an uncle who was a *cure* in the Black Forest. Here he was educated with another boy of his own age who excelled him in learning his lessons. The two youths passed on to school at Baden, and Gall discovered that, when it was a question of learning by heart, he was beaten by those who were greatly inferior to him in written composition. Two of his new schoolfellows surpassed even his first companion in the ease with which they learnt by heart, and because they had *large and prominent eyes* [italics added] . . . they received the nickname of "Ox eyes." Three years later at Bruchsal and again at the University of Strasbourg he continued to notice that those who learnt easily by heart had the same sort of eyes. He began to associate this conformation with a good verbal memory, and so arrived at the conclusion that this faculty was situated in that part of the brain which lay behind the orbits. From such fantastic beginnings sprang the idea that memory for words was situated in the frontal lobes. (Head, 1963, p. 9)

Here we have a classic example of a person arriving at a correct conclusion—i.e., formulating a valid hypothesis—on the basis of observations that were made in a manner inconsistent with the scientific method. Historians of science have reported a number of such cases (Bush, 1974; Kuhn, 1962).

If one can arrive at valid conclusions by using procedures that are not compatible with the scientific method, why is it important to use procedures that are compatible with it? The use of such procedures *maximizes the probability* that answers to questions will be "accurate" and hypotheses formulated, or conclusions drawn, from these answers will be plausible and testable. While these results can also be achieved when the scientific method is not rigorously applied, they are more likely to be achieved when it is. For this reason, researchers usually design and conduct their studies in such a way that their methodology is compatible with the scientific method.

THE SCIENTIFIC METHOD AS A SET OF RULES
FOR ASKING AND ANSWERING QUESTIONS

The objective of this final section will be to demonstrate that the scientific method as applied to research can be viewed as a set of rules for asking and answering questions.

The characteristics of the scientific method discussed implicitly or explicitly suggest rules or criteria for formulating questions, making observations to answer them, and relating the answers to the existing body of knowledge. The criterion we referred to as "intersubjective testability," for example, suggests that the observational procedures used to answer questions should be described in sufficient detail that they can be repeated by others. That is, the methodology used to arrive at an answer should be described in sufficient detail that someone else could attempt to replicate the answer—i.e., arrive at the same answer.

The second criterion of the scientific method which we discussed, "reliability," in this context suggests that a sufficient number of observations should be made before we attempt to answer a question so that we can have a reasonable degree of confidence in the accuracy of the answer. It further suggests that we should incorporate into our studies some way of estimating the reliability of the observations we use to answer questions so that we can judge the maximum degree of confidence we can reasonably have in the accuracy of an answer.

The criterion we referred to as "definiteness and precision" also is relevant to the asking and answering of questions. It suggests that concepts referred to in questions formulated for research purposes should be as definitely delimited as possible. If such concepts are not defined precisely (i.e., with minimum borderline vagueness), questions which deal with them may not be answerable. (What makes a question answerable will be discussed in Chapter 5.) It also suggests that the language used to *answer* questions should be as unambiguous as possible. Concepts referred to should be clearly defined. Likewise, it suggests that the language used for *interpreting* answers to questions should be as unambiguous as possible with theoretical constructs clearly defined.

The criterion we referred to as "coherence or systematic structure" also has relevance here. Before we attempt to answer a question, we should organize the pieces of relevant information resulting from the observational process to make them coherent. This increases the probability of a correct answer. (Strategies for organizing qualitative and quantitative information to answer questions are discussed in Chapters 9 and 10.)

The final criterion of the scientific method we discussed was "comprehensiveness or scope of knowledge." It indicates that answers to questions should be regarded as tentative and subject to change when new information becomes available.

I have attempted to demonstrate in this chapter why the scientific method can be viewed as a set of rules for asking and answering questions. From this frame of reference, how might research be defined? For our purposes, we will define research as a *process of asking and answering questions that is governed by a set of rules referred to as the scientific method.*

EXERCISES AND DISCUSSION TOPICS

1. You are an audiologist who fits hearing aids. Indicate how each of the following assumptions which underlie the scientific method would be relevant when performing this task.

   a. The principle of causality

   b. The principle of uniformity

   c. The principle of the finitude of relevant factors

2. You are asked to evaluate Mary, a six-year-old who is reported by her parents to be saying some speech sounds incorrectly. You, therefore, have to make the observations necessary for answering the question: "What articulation errors is Mary making?" How might each of the following characteristics of the scientific method influence the manner in which you would make the observations needed to answer this question?

   a. Intersubjective testability

   b. Reliability

   c. Definiteness and precision

   d. Coherence or systematic structure

   e. Comprehensiveness or scope of knowledge

3. How can a knowledge of the scientific method be helpful when making statements of prognosis?

4. Research is viewed in this chapter as a process of asking and answering

questions. Can clinical evaluation (diagnosis) also be viewed from this perspective? Why?

5. A speech-language pathologist determined the level of phonological development of 100 children between the ages of six months and 12 years. He also measured the length of each child's foot. The correlation between the measures of foot length and phonological development was very high (over 0.85). Based on the strength of this correlation he concluded that foot length is a valid measure of phonological development. Do you agree or disagree that the correlation he obtained warrants this conclusion? Why?

4

Searching the Literature

Speech-language pathologists and audiologists—whether functioning as consumers or producers of research—have to be able to locate information efficiently. As consumers of research they have to be able to do so to maximize the effectiveness of their intervention strategies. That is, they have to be able to locate information bearing directly or indirectly on the "impacts" of those they are considering using. And as producers of research, they have to do a systematic search for relevant literature whenever they begin (or contemplate beginning) a research project. Since the literature on most communicative disorders is relatively large and widely scattered, information in it usually cannot be located efficiently without using an *index.* Trying to do so would be as inefficient as trying to find specific information in a book by "thumbing through the pages." Several types of indexes to *portions* of the communicative disorder literature are described in this chapter. Unfortunately, there isn't a single index to all of it, and those that are available may not identify all relevant papers. However, if you use them, you are likely to find the information you want more quickly than you are otherwise.

There are two main types of indexes that can be used for accessing the literature in a particular field (e.g., communicative disorders): abstracts journals and online, interactive computer-based information retrieval systems. Abstracts journals contain abstracts of papers that have been published in other journals rather than original papers. Each of them abstract papers in a particular field—e.g., *Psychological Abstracts* abstracts papers in the field of psychology, and *Index Medicus* abstracts ones in the field of medicine. In the final issue of each volume (usually the last issue for the year), there is an index to all of the abstracts in that volume. You can use this index for identifying papers that are likely to contain the information you are seeking.

Online, interactive computer-based information retrieval systems are "tools" for retrieving information from computer databases (Borgman, Moghdam, and Corbett, 1984). They are *online* because the user is in direct communication with the computer containing the database through a terminal or a microcomputer that has been programmed to function as one. And they are *interactive* because the user and computer engage in a "conversation" in which the computer responds quickly. The databases they access contain information similar to that in abstracts journals. In some cases, the information in an abstracts journal is essentially the same as that in a database. For example, the information in the Medline database (Albright, 1988; *PlusNet2 Medline System: End-user Introduction*, 1990; Reiner and Ludlow, 1979a, 1979b, and 1981) is essentially the same as that in the abstracts journal *Index Medicus*, and that in the PsycLIT one (Gosling, Knight, and McKenney, 1989) is essentially the same as that in the abstracts journal *Psychological Abstracts*. However, the contents of these abstracts journals and databases are not identical (Pfaffenberger, 1990). The "index" you would use for identifying relevant papers with such a database is accessed by inputting one or more terms from it into the computer via the keyboard. Printouts of the terms the index for a particular database will recognize have been published for most of them, including the Medline and PsycLIT ones. Partial printouts of this index for the Medline database have been published for specialists in communicative disorders (Reiner and Ludlow, 1979a, 1979b, and 1981).

While abstracts journals and online, interactive computer-based information retrieval systems are the most frequently used "tools" for doing literature searches, they are not the only ones. Two others that can be used for supplementing them are published and unpublished bibliographies and reference lists in books and papers (particularly review papers). Bibliographies have been compiled for a number of topics relevant to communicative disorders, including the following: aphasia (Sarno and Sands, 1967), augmentative communication (Lloyd, 1980; Rabush, Lloyd, and Gerdes, 1982, 1983; Silverman, 1977a, 1989; Villarruel, Mathy-Laikko, Ratcliff, and Yoder, 1987), microcomputer applications (Silverman, 1987), and stuttering (Elliott, 1951; Silverman, 1978; Silverman, Silverman, and Meagher, 1979; Silverman and Trotter, 1973a). Bibliographies and reference lists can be particularly helpful when searching for information in books, convention (and other unpublished) papers, and "older" published papers and monographs.

LITERATURE SEARCHING WITH ONLINE, INTERACTIVE COMPUTER-BASED INFORMATION RETRIEVAL SYSTEMS

There are several computer databases that can be used with online, interactive information retrieval software for searching portions of the international communicative disorders literature. The one that probably has been used most often for this purpose by speech-language pathologists and audiologists is Medline (Reiner and Ludlow, 1979a, 1979b, and 1981). This database indexes papers in more than 3000 journals (including those of the American Speech-Language-Hearing Association) dealing with medicine and related subjects from 1966 to the present. It is available in two forms: one that is stored on tape and requires the use of a mini- or mainframe computer (Silverman, 1987) to access and one that is stored on compact disks (CDs) and can be accessed with a microcomputer. A single compact disk can store as many as 275,000 pages of typed information (Pfaffenberger, 1990). One CD-based database—CD + Medline—stored the entire Medline database on eight CDs when this chapter was written. While the 3000 + journals indexed by this database include most that publish papers on communicative disorders, it does not include them all. The *Journal of Fluency Disorders,* for example, was not indexed when this chapter was written.

Another computer database that indexes a portion of the communicative disorders literature and is available on CDs is PsycLIT (Gosling, Knight, and McKenney, 1989). This database, which is produced by the American Psychological Association, indexes papers on psychology and related subjects in more than 1300 journals from 1974 to the present. Among the journals indexed are ones published by the American Speech-Language-Hearing Association. Since some journals that publish papers on communicative disorders are indexed by PsycLIT but not by Medline and vice versa, using both is likely to result in a more complete search than using only one.

There are a number of other computer databases available in one or both of these forms that index portions of the communicative disorders literature. Three that speech-language pathologists and audiologists are likely to find particularly helpful are the following:

- *ERIC* (Educational Resources Information Center) indexes papers in 700 + educational journals from 1966 to present.
- *Dissertation Abstracts* indexes titles and abstracts in dissertations from 1980 to the present and titles only prior to that.
- *PsycINFO,* which like PsycLIT is produced by the American Psychological Association, indexes papers dealing with psychology and related areas from 1967 to the present. It differs from PsycLIT in that it is not available on CDs, includes both dissertations and published papers, and is updated monthly rather than quarterly (Gosling, Knight, and McKenney, 1989).

Most college and university libraries employ at least one research librarian who is knowledgeable about such databases and can recommend ones that would be worth searching for particular topics.

Deciding When to Use an Online, Interactive Computer-Based Information Retrieval System

It may be possible to do a literature search for a particular topic using either an abstracts journal or a computerized database. The same information may be in both. Topics with one or more of the following characteristics are likely to utilize the capabilities of computerized literature searching to their fullest (Borgman, Moghdam, and Corbett, 1984, pp. 21–22):

1. Searches that require the coordination of two or more distinct concepts; for example, "the effect of vitamin C on the common cold." The two concepts are "vitamin C" and "the common cold."
2. Searches on topics so new or obscure that they may not yet appear as subject headings in printed indexes.
3. Searches for information which is known to be more recent than the printed index, and it is known that the online database is current.
4. Searches on topics which may be stated in so many synonymous terms that manual searching of indexes would be unreasonably time-consuming.
5. Searches which are relatively narrow in scope and are likely to result in rather small retrieval.
6. Topics covered in databases that do not have a corresponding printed index. While many databases include information which duplicates printed indexes [abstracts journals], some databases have no printed counterpart.

Literature searching using online, interactive computer-based information retrieval systems tends to be faster than doing so using abstracts journals because a number of years can be searched simultaneously. For example, with the PlusNet2 Medline database relevant papers published between 1986 and 1991 can be identified from a single search. On the other hand, it usually is not possible to search as far back using a database as it is using an abstracts journal. With the PsycLIT database, for example, it is only possible to search from 1974 to the present (Gosling, Knight, and McKenney, 1989). However, with the journal *Psychological Abstracts* it is possible to do so as far back as 1927.

Planning the Search

Before performing a search using a computerized database, it is necessary to decide the following:

1. The keywords that will be included in the search and the manner in which they will be "linked." Ways in which they can be linked are discussed in the next section.

2. The database(s) that will be searched.
3. The range of years that will be included in the search.
4. Whether the search should be limited in any way(s), e.g., English language only, children only, females only, human subjects only, or review articles only.
5. Whether abstracts, if available, will be printed.

After these have been decided, the search can be performed by either a research librarian or the enduser (You!). If a database to be searched is on CDs or tape at one of the college's or university's computer facilities, it should be possible for the enduser to do the search himself or herself. However, if the database is on a mini- or mainframe computer that does not belong to the institution and is accessed via a terminal and modem over telephone lines, the institution may require that searches be performed by a research librarian. If this is the case, then information defining the search usually will be communicated to the librarian on a special form (see Figure 4.1).

Doing the Search

Search Strategies. Most computer databases are searched in a similar fashion—through the use of <u>keywords</u> and the <u>Boolean logic connectors</u> AND, OR, and NOT (Berkman, 1990). (Boolean logic was named after the mathematician who invented it, George Boole.) The manner in which this is done is illustrated in Figures 4.2 through 4.9. Let's represent the keywords "hearing loss," "otitis media," and "children" by A, B, and C respectively. The strategy diagrammed in Figure 4.2 is one in which we are searching for all references containing a particular keyword (which can consist of more than one word). We would use this strategy, for example, if we were interested in retrieving from a database all references containing the keyword "hearing loss."

The strategy diagrammed in Figure 4.3 is one in which we are searching for all references containing two keywords. We could use this strategy, for example, if we were interested in retrieving from a database all references containing the keywords "hearing loss" <u>AND</u> "otitis media." That is, we would use it if we were only interested in retrieving references dealing with hearing loss resulting from otitis media.

The strategy diagrammed in Figure 4.4 is referred to as the *inclusive* OR strategy because it not only will retrieve references containing one of two keywords, but also those containing both of them. We could use this strategy, for example, if we were interested in retrieving from a database all references containing the keywords "hearing loss" OR "otitis media" OR both of these. All computer databases support an OR search strategy that functions in this manner.

FIGURE 4.1   A representative search request form.

COMPUTER SEARCH REQUEST—MARQUETTE UNIVERSITY LIBRARIES

DATE _____   FACULTY ____ STAFF ____ GRADUATE ____
Name _____   UNDERGRAD ____ ID NUMBER _____
School or Dept _____
Address _____   ___ Dissertation/thesis
Phone   Day _____ Night _____   ___ Coursework
(In case further information is needed)   ___ University research
                                           ___ Other (specify)

SEARCH TOPIC   Please explain in sentences exactly what you want covered. Be specific!
Define terms that have special meanings. Feel free to attach another
page.

SUGGESTED KEYWORDS/DESCRIPTORS	Which indexes or abstracts have you searched? Which subject headings were useful?
Please list a few recent relevant articles or books (authors, titles, journals, dates). Can you think of an ideal journal article title on the subject?	How many citations do you need? ___ A few relevant articles (under 25) ___ An exhaustive search which may retrieve a substantial number of irrelevant citations ___ Something in-between Time period to be covered ___ Current (last 2–3 years) ___ All years possible ___ Other time period (specify) ___ English _____ All languages ___ Other languages (specify) _____ _____

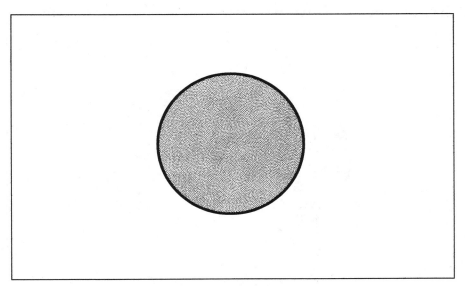

FIGURE 4.2   A single keyword search strategy.

FIGURE 4.3   A single AND search strategy.

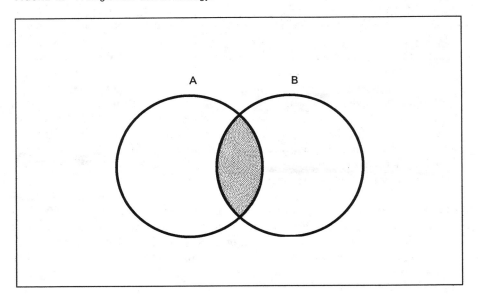

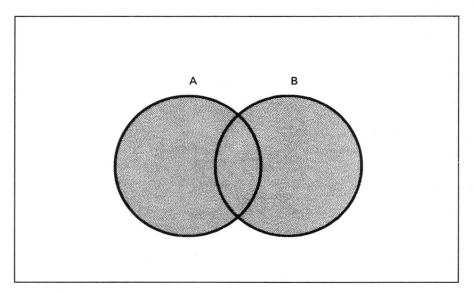

FIGURE 4.4   An inclusive OR search strategy.

Some of them also support an *exclusive* OR search strategy (see Figure 4.5) which will not retrieve references containing both keywords. Because you usually would not want to exclude such references, the *inclusive* OR strategy is used far more often than this one. An example of where you might want to use the *exclusive* OR strategy is for retrieving references dealing with "dysarthria without aphasia" and "aphasia without dysarthria: The two keywords here would be dysarthria and aphasia.

The AND NOT search strategy is illustrated in Figure 4.6. (In some systems it may be referred to as the NOT or BUT NOT one). It will retrieve references that mention one keyword that do not mention a second keyword. It can be used, for example, to retrieve all references on hearing loss that do not mention otitis media. This strategy should be used with caution because it will eliminate all references that mention the excluded keyword, including those that only do so in passing.

A search strategy can involve more than two keywords. A multiple AND search strategy that involves three keywords is illustrated in Figure 4.7. It can be used for retrieving references in which three keywords are mentioned. It could be used, for example, for finding papers dealing (at least in part) with "hearing loss" in "children" resulting from "otitis media." This search strategy—which can use more than three keywords—is one of the most useful ones.

Another type of search strategy that involves more than two keywords combines the AND and AND NOT logical connectors (see Figure 4.8). It can be used for retrieving references that mention two keywords that do not mention a third. It could be used, for example, for finding papers dealing

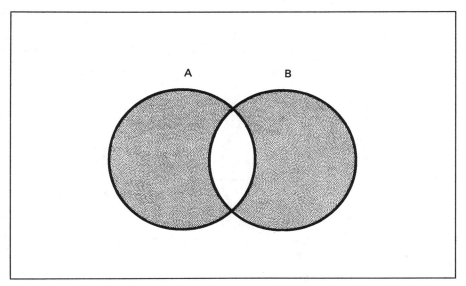

FIGURE 4.5 An exclusive OR search strategy.

FIGURE 4.6 An AND NOT search strategy.

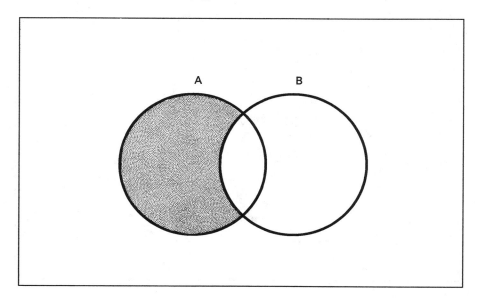

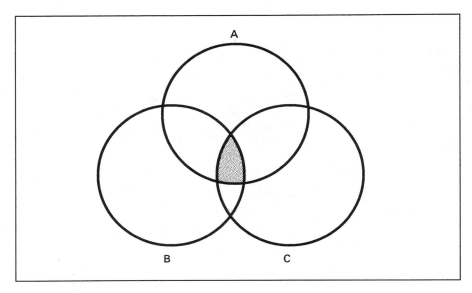

FIGURE 4.7   A multiple AND search strategy.

FIGURE 4.8   A compound AND and AND NOT search strategy.

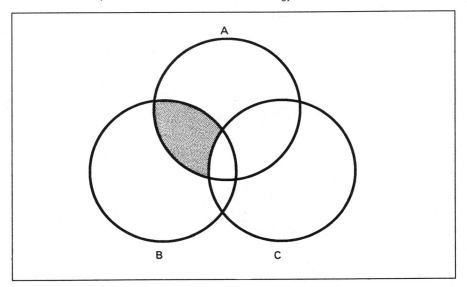

with "hearing loss" in "children" that do not mention "otitis media." The problem mentioned in the discussion of the AND NOT search strategy affects this one also.

A third type of search strategy that involves more than two keywords combines the AND and OR logical connectors (see Figure 4.9). When using it, two keywords are connected to each other by OR and these in turn are connected to another keyword by AND. This strategy could be used, for example, to locate papers dealing with "children" in which either "otitis media" or "hearing loss" is mentioned.

Conducting an Online Search. If a database you decide to search is one that can be searched at your institution by an enduser, you can begin the search after you have formulated a strategy for doing so. The first step in the process is "logging on," or "signing on," to the computer on which the database is stored. If the database is stored on CDs on a microcomputer that cannot be accessed remotely, the enduser would log on to that computer. On the other hand, if the database is stored on a mini- or mainframe computer, the enduser would log on to it using a terminal or a microcomputer that was programmed to simulate one. Most logon procedures involve keyboarding your name and a password when requested to do so. The password, which is issued by the institution where the computer being accessed is located, may not be displayed on the screen while it is being keyboarded for security reasons.

FIGURE 4.9 A compound search strategy in which two keywords are connected to each other by OR and these in turn are connected to another keyword by AND.

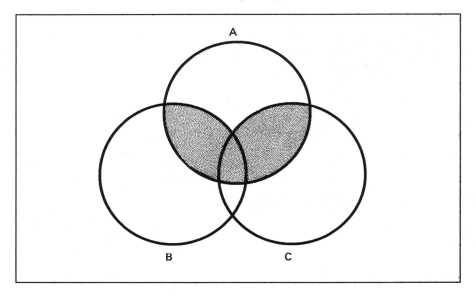

When the logon procedure is completed, you are given access to the database's main menu (see Figure 4.10). This menu may also give you access to a tutorial that provides basic information about the commands and procedures used for searching that database (see Figure 4.10). It is a good idea to go through the tutorial at least once, particularly if you do not have access to a manual that provides this information.

The second step in the process is actually executing the search. This is done by selecting the appropriate item from the main menu (it would be "search for information" in Figure 4.10) and by sending commands to the computer. Commands may be sent by activating single keys or combinations of ESCAPE or CONTROL keys and other keys. For example, X may be used for highlighting an option on a menu (see Figure 4.10), CONTROL J (abbreviated as ^J) for instructing the computer to browse through a set (see Figure 4.11), and ESCAPE E for instructing it to move to the last line of a citation. Unfortunately, the commands used for accessing databases have not been standardized. The same command may be used in two databases but have a different meaning in each.

The search is initiated by entering the "string" containing the keywords that are to be used for it (see Figure 4.11). The string entered for the example diagrammed in Figure 4.12 would be the following:

hearing loss

FIGURE 4.10   A representative main menu screen for a computer database intended for enduser searching.

Options
Search for information
Review search results
File management
Print or copy search results
Maintenance functions
Introduction
Tutorial
Copy tutorial and editor
Exit

CD PLUS

Use ^ or v to position cursor.

Press 'x' to highlight an option,.
then press ENTER to select that option.

Copyright (C) 1990 by CD Plus

```
┌──────────┬─────────────────────────────────────────────────┬──────────────┐
│ Number   │ Search Sets                                     │ Results      │
├──────────┼─────────────────────────────────────────────────┼──────────────┤
│          │                                                 │              │
│          │                                                 │              │
│          │                                                 │              │
│          │                                                 │              │
│          │                                                 │              │
│          │                                                 │              │
├──────────────────────── Medline <1987 forward> ───────────────────────────┤
│                                                                            │
│          Enter subject, then press ENTER                                   │
│                                                                            │
│       _: hearing loss                                                      │
│                                                                            │
├────────────────────────────────────────────────────────────────────────── ┤
│   ^A  Help              ^F  Limit Set          ^J  Browse Set              │
│   ^B  Search Text Words ^G  Combine Sets       ^K  Print/Download Set      │
│   ^E  End Session       ^I  Save/Change Files  ^L  Additional Options      │
└────────────────────────────────────────────────────────────────────────── ┘
```

FIGURE 4.11   A representative screen for entering the subject of a search.

FIGURE 4.12   A representative screen menu of subject headings for limiting a search by adding a Boolean AND and a keyword.

```
┌──────────────────────────────────────────────────────────────────────────┐
│          Medical Subject Headings          Line 1 of 10                    │
├──────────────────────────────────────────────────────────────────────────┤
│       hearing loss, sensorineural                                          │
│       hearing loss, noise-induced                                          │
│       hearing loss, partial                                                │
│       hearing disorders                                                    │
│       cochlea                                                              │
│       neomycin                                                             │
│       evoked potentials, auditory                                          │
│       audiometry, evoked response                                          │
│       occupational disease                                                 │
│       middle age                                                           │
├──────────────────────── Medline <1987 forward> ───────────────────────────┤
│                                                                            │
│       Press 'x' to mark the single most relevant subject heading, then     │
│       press ENTER.  Or press ENTER to pick no heading, or ^A for help.     │
│                                                                            │
├──────────────────────────────────────────────────────────────────────────┤
│   ^A  Help                                                                 │
│   ^B  Scope Note                                                           │
└──────────────────────────────────────────────────────────────────────────┘
```

The computer after searching will indicate whether there are any items in the database that can be indexed by the string and, if so, how many. If there are many, it may indicate ways that you can eliminate some (i.e., narrow the search) by focusing more directly on the specific information you want. It may do this by adding a Boolean AND and keyword to the search. For example, it may permit you to limit the items selected to those dealing with partial hearing loss or hearing loss occurring during middle age (see Figure 4.12). After you have made a decision about whether you are interested in all the items or a more limited set, you will be informed how many items there are and possibly given the opportunity to limit the search further by restricting it to articles in which the keyword (index term) is a main focus (see Figure 4.13). After making this decision you may be presented with another menu of subheadings that will allow you to further limit (focus) the search if you want to do so (see Figure 4.14). After you respond to this menu, the number of items in the search set is indicated and you are given the opportunity to "browse" through them (see Figure 4.15)—ie., to view them one at a time on the screen (see Figure 4.16). If you want an item included in the printout, you can issue a command (e.g., ^E) after viewing it (see Figure 4.16).

If the computer indicates that there are no items containing the keywords you selected, the reason may be that you have chosen the wrong ones. Each database has a printed thesaurus, as a reference tool, which lists the keywords to which it will respond—i.e., ones that are in its index.

The final steps in the search process are printing relevant items and

FIGURE 4.13   A representative screen for limiting a search by restricting it to articles in which the keyword (index term) is a main focus.

```
:----------------:----------------------------------------------------:---:
:                : Index Term Selected                                :   :
:----------------:                                                     :---:
:                : *hearing loss, partial                             :   :
:                :                                                     :   :
:                :                                                     :   :
:                :                                                     :   :
:                :                                                     :   :
:                :                                                     :   :
:                :                                                     :   :
:                :                                                     :   :
:                :                                                     :   :
:----------------:-----------------------------------------------------:---:
:------------------------------Medline <1987 forward>---------------------:
:             565 articles contain the above index term.                  :
:             In 456 articles this term is the focus of the article.      :
:                                                                         :
:             Restrict to focus?  Enter 'y' or 'n', then ENTER _:         :
:-------------------------------------------------------------------------:
:      ^A  Help                                                           :
:                                                                         :
:                                                                         :
:-------------------------------------------------------------------------:
```

```
+-----------------------------------------------------------------+
| Subheadings          Line 1 of 20              : Results        |
+-----------------------------------------------------------------+
|    chemically induced                             33            |
|    complications                                  15            |
|    congenital                                      7            |
|    diagnosis                                      69            |
|    drug therapy                                    9            |
|    epidemiology                                   11            |
|    etiology                                      113            |
|    genetics                                       16            |
|    history                                         1            |
|    immunology                                      1            |
|       v More v                                                  |
|----------------------Medline <1987 forward>--------------------|
|    The subheadings shown above may be applied to refine your    |
|    search.                                                      |
|    Press 'x' to mark as many as are relevant, then press ENTER. |
|    To restrict to no particular subheading, simply press ENTER. |
|-----------------------------------------------------------------|
|  ^A  Help                                                       |
|  ^B  Explain subheading                                         |
+-----------------------------------------------------------------+
```

FIGURE 4.14 A representative screen menu of subheadings for further limiting a search by adding a Boolean AND and an additional keyword.

FIGURE 4.15 A representative screen for selecting a search set to browse.

```
+-----------------------------------------------------------------+
| Number : Search Sets            Line 1 of 1       : Results     |
+-----------------------------------------------------------------+
|  01    : *hearing loss, partial                      456        |
|                                                                 |
|                                                                 |
|                                                                 |
|                                                                 |
|                                                                 |
|----------------------Medline <1987 forward>--------------------|
|    Mark set to browse, then press ENTER.                        |
|    Press ENTER to browse last set.                              |
|-----------------------------------------------------------------|
|  ^A  Browse Selected Fields                                     |
+-----------------------------------------------------------------+
```

```
..................................................................................
:               | Citation 4 of  456                              |             :
:................................................................................:
: Unique Identifier                                                              :
:      91073233                                                                  :
: Author                                                                         :
:      Hasegawa S.                                                               :
: Title                                                                          :
:      Hearing and language ability in mild and moderate hearing impaired children:
:      [Jpn]                                                                     :
: Institution                                                                    :
:      Department of Otolaryngology, Nagoya University School of Medicine.       :
: Journal                                                                        :
:      Nippon Jibiinkoka Gakkai Kaiho [JC:jjz] 93(9): 1397-409, 1990 Sep.        :
: Abstract                                                                       :
:      102 children (mean age-7 years 9 mo.) with mild and moderate perceptive   :
:      hearing impairment who had neither any auditory training nor had used a   :
:      hearing aid were studied. Mean hearing level was 51.9 dB. Our findings: (1):
:      Speech discrimination score (SDS) correlated with the hearing level at 2, 4:
:      and 1 kHz, in that order. In all patients SDS gradually worsened to 60 dB :
:--------------------------------------------------------------------------------:
:      ^A  End Browsing         ^F  Skip to Citation      n  Next Citation        :
:      ^B  Find Similar Citations ^G  Flag Citations       p  Previous Citation    :
:      ^E  Print Citation                                                         :
:................................................................................:
```

FIGURE 4.16   A representative screen when citations are being browsed. You could have the remainder of the abstract displayed by typing a command.

logging off. You may be given choices about the format in which you want the bibliography printed, including whether you want abstracts included, if available. If you are using a microcomputer as a terminal, you probably will be given the option of downloading the bibliography to it for saving as a file that can be edited and printed with a word-processing program. After the bibliography is printed or transferred to the microcomputer and saved as a file, you are expected to log off unless you plan to do another search immediately. Doing so usually involves sending a command indicating that you want to quit and possibly keyboarding a sequence of characters such as LO (for "logging off").

Some computerized databases support searches other than keyword topic ones. For example, they may allow you to identify items by a particular author or those published by authors at a particular institution.

LITERATURE SEARCHING USING ABSTRACTS JOURNALS

The abstracts journals that cover the field of communicative disorders include *dsh Abstracts* (1960–1984), *Dissertation Abstracts* (1952–), *Index Medicus* (1916–), *Linguistics and Language Behavior Abstracts* (1967–), and *Psychological Abstracts* (1927–). There was no abstracts journal when this chapter was written (1991) that comprehensively covered the field. The journal *dsh [deafness, speech, and hearing] Abstracts* did so between 1960 and 1984 and, hence, is a valuable resource for doing literature searches that include these years.

1678. SEMPLE, J. E. Hearing-impaired preschool child. Springfield, Ill.: Charles C Thomas, 1970. Pp 86.

Designed for parents, the book first describes the problems parents face in coping with their hearing-impaired child and suggests some solutions to these problems. The next two chapters deal with hearing aids and with language and speech development. The last and major chapter presents a series of daily home lesson plans to be used by the parent to assist the child in developing speech and language. The appendixes include reading materials, children's books, an outline for an auditory training program, and suggestions for auditory training.—*I. M. Ventry*

1679. SHARRATT, J. Teaching deaf children to read. *Teacher Deaf*, 68, 1970, 42–44.

Some of the experiences of a teacher of young deaf children during her first three years' teaching.—*K. W. Kritz*

1680. THAN, A. M. (Roy. Nat. Inst. Deaf, 105 Gower St., London W.C. 1, England) **Education of the deaf in Burma.** *Hearing*, 25, 1970, 108–111.

After a very brief geo-political description of the Union of Burma, the history of services to handicapped children in that country are described. Considers present audiological and educational facilities, and indicates "that by late 1970, two E.E.N.T. specialist doctors and the author will open the first audiology clinic in the country . . ." Goes on to provide some statistics on incidence and services.—*S. E. Gerber*

1681. TRUFFAUT, B. La préparation des jeunes sourds au C.A.P. de dessinateur en construction mecanique. (Training of young deaf as draftsmen.) *Rev. gen. Enseigne. deficients auditifs*, 61(4), 1969, 28–31.

For 10 years the Institute of Saint-Jean-de-la-Ruelle has trained draftsmen, both hearing and deaf. The average age of admission is 16 years. Selection is empirical. The course is of three years' duration. Despite certain difficulties, most deaf graduates obtain satisfactory employment.—*P. J. Wevrick*

1682. VAN UDEN, A. (U. St. Michielsgestal, The Netherlands) **Johann Vatter, a German teacher of the deaf.** *Teacher Deaf*, 68, 1970, 21–34.

The work and philosophy of this teacher of the deaf is discussed. Pure oral instruction in a residential setting is advocated. Language learning is based on conversation.—*K. W. Kritz*

1683. WRIGHT, D. Deafness. New York, N.Y.: Stein and Day, 1969. Pp 213.

David Wright, the author of this book, is a poet who became profoundly deaf at age seven. In the first section of the book (eight chapters) he provides a biographical account of the impact of deafness on his life, with special emphasis on conveying the feelings of a deaf person as he participates in a variety of activities. The second section (five chapters) is a history of education of the deaf. A short appendix by K. Murphy summarizes basic hearing physiology, hearing pathology, and related research trends. The author indicates that when he wrote this book he had in mind the predicament of parents who have a deaf child.—*J. B. Chaiklin*

ETIOLOGY AND PATHOLOGY

1684. ANDERSON, H. (Karolinska Hosp., Stockholm, Sweden), **FILIPSSON, R., FLUUR, E., KOCH, B., LINDSTEN, J. and WEDENBERG, E. Hearing impairment in Turner's syndrome.** *Acta otolaryngol.*, Suppl. 247, 1969. Pp 26.

The hearing was studied in 79 clinically and cytogenetically analyzed patients with Turner's syndrome. Middle ear infections had occurred in 68% of the patients. Conductive or mixed losses were found in 22%. Cephalometric analysis showed the external auditory meati to be caudally displaced which resulted in abnormal orientation of the Eustachian tube, a condition that may explain the predisposition to middle-ear infections. Sensorineural hearing impairment with recruitment was found in 64% of the patients. Vestibular findings were normal for the nine patients who were given vestibular tests. The etiological significance of the abnormal sex chromosome constitution for the hearing impairment is discussed.—*Authors, edited*

FIGURE 4.17 A representative page of abstracts from an abstracts journal.

Communication, Manual 131, 142, 144, 631, 642, 774, 833, 1089, 1094, 1095, 1179, 1662, 1669, 1672, 1676
Communication, Theory 281, 282, 300, 305, 309, 386, 434, 790, 792, 793, 807, 809, 833, 1451, 1669, 1820, 1821, 1824, 1965
personality 434, 1824
research 386
Conditioning 16, 382, 764, 831, 885, 932, 1198, 1217, 1251, 1461, 1475, 1531, 1644, 1849, 1852
operant 764, 831, 885, 932, 1198, 1251
verbal learning 1849
Cortex 958, 959, 962, 967, 968, 982, 1033, 1464, 1473, 1474, 1486, 1493, 1501, 1511, 1512, 1517, 1521, 1528, 1548, 1571
auditory response 958, 959, 962, 967, 968, 982, 1474, 1486, 1493, 1501, 1511, 1512, 1517, 1521, 1529, 1548, 1571
lesions 1033
single cells 1464, 1473
Deafness 19, 33, 48, 53, 55, 74, 93, 94, 96, 97, 98, 100, 103, 104, 105, 110, 114, 115, 117, 119, 123, 124, 126, 128, 129, 130, 131, 135, 136, 137, 138, 140, 145, 147, 149, 150, 152, 154, 155, 157, 158, 159, 160, 161, 163, 164, 166, 167, 168, 169, 170, 171, 172, 173, 174, 175, 176, 177, 178, 179, 180, 181, 183, 184, 185, 186, 187, 188, 189, 192, 194, 195, 196, 197, 198, 203, 206, 212, 215, 221, 223, 225, 227, 229, 234, 239, 241, 246, 247, 248, 249, 250, 252, 253, 257, 259, 261, 262, 263, 264, 265, 266, 267, 268, 269, 271, 373, 382, 395, 441, 442, 480, 512, 528, 562, 563, 565, 566, 567, 568, 569, 571, 573, 576, 578, 580, 581, 584, 589, 593, 595, 598, 599, 600, 602, 603, 606, 608, 609, 614, 616, 617, 620, 623, 625, 633, 635, 640, 641, 646, 648, 650, 655, 656, 658, 662, 665, 667, 670, 671, 673, 674, 675, 678, 681, 682, 685, 688, 689, 690, 691, 692, 693, 697, 699, 702, 703, 704, 706, 708, 709, 711, 714, 717, 719, 720, 725, 727, 728, 729, 733, 741, 742, 743, 745, 751, 752, 753, 758, 764, 766, 767, 768, 769, 770, 771, 772, 778, 779, 780, 820, 888, 947, 1064, 1067, 1068, 1069, 1071, 1074, 1077, 1078, 1079, 1081, 1082, 1083, 1084, 1086, 1087, 1088, 1089, 1090, 1091, 1092, 1093, 1095, 1101, 1102, 1103, 1105, 1106, 1107, 1108, 1111, 1112, 1113, 1115, 1117, 1121, 1123, 1127, 1128, 1130, 1132, 1133, 1134, 1136, 1141, 1142, 1143, 1145, 1146, 1147, 1150, 1162, 1166, 1167, 1172, 1176, 1178, 1179, 1180, 1181, 1182, 1183, 1184, 1185, 1186, 1187, 1188, 1189, 1190, 1191, 1192, 1314, 1346, 1418, 1422, 1431, 1478, 1516, 1518, 1570, 1583, 1587, 1590, 1591, 1595, 1597, 1598, 1599, 1601, 1602, 1603, 1608, 1610, 1611, 1612, 1613, 1614, 1618, 1622, 1627, 1628, 1629, 1630, 1631, 1632, 1633, 1639, 1640, 1641, 1642, 1643, 1644, 1647, 1648, 1650, 1651, 1653, 1656, 1658, 1659, 1660, 1661, 1664, 1667, 1669, 1670, 1672, 1673, 1674, 1678, 1679, 1682, 1683, 1684, 1685, 1686, 1687, 1688, 1689, 1692, 1694, 1696, 1697, 1698, 1699, 1700, 1702, 1703, 1704, 1707, 1708, 1709, 1710, 1711, 1712, 1713, 1715, 1716, 1717, 1719, 1720, 1723, 1724, 1725, 1733, 1734, 1735, 1736, 1740, 1742, 1743, 1744, 1745, 1746, 1747, 1748, 1750, 1751, 1754, 1759, 1761, 1765, 1767, 1772, 1775, 1780, 1781, 1782, 1786, 1787, 1790, 1791, 1792, 1793, 1794, 1795, 1796, 1797, 1798, 1799, 1800, 1801, 1803, 1804, 1805, 1920, 1956, 1958, 1960, 1964
acromegaly 673
adolescents 593
adults 569
allergy 168
and aging 33, 74, 123, 149, 163, 172, 173, 176, 177, 178, 188, 192, 263, 562, 656, 667, 699, 702, 706, 1112, 1142, 1602, 1612, 1613, 1673, 1687, 1689, 1692, 1694, 1719, 1767
assessment 1190
audiometric patterns 1692
auditory training 563, 565, 703
bilateral 578
chemically induced 1123
in children 117, 128, 138, 140, 145, 225, 573, 580, 608, 623, 648, 1074, 1078, 1079, 1081, 1084, 1087, 1103, 1121, 1127, 1128, 1141, 1146, 1172, 1570, 1591, 1601, 1603, 1631, 1647, 1653, 1685, 1746, 1748
classification 1106
cleft palate 1733
communication 1516
conductive 395, 617, 675, 721, 725, 1640, 1684, 1710, 1761, 1782, 1787
congenital 114, 115, 150, 164, 174, 184, 189, 614, 1084, 1127, 1711, 1717
counseling 1664, 1683, 1772
diabetes 674, 1622
differential diagnosis 722, 1068, 1597, 1610, 1611, 1614
diving 1708
and drugs. See *Drugs: and hearing*
and dying 5
education 1792
emotional instability 262
encephalitis 195
in England 129
etiology 617, 1136, 1478, 1684, 1689, 1707, 1711, 1759, 1786
evaluation 752
in France 137
functional 104, 105, 609, 768, 1650
and head injury 1696
hereditary 114, 157, 166, 180, 183, 197, 568, 670, 678, 690, 691, 1150, 1587, 1608, 1697, 1698, 1703, 1711, 1715, 1717, 1724, 1798
hidden 581, 685
high frequency 1077
identifications 608
incidence 633
in India 1105

FIGURE 4.18 A representative index page from an abstracts journal.

The journal *Linguistics and Language Behavior Abstracts* was titled *Language and Language Behavior Abstracts* between 1967 and 1984.

Representative abstracts and index pages from abstracts journals are reproduced in Figures 4.17 and 4.18 respectively.

Begin a literature search with the last issue of the most recent complete volume of the journal. An index in the back of this issue covers the entire volume (i.e., all four issues for a quarterly journal). You look up your keywords in this index. If you do not find them, you look up synonyms. Then you scan the abstracts of papers that may contain relevant information. Finally, you write down references to those that appear to contain such information.

This process is repeated with the next most recent volume of the abstracts journal and continues until you have covered the number of years you want to include in your search. If the most recent volume of the abstracts journal is *incomplete*, you can check the "Table of Contents" of each issue for sections in which there may be papers that contain relevant information.

EXERCISE

Search the literature on a topic using both an abstracts journal and a computerized database. How similar are the bibliographies yielded by each?

5

Asking Questions That Are Both Relevant and Answerable

The first four chapters were intended to "set the stage" for our discussion of research design. My primary objective in this chapter and the seven that follow is to provide basic information about the process of asking and answering questions that a speech-language pathologist or audiologist needs to function as a clinician-investigator. This chapter will deal with selecting and formulating questions for research. It also will be concerned with selecting a topic, or area, to research. The topic selected, of course, determines the questions asked.

A speech-language pathologist or audiologist who chooses to function as a clinician-investigator must first decide what to investigate—what question or questions to try to answer. This decision is important because it will influence both the impact of his or her research and the likelihood that the research will be completed. By *impact* here we mean the effect that answering a particular question or group of questions is likely to have on clinical process in speech-language pathology and audiology. Unfortunately, the amount of impact that answering a particular question is likely to have on clinical process is quite difficult to predict. As Murray Sidman has pointed out,

> It is necessary . . . to be wary about using the presumed importance of data as a criterion for evaluating them. Science, like fashion, has its fads and cycles. A discovery that lies outside the current stream of interest may be unrecognized and eventually forgotten, perhaps to be rediscovered at some later date. On the

other side of the coin, we often find experiments acclaimed as significant because they resolve a problem of great contemporary concern, but of little lasting
interest. It is a characteristic of science that we are seldom able to predict its
future course of development. Many of the exciting issues of today will be
forgotten tomorrow as the stream of scientific progress shifts into new chan-
nels. (Sidman, 1960, p.2)

Sidman's comments obviously have relevance for assessing the probable impact of answers to questions (i.e., experimental results) on clinical process in
speech-language pathology and audiology. While the criterion of "importance" will always be of concern to investigators, it will not be particularly
useful either for selecting questions to answer or for evaluating answers to
questions.

An investigator's choice of questions to answer influences the likelihood
that he or she will complete the research, for several reasons. The first is the
time required to make the necessary observations. The longer you take to make
these observations, the less likely you are to complete your research. As long
as the time necessary does not exceed a year, this probably would not be an
important consideration. While I do not wish to imply here that investigators
should avoid questions that take longer than a year to answer—since there
are probably many such questions that would be worthwhile answering—you
should realize that when you attempt to answer such questions you are less
likely to complete your research. This may be one of the reasons, incidentally,
why so little longitudinal research has been reported.

A second factor likely to influence the probability that research will be
completed is the *complexity of the procedures required to make the necessary
observations.* The more complex such procedures, the less likely an investigator is to complete the research. If you need electronic instrumentation (particularly, complex electronic instrumentation) to make your observations, you
may have difficulty getting the instrumentation to function well enough to
make them. The author experienced such difficulty in his own research with
a miniature voice-actuated white-noise generator that was designed to be
used with stutterers. About 50 percent of the time the device would not function properly, and several electronics technicians who tried to repair it were
unsuccessful. While we are not attempting to discourage investigators from
answering questions that require instrumentation to answer, you should realize that problems can arise when you attempt to answer such questions.

A third factor is the *availability of subjects.* If subjects are not available
in sufficient numbers *within a reasonable time period,* the probability that the
research will be completed can be reduced. It should be noted, however, that
speech-language pathologists and audiologists have successfully completed
research which has taken a number of years to observe a sufficient number
of subjects. Berry *et al.* (1974), for example, required 15 years to observe a
sufficient number of persons with Wilson's disease to be able to describe the
speech deviations associated with it.

A fourth factor is the *time available for the purpose.* Some questions require more time to answer than others. Before beginning a piece of research, therefore, you should at least roughly estimate both the time required to complete it and the time you are likely to have available for the purpose.

A fifth factor is the *availability of supporting personnel (including consultants) and services.* To make the observations necessary to answer a question may require the cooperation or assistance of persons with expertise in various areas, and such persons may not be available. For example, a study of the effect of a therapy program on persons who have vocal nodules may require the services of an otolaryngologist to do indirect laryngoscopy on the subjects before and after participating in the program. The investigator may be unable to locate an otolaryngologist who would be willing to provide this service. This possibility should be considered before beginning a piece of research.

The sixth, and final, factor that should be considered is *available funding.* To answer some questions, a research grant would be needed, and to answer others, only minimal funding (less than $100) would be required. Many questions of interest to speech-language pathologists and audiologists, incidentally, would require only minimal funding to answer: Funding may only be needed for supplies, such as postage stamps, recording tapes, or test forms. Before you commit yourself to answering a particular question, or questions, you should be reasonably certain that available funding will be adequate.

GENERATING RELEVANT QUESTIONS FOR RESEARCH

Now that we have considered some factors to think about when choosing questions to answer, we will consider some strategies that can be used to generate relevant questions for research. By a "relevant question" we mean one for which a response to the "so what" or "who cares" question can be provided—in other words, a question for which *a need* for answering can be established.

Need for Selecting Relevant Questions

Though the scientific method does not require it, you will find it advantageous to select questions to answer that you feel are relevant and that others will think are relevant, for several reasons. First, your research is more likely to be publishable if you select such questions. In the introductory section of a research report for a professional journal such as the *American Journal of Audiology: A Journal of Clinical Practice,* the *American Journal of Speech-Language Pathology: A Journal of Clinical Practice,* the *Journal of Speech and Hearing Research* and *Language, Speech, and Hearing Services in Schools,* the author is expected to establish *scientific justification* for the research reported. That is, the author is expected to demonstrate the importance of answering the question or questions proposed. If you understand why it is important and can communicate this to readers of your report, you will increase the probability that your report will be accepted for publication.

A second reason to select questions that both peers and administrators to whom you are responsible will regard as relevant is to increase the possibility that you will receive the support you need for your research. You are more likely to secure funding for research you can justify as relevant than for research for which you can provide no such justification. Also, you are more likely to receive approval from administrators for "released time" for research if they view your research as satisfying an important need. Such approval would be particularly important for speech-language pathologists and audiologists who are employed in clinical settings and whose primary responsibilities are clinical.

Identifying a Problem Area

What should a speech-language pathologist or audiologist take into consideration when attempting to identify a problem area from which to generate relevant questions for research? Several factors need to be considered. These factors include: (1) personal interests, (2) competencies, (3) the potential value of the research, (4) the available equipment and facilities for making observations and analyzing data, (5) the "populations" available for study, (6) the financial resources available, (7) the amount of time available, and (8) the possibilities for consultation. Several of them are discussed in a different context earlier in this chapter.

The first factor a speech-language pathologist or audiologist should consider when attempting to identify a problem area for research is *personal interests*—you should attempt to identify the problem areas within the field of communicative disorders that are of most interest to you. An area could be defined partially by a symptom complex such as aphasia, stuttering, defective articulation, or conductive hearing loss. An area could also be defined partially by a technique such as impedance audiometry, operant conditioning, or language testing. You should attempt to identify as many such areas as you can and roughly order them on the basis of your interest in them. It is desirable to identify more than one area initially since factors may be present that would make it quite difficult to pursue certain areas. Several such factors will be discussed in this section.

You should select an area to research in which you have some interest. Your interest in the research will influence both how positively reinforcing you will find the experience and the probability that you will complete it. We all tend to pursue activities we find positively reinforcing and avoid those we find "punishing."

A second factor a speech-language pathologist or audiologist should consider when selecting a problem area for research is *competencies*. Because of your training and experience, the probability that you will be successful in your research endeavors may be greater if you avoid certain problem areas. If you had no training or experience in aphasia testing, for example, you might be wise to avoid questions that required the administration of aphasia tests to answer. While you could probably learn to administer such tests, it might require a considerable investment of time before you would be sufficiently competent to administer them with adequate reliability for your purposes. Of course, you might be able to find someone with whom to collaborate on the research who is competent in aphasia testing. This illustrates one way an investigator can reduce the consequences of a "deficiency" in training or experience. It is not unusual, incidentally, for two or more persons to collaborate on a piece of research. In fact, 48 percent of the papers in five randomly selected issues of the *Journal of Speech and Hearing Disorders* were authored by two or more persons. It is desirable, therefore, when attempting to evaluate a potential problem area for research, to specify as completely as you can the competencies necessary to pursue the research and to judge whether you possess each one. If you do not possess some necessary competencies and cannot find a collaborator (or collaborators) who does, you might be wise not to pursue research in the area, particularly if overcoming such deficiencies would require large investments of money and/or time.

A third consideration when attempting to identify a problem area for research is the *potential value of the research*. As already indicated, it is difficult to predict the impact a piece of research will have on a discipline. Nevertheless, this is almost always a consideration when an investigator chooses an area of research. You will usually choose a problem you regard as worthwhile to investigate. For this reason, you may choose a problem with immediate relevance—e.g., you may attempt to evaluate a therapy program that you are presently using or are contemplating using. Such research could have considerable impact on your own caseload and, if it is communicated to other clinicians, on their caseloads as well.

A fourth factor is the *availability of equipment and facilities for making observations and analyzing data*. An investigator may not be able to pursue a research area of interest because the necessary facilities, equipment, or both, are lacking. From one frame of reference this factor could restrict an investigator in exploring certain problem areas. From a second frame of reference additional possible problem areas for research might be suggested. An investigator with equipment and facilities that are not generally available may wish to exploit them—that is, to define a problem area based on questions they would permit to be answered. An audiologist, for example, who possessed some pieces of testing equipment not generally available might choose to ask questions that could be answered through the use of this equipment. Or a speech-language pathologist who is employed in a clinic that has sophisticated instrumentation for augmentative communication might choose to exploit it in a similar manner. As an investigator, therefore, you might find it worthwhile to prepare an inventory of the equipment and facilities available to you as a preliminary step in defining a problem area for research. Such an inventory could assist you in assessing problem areas you are considering and in identifying additional possible problem areas.

A fifth factor is the *"populations" available for study.* Before you begin to try to identify such an area, you might find it worthwhile to inventory relevant attributes of persons who might be available and willing to serve as research subjects. Relevant attributes might include: (1) sex, (2) whether or not they have particular communicative disorders, (3) chronological age, (4) physical status, (5) intellectual and emotional status, (6) socioeconomic status, and (7) therapy history—whether or not they have previously had therapy and if they have, what kind or kinds. Such an inventory could provide two types of input into the selection process. First, it could alert you, the investigator, to research areas you would be wise to avoid because subjects who have the necessary attributes would probably not be available to you in sufficient numbers. A speech clinician employed in a school setting, for example, might have a difficult time obtaining adequate numbers of laryngectomized geriatric subjects for a research project. Second, the inventory could suggest problem areas you might want to consider. If you had subjects available in fairly large numbers who were relatively homogeneous in some attribute (e.g., deaf children or mentally retarded children) or if you had small numbers of subjects available who were unusual in some way (e.g., persons with rare diseases or conditions that influence communicative behavior), you might be able to define a problem area in which you could use observations made on such subjects to answer questions. A single subject, incidentally, who is unusual in some regard might be used in this manner for an individual case study.

A sixth factor is the *financial resources available.* As previously mentioned, while some research requires only minimal funding, other research can be quite costly. To do research that required more than minimal funding, an investigator would probably have to secure a research grant from a government (state or national) agency, private organization, or private foundation. Many such agencies, organizations, and foundations have funded research on communicative disorders. Nevertheless, a person who is considering applying for such a grant should be aware that they are usually quite competitive. More applications are ordinarily submitted than can be funded. Investigators who have demonstrated research competence by publishing are usually favored for the larger grants; they also are favored for many relatively small grants. A beginning investigator, therefore, would probably be wise to select a project that only requires minimal funding. However, after demonstrating research competence by publishing the results of several such projects, you can consider projects that require external funding if you so desire.

A seventh factor is the *amount of time available.* Before you decide to do a particular research project, it is a good idea to estimate roughly both the amount of time it would take to complete and the amount of time that is likely to be available. If the amount of time necessary grossly exceeds the time available for the purpose, you have several options as an investigator: (1) you can try to locate one or more professional colleagues who would be interested in collaborating with you on the project and sharing the work; (2) you can enlist the aid of persons who are not speech-language pathologists or audiologists, such as spouses or secretaries, for parts of the project that do not require competence in these areas; (3) you can secure a grant and hire full- or part-time research assistants to gather data and assist with data analysis; (4) you can attempt to arrange your schedule to have adequate time available for the project; or (5) you can decide not to pursue the project. Many projects, incidentally, require a time investment that would not exceed that available to most clinicians. Among these are projects for which data could be gathered in conjunction with ongoing clinical activities, e.g., therapy evaluation studies.

The eighth, and final, factor is the *possibilities for consultation.* If, to do a research project, you must consult with persons who have expertise in certain areas such as electronics, computer programming, or mental measurement, you should be reasonably certain before beginning that such persons will be available for consultation. As previously mentioned, faculty members at local colleges and universities who have the required expertise may be willing to serve as consultants.

Generating Relevant Research Questions

After a problem area has been selected, the next task is to generate one or more questions to answer that are relevant to the area. These questions, implicitly or explicitly, define the research topic. They indicate what the investigator is trying to find out. They also indicate the kinds of information that are apt to result from the research. Since most research questions only can be answered in a finite number of ways, we usually can infer from a question what the possible answers could be. If, for example, the question we sought to answer was, "Do most elementary-school stutterers avoid talking?" our research could lead to three possible answers: (1) it could indicate unequivocally that the majority of elementary-school stutterers avoid talking; (2) it could indicate unequivocally that the majority of elementary-school stutterers do not avoid talking; or (3) it could lead to an equivocal result. Finally, the questions asked specify, at least partially, what has to be done to answer them. Suppose, for example, we asked the question, "How likely are persons who are employed as firemen for more than 10 years to develop noise-induced hearing losses?" To answer this question, we would have to measure the hearing acuity of persons who have been employed as firemen for more than 10 years using methods that were sufficiently reliable and valid to detect noise-induced hearing losses if they were present.

What approaches can be used for selecting a research topic—i.e., generating questions to answer? A number of approaches can be used for this purpose, including the following:

You can do a careful review of the literature in the area selected to identify: (1) questions that have been formulated but only partially answered, (2) questions that have been formulated but not answered, and (3) questions that have not been formulated but should be.

Many questions about communicative disorders have been formulated but only partially answered. A question is rarely answered unequivocally on the basis of a single set of observations for several reasons. First, in many cases the observations that have been used to answer questions of concern to speech-language pathologists and audiologists were *not* made on a *random sample* of subjects from the population referred to by the question. To illustrate this point, let us again use the question, "How likely are persons who are employed as firemen for more than 10 years to develop noise-induced hearing losses?" The population referred to by this question consists of all firemen who have more than 10 years' experience. For a sample from this population to be random, all such firemen would have to have an equal chance of being selected. However, it would be unusual for an investigator who sought to answer this kind of question to use a random sample. You would most likely base your observations on a "nonrandom" sample, such as a local group of firemen with more than 10 years' service who volunteered to have their hearing tested. The likelihood of the subjects in such a sample having noise-induced hearing losses may differ systematically from that for firemen in general. In other words, the answer to the question could be different for this sample than it would have been for a random sample. Hence, the generality of an answer based on nonrandom sample would be uncertain. In cases where a question has been answered through the use of a nonrandom sample, therefore, the answer should be regarded as equivocal until the observations have been replicated on other samples of subjects from the population. This would be true even if the results were statistically significant. One assumption that underlies almost all tests of statistical significance is that the subjects observed were a random sample from the population of interest. (This concept is further discussed in Chapter 11.)

A second reason why a question may not have been answered unequivocally on the basis of a single set of observations is that they were *not* adequately *reliable, valid,* or both. If the observations were not sufficiently reliable, the investigator may not have been able to observe the phenomenon with sufficient clarity to answer the question accurately. Returning to the fireman example again, if the audiometer used had not been properly calibrated, or if the person who administered the test or tests had not been sufficiently proficient, or if the room in which the testing was done had not been adequately sound treated, the thresholds recorded could have been sufficiently in error that the effect of noise on firemen's hearing might not be detected. Also, if the observations used to answer a question were not sufficiently valid, the answer *might* be incorrect. We use the word *might* here because an investigator could arrive at the right answer for the wrong reason (e.g., Gall's conclusion that the anterior portion of the brain is dominant for speech, discussed in Chapter 3). In our fireman example, an investigator could conclude through the use of an invalid testing procedure (e.g., one that was thought to be able to detect noise-induced hearing losses but was not sensitive to such losses) that the firemen did not have noise-induced hearing losses when they did, or that they had noise-induced hearing losses when they did not.

A third reason why a question may not have been answered unequivocally on the basis of a single set of observations is *random*, or chance, *sampling error*. This can influence research results derived from random samples of subjects by methods which were adequately reliable and valid. What happens here is that by chance the behavior of the subjects in the sample is not representative of that in the population from which they were selected, even though appropriate sampling procedures were used. While random sampling is more likely to result in a sample that is representative of the population than are other sampling procedures, it does not always result in such a sample. The sample selected will not be representative of the population from which it was selected a certain percentage of the time. (The reason for this phenomenon is discussed in Chapter 11.) The observations that were made on such a sample of subjects could be sufficiently biased to cause an investigator to answer a question incorrectly. Because of this possibility, research findings should be regarded as suspect until they have been replicated. A question should not be regarded as having been answered unequivocally until the same answer has been obtained with several samples of subjects.

A fourth, and final, reason why a question may not have been answered unequivocally on the basis of a single set of observations is *experimenter bias*. A number of studies have demonstrated that an investigator's expectations and theoretical biases can influence his or her observations without the investigator being conscious of it (Barber, 1976; Rosenthal, 1969, 1976). If you expect a question to be answered in a particular way or if your theoretical biases suggest that a question should have a particular answer, you may unconsciously "filter" your observations to obtain the answer you expect. This is particularly apt to be a problem when an investigator has considerable ego-involvement in a theoretical position relevant to the questions he or she is attempting to answer. This problem is extremely difficult to deal with. With regard to our concern here—selecting questions to answer—the relevance of experimenter bias is that if a question has only been answered by a single investigator (particularly one with an ego-investment in the answer), the answer should probably not be regarded as unequivocal unless it has been replicated by other investigators unlikely to have the same theoretical biases.

In addition to helping identify questions that have been formulated but only partially answered, a search of the literature in the area of interest may reveal questions that have been *formulated but not answered*. There are several places in which such questions might be found. One is the "discussion" section of research reports in the area. Frequently in this section the author or authors will indicate some implications they feel their findings have for future research. They may even indicate what specific questions they feel should be answered, for a piece of research often raises more questions than it answers.

Another source of questions that have been formulated but not answered is review papers in the area of interest. A review paper is one that summarizes and integrates the research in a particular area. Such papers usually suggest some information that is needed to improve our understanding of the area, thus indicating questions that need to be answered. Review papers have been published for many areas of interest to speech-language pathologists and audiologists. They have appeared in journals and monographs as well as in books. One way to locate a review paper on a topic of interest that was published in a journal or monograph (if one has been written) is to use an abstracts journal or computer database (see Chapter 4). Abstracts of papers relevant to the topic can be scanned to determine if they are review papers. If you are using an abstracts journal rather than a computer database (e.g., Medline), it would be wise to begin a literature search with the most recent volume and work backward. This procedure would maximize the odds of finding the most recent review paper on a topic, if there has been more than one.

Thus far, we have considered how a review of the literature in the area of interest can help to identify questions that have been formulated but only partially answered and questions that have been formulated but not answered. We now will consider how such a review can suggest *questions that have not been formulated but should be.* The strategy here would be to: (1) do a careful search of the literature in the area to determine what is known (what questions have been answered), and (2) formulate questions which, if answered, would be likely to increase our understanding of the area.

The first task, the literature search, can be expedited by the use of abstracts journals and computer databases (see Chapter 4). The reference lists of all papers found should be checked for relevant research reports that were not identified. Such reports would include those published prior to the year in which the literature search began; those that appeared in limited circulation journals such as state speech and hearing journals; those that were presented orally at state, national, and international professional and scientific meetings; those that were reported in unpublished master's theses and doctoral dissertations; and those that were reported in unpublished papers, including technical reports.

The research reported should be organized in a manner to make it apparent what is known about the area. One approach that can sometimes be used for this purpose is to define *a dependent variable* and indicate what *independent variables* have been shown to influence it. One example of a dependent variable is speechreading ability; examples of independent variables that have been shown to influence it include visual acuity and training in speech-reading. Another example of a dependent variable is extent of recovery from aphasia. Independent variables that would be expected to influence it include chronological age, extent and location (e.g., right or left hemisphere) of lesion, and amount of language stimulation received.

After the available data has been organized to make it apparent what is known about the area, the next task is to formulate questions which, if answered, would be likely to increase our understanding of it. What is required here is first to formulate as many questions as possible that have not been answered, and then to select from these one or more to answer. Organized in this way, the information available on a topic would facilitate the question formulation process. This would be particularly true if a dependent variable had been defined and independent variables that have been shown to influence it cataloged. One would then attempt to identify independent variables not yet studied that might be relevant. A question, or questions, could be formulated about each such variable. If the dependent variable, for example, were speechreading ability and an independent variable that had not been investigated were telepathic ability, one question that might be asked would be, "Do persons who earn relatively high scores on a Duke University card-guessing telepathy task exhibit greater speechreading ability than those who earn relatively low scores on this task?"

How can we identify uninvestigated independent variables that may influence a particular dependent variable? This question is difficult to answer since the process of discovery is not fully understood. Perhaps our ability to identify such independent variables involves what Michael Polanyi (1967) has referred to as "tacit knowing." According to Polanyi,

> . . . *we can know more than we can tell.* This fact seems obvious enough; but it is not easy to say exactly what it means. Take an example. We know a person's face, and can recognize it among a thousand, indeed among a million. Yet we usually cannot tell how we recognize a face we know. (Polanyi, 1967, p.4)

Polanyi states that tacit knowing guides the scientist to problems worth investigating—i.e., to questions worth answering. Hunches and intuitions resulting from tacit knowing may be the mechanism by which we identify relevant independent variables.

While the process used to identify relevant independent variables is not fully understood, there is a strategy which may facilitate it. This strategy is to identify independent variables that have been shown to influence other dependent behavioral variables that have not been investigated with regard to the dependent variable of interest. Chronological age is an example of an independent variable that has been shown to influence many dependent behavioral variables of interest to speech-language pathologists and audiologists. If such an independent variable had not been investigated with regard to the dependent behavioral variable in which you are interested, it might be worthwhile for you to do so. The author worked for several years as a research associate on a project which investigated the variability of stuttering frequency (dependent variable) in school-age children under the same conditions it had previously been investigated in adults. The question we sought to answer was, "Do conditions which have been shown to influence (reduce or increase) stuttering frequency in adults also do so in school-age children?"

A second general approach for identifying relevant research questions is to examine your clinical experience in the area of interest for questions that seem worth answering and then to search the relevant literature to determine whether they have been answered. You should ask yourself the following question: "To what clinically relevant questions have I sought answers for which I know of no data to answer?" You also should ask yourself, "To what clinically relevant questions do I feel I have answers where the validity and reliability of the data on which the answers are based is uncertain?" That is, "What questions am I assuming have been adequately answered empirically that may not have been?" Things are frequently done clinically not because they have been shown to be effective empirically, but because they have either been recommended by an authority, "make sense" theoretically, or are *traditional*. What I mean by being traditional can be illustrated by the frequency and duration of therapy sessions assigned to clients. It may be traditional in a particular clinical setting for clients with a particular communicative disorder to be scheduled for therapy a particular number of sessions per week, each of which is a particular number of minutes in duration. One might ask whether this number of sessions per week of this length is optimal for reducing the severity of these clients' communicative disorders. Perhaps the sessions either are: (1) longer and more frequent than necessary, or (2) longer but not more frequent than necessary, or (3) less frequent but longer than necessary, or (4) shorter and less frequent than necessary. One way to answer this question—to determine whether the frequency and duration of therapy sessions are optimal—would be to vary systematically the frequency and duration of sessions for clients who have a given communicative disorder and observe whether better results are obtained when a different frequency or duration is used.

One approach that can be used for identifying questions that have answers based on "authority" or "tradition" rather than on empirical data is to subject information on which we operate clinically to the "How do we know?" question. How do we know, for example, that a therapy procedure does what it is supposed to do? If there were no unequivocal empirical evidence that a therapy procedure did what it was supposed to do, this circumstance would suggest questions for research.

The available data on clinical procedures of interest can be located through the use of computer databases and abstracts journals (see Chapter 4).

A third approach for generating questions that might be worth answering is "brainstorming" with colleagues about their clinical experience in the area and then searching relevant literature to determine whether the questions suggested have been answered unequivocally. The procedure here is much the same as that described for the second approach. The only difference is that questions are abstracted from informal discussions with colleagues about their clinical experience rather than from the clinician's own experience. If you adopt an appropriate set, many potential research questions probably can be abstracted from informal conversations with colleagues.

What specifically might colleagues say that would suggest potential research questions? They might indicate concern over the effectiveness of a particular diagnostic or therapeutic procedure. They might state that they failed to obtain the results reported for this procedure in the literature. Assuming that they appeared to have applied it as described in the literature, one might ask whether the results reported in the literature can be replicated. Such could be the genesis of a piece of clinical research.

A colleague might raise questions concerning the organization of clinical programs for which no data-based guidelines exist in the literature. Such questions may relate to any of a number of areas, including intake procedures, dismissal procedures, follow-up procedures, and the utilization of paraprofessionals.

A colleague might also raise questions concerning the validity of research results reported in the literature. He or she may state, for example, that the incidence of a particular communicative disorder appears to be considerably higher or lower than reported in the literature. Or he or she may indicate that most of those clients who have a particular communicative disorder fail to exhibit some aspect or aspects of the symptomatology reported in the literature as characteristic of this disorder.

STRUCTURING RESEARCH QUESTIONS
TO MAKE THEM ANSWERABLE

The question considered thus far in this chapter has been, "How can we generate relevant questions for research?" In this section we will consider the question, "How can we structure research questions to make them as 'answerable' as possible?" By an answerable question we mean one that can be answered by observations and that implicitly or explicitly (preferably the latter) specifies the observation or observations necessary to answer it.

Not all questions of interest to speech-language pathologists and audiologists are equally answerable empirically. One reason is that a question may be formulated in a way that makes it uncertain what observations have to be made to answer it. Consider, for example, the following questions:

1. Is hypnosis effective in treating stuttering?
2. Is the post-hypnotic suggestion, "You will not stutter anymore," effective in reducing stuttering frequency?

These questions are not equally answerable. The second specifies the observations that would have to be made to answer it more explicitly than the first and hence is more answerable empirically.

A question may not be answerable empirically because it is not possible to make the observations necessary to answer it. In some cases the reason is that the necessary observational procedures have not been developed. When they are, the question would no longer be unanswerable. In other cases, a question may be unanswerable because the instruments required to make the observations are not available to the investigator. While such a question would be unanswerable for him or her, it might not be for someone else (someone who has the necessary instruments).

How does one structure a question to make it answerable? According to Wendell Johnson,

> One cannot get a clear answer to a vague question. The language of science is particularly distinguished by the fact it centers around well-stated questions. If there is one part of a scientific experiment that is more important than any other part, it is the framing of the question that the experiment is to answer. If it is stated vaguely, no experiment can answer it precisely. If the question is stated precisely, the means of answering it are clearly indicated. The specific observations needed, and the conditions under which they are to be made, are implied in the question itself. (Johnson, 1946, pp. 52–53)

For a question to be answerable, therefore, it cannot be vague or ambiguous. The meanings of all words must be made explicit and, if possible, defined operationally. If a question we wished to answer were "Do persons with cleft palates have normal intelligence?" we would have to specify as precisely as possible what segment of the cleft palate population we were referring to (i.e., those with a cleft of the soft palate only, or those with clefts of both hard and soft palates, or both groups) and what we meant by intelligence (i.e., performance on what task or test). The question would be more answerable, for example, if it were structured as follows: "Are five-year-old children who have clefts of the palate only more likely to have below normal intelligence as measured by the Stanford-Binet than five-year-old children who do not have this condition?"

To develop further your intuitive understanding of what an answerable question consists of, pairs of questions are presented in Table 5.1 in which the members of each pair differ in the degree to which they are answerable. The member in column one is less answerable than that in column two. The

TABLE 5.1   Pairs of questions that differ in the degree to which they are answerable.

Less Answerable Version	More Answerable Version
How much can aphasics be expected to improve between one month and one year following trauma?	How many points can receptive aphasics be expected to gain, on the average, on the Minnesota Aphasia Test between one month and one year following trauma?
Does drinking alcoholic beverages reduce stuttering?	Does drinking five highballs in a period of two hours reduce the stuttering frequencies of most adult stutterers?
Are home assignments helpful for correcting articulation errors?	Is a particular home assignment at a particular stage of therapy for a particular articulation error helpful for correcting this error?
Is a particular ear-protector effective in preventing noise-induced hearing loss?	Is a particular ear-protector effective in preventing a temporary threshold shift if used in the presence of noise of a particular intensity with a particular spectrum for a particular period of time?

two versions presented are not necessarily the least and most answerable possible.

EXERCISES AND DISCUSSION TOPICS

1. Determine whether each of the following questions is answerable by attempting to specify the observations necessary for answering it. If you feel that a question is not as answerable as it could be, rewrite it to make it more answerable and specify the observations you would make to answer the question as you have rewritten it.

   a. Do aphasics benefit from therapy?

   b. Can lateral emission during /s/ production be eliminated by training in auditory discrimination?

   c. How accurately can classroom teachers identify children in their classrooms who have hearing losses?

2. Formulate an answerable question about clinical process (i.e., evaluation or therapy) you could answer using observations you made while working with a specific client during your practicum experience. Describe these observations.

6

Single Subject
and
Group Designs

After an investigator has formulated research questions, the next task is to select an appropriate design for making the observations needed to answer them. There is no one design appropriate for gathering the data needed to answer all questions. This chapter will describe the two main types of designs that are used for this purpose: those in which the data are descriptions of the attributes of *single* subjects or those in which they are descriptions of the attributes of the *typical* member of a group. Before doing so, we will consider some of the terminology used for describing them.

TERMINOLOGY USED FOR DESCRIBING GROUP
AND SINGLE SUBJECT RESEARCH DESIGNS

Group and single subject research designs have been categorized in a number of ways and a terminology has developed for describing them. Some terms that have been used for this purpose are defined below. Others are defined elsewhere in the chapter.

Counterbalanced design. A group experiment design in which all the conditions are administered to all subjects, but not in the same order. Subjects are divided into approximately equal size groups, the number being equal to the number of conditions. For example, suppose we wanted to determine in which of two conditions (A or B) stutterers tended to stutter most severely. We would obtain a speech sample from each stutterer under each condition. Half would speak under *Condition* A first and half under *Condition* B. This design allows us to control for *order effects* which are described elsewhere in this chapter.

Ex post facto design.   A group or single subject research design in which causation is studied by an analysis of past events. This has also been referred to as both a *causal-comparative* and a *correlational* design. The latter term is used when the analysis involves the computation of correlation coefficients (see Chapter 9). This is the type of design that was used for generating the data indicating that smokers are more "at risk" than nonsmokers for developing a number of health problems. The data used were from medical case *histories* of smokers and nonsmokers. It is also the type of design that is used for studying causation (e.g., inferring the impacts of a therapy program) in individual case studies in which the data utilized are abstracted from material in the client's clinic file.

Experiment.   A group or single subject research design in which an investigator *manipulates* one variable and watches the effect on another. An example would be watching the effect on stuttering frequency of manipulating stress level.

Factorial design.   A group research design in which it is possible to determine the impacts of more than one independent variable (factors) on a dependent variable. Real-world outcomes usually are the result of a number of factors. In research on the effect of an aphasia therapy, for example, we might want to assess the impacts of two independent variables: age and number of months posttrauma. This would allow us to determine whether the age of the client and/or the length of time he or she has been aphasic influences therapy outcome.

Longitudinal design.   A group or single subject research design in which observations are made of the same persons for a relatively long period of time, usually years. An example would be observing for a number of years young children judged to be "at risk" for developing a particular communicative disorder to determine how many develop it.

Natural experiment.   A group or single subject research design in which it is possible to observe the effect that one variable (usually some type of abnormality) has on others without having to produce it. It is also referred to as an *investigation.* An example would be determining the function of a part of the right cerebral cortex by observing the behavior of one or more persons who have a lesion in it.

Pretest-posttest design.   A group or single subject research design in which the impact of an intervention strategy is judged from the difference between pretreatment and posttreatment measures.

Randomized controlled trials (RCTs).   A group design used for treatment outcome research in which clients are randomly assigned to two groups—those in one receive the treatment being assessed and those in the other do not. The person doing the assigning is not told to which group a particular client is assigned until after the assignment is made in order to prevent any of his or her conscious or unconscious biases from influencing assignment decisions (e.g., wanting the therapy to be effective and, therefore, assigning clients with the best prognosis to the treatment group). This methodology has been used for evaluating aphasia therapies (Howard, 1986).

Replication.   A research design that is the same as that of an earlier study. It is used for evaluating the reliability and/or generality of the findings of that study. A *systematic replication* is the same as a replication except that one aspect of the design is changed—e.g., males are used instead of females. If the findings from the modified design are the same as those from the earlier study, their generality is increased. If the findings are not the same, it could be either because those of the earlier study are not reliable or that the change in design made a real difference. Hence, systematic replications are risky!

Retrospective design. A group or single subject research design for collecting reports of observations made at an earlier point in time. An example would be the parental interview data reported by Johnson and Associates (1959) on the speech of children at the "moment" they were initially regarded as beginning to stutter by their parents. It differs from the *ex post facto design* in that the data generated may be used to describe events rather than explain them.

Static-group comparison design. This design compares the status of a group that has received an experimental treatment to one that has not. The first is referred to as the *experimental group* and the second the *control group*. This is one of the most frequently used designs in speech, language, and hearing research.

Time-series design. A group or single subject research design in which observations (e.g., measurements) are made at periodic intervals and there is an experimental treatment between two of them. The treatment is judged to have had an effect if there is a change from the observation immediately before to the one immediately after its introduction. These designs are used frequently in therapy outcome research.

THE SINGLE SUBJECT VERSUS THE GROUP RESEARCH DESIGN

There are two basic types of designs that are used in speech, language, and hearing research: the single subject and the group design. What are these two types of designs? In what ways are they different? What are their advantages and disadvantages? What variations are possible within each type? Can they be combined? These questions will be dealt with in turn to help the reader develop an intuitive understanding of the attributes of these two basic types of designs.

A single subject design permits the performance of single subjects under the experimental condition or conditions to be *reliably* determined. Reliable conclusions can be reached concerning the effects of an experimental condition on the behavior of a single subject. The question, "Has a client improved following a period of therapy?" would require a single subject design to answer. The simplest such design would be one that permitted relevant "before and after" measures (e.g., pretherapy and posttherapy measures) to be made.

Single subject designs are *not limited to studies in which there is only one subject.* They can be used in studies in which there is almost any number of subjects. However, when they are used, the data from each subject is reported separately (usually in a graph or table). That is, the data generated by individual subjects are not combined and manipulated arithmetically.

A group design *reliably* permits the average (mean, median, or mode) performance of the subjects in a group under the experimental condition or conditions to be determined. Reliable conclusions can be reached concerning the effects of an experimental condition on the behavior of the average, or "typical," member of a group. The question, "Are elementary-school stutterers able to predict their moments of stuttering as accurately as adult stutterers?" would require a group design. To answer it, the average (i.e., mean or median) performance of a group of elementary-school stutterers on a stuttering prediction task could be compared to that of a group of adult stutterers on the same task.

Thus far, these two types of designs have been discussed as if they were mutually exclusive. This is not the case. Some studies use designs that generate both types of data. They permit the average performance of a group as well as the performance of the individual subjects in that group under the experimental condition or conditions to be *reliably* determined. Such designs are useful when it appears likely that subjects will respond differently to an experimental condition. In fact, they permit the investigator to determine whether subjects do, in fact, respond differently to such a condition. It might be suspected, for example, that a particular approach to teaching speechreading would be more effective with some hard-of-hearing persons than with others. It probably would be worthwhile, therefore, to gather sufficient data on each person with whom the approach is used so that the amount each learned could be *reliably* estimated. From these data could be determined: (1) the amount the "average" person in the group learned, and (2) the degree of variability in the amount learned. Also, if considerable variability occurred, an attempt could be made to identify the factor or factors responsible through the use of correlational procedures. (These are described in Chapter 9.)

Considerable emphasis has been placed here on the word *reliability*, particularly with regard to the single subject design. The types of data usually gathered when group designs are used—i.e., each subject run only once under each experimental condition—usually are not sufficiently reliable for determining the responses of single subjects to experimental conditions. A subject may not always respond to an experimental condition in the same manner, because of the effects of extraneous variables that have not been controlled and in many cases would be quite difficult to control even if we wished to. A subject's emotional state and degree of motivation would be examples of such variables.

Another reason for the lack of reliability of such data is that descriptions of behavior (both numerical and verbal) are subject to error of various kinds. The human observer is not an error-free describer of events. The more observations on which a description is based, the more reliable it is apt to be (Kraemer and Thiemann, 1989). Suppose that we wished to determine the effect of speaking in the presence of masking noise on stuttering. Our description would probably be more reliable if each stutterer spoke five times without masking noise and five times with masking noise and stuttering frequencies during the five speeches under each condition were averaged than it would be if each spoke only once under each condition.

To clarify the distinction between single subject and group designs, we have indicated in Table 6.1 eight of the more important differences between them. The order in which they appear in the table is not necessarily related to their importance.

TABLE 6.1 Differences between single subject and group designs.

Single Subject Designs	Group Designs
Provide data concerning the "typical" behavior of an individual subject under an experimental condition	Provide data concerning the behavior of the "typical" member of a group under an experimental condition
Not necessary to assume that subjects respond similarly to an experimental condition	Necessary to assume that subjects in a group respond similarly to an experimental condition
Necessary for subjects to be run more than once under each experimental condition	Not necessary for subjects to be run more than once under each experimental conditions
Generalize to "typical" behavior of individual studied under experimental condition	Generalize to "typical" behavior of mean or median group member under experimental condition
May not be relatively easy to control for order and sequence effects	Usually relatively easy to control for order and sequence effects
Statistical procedures for assessing the reliability of research findings are not as well developed as for typical subject designs	Statistical procedures for assessing the reliability of research findings are well developed
Minimum number of subjects necessary is 1	Minimum number of subjects necessary is usually more than 10
Generalize to population from which subjects are selected on logical basis	Generalize to population from which subjects are selected on statistical basis

One of the more important differences between these two designs is the nature of the data provided. Single subject designs provide data on the *typical* response of *one person* to an experimental condition. The typical response referred to here would be the mean, median, or most frequently occurring (modal) response. Group designs, on the other hand, provide data on the mean, median, or most frequently occurring (modal) response of the *members of a group.*

With both designs, it is possible for the typical response to an experimental condition not to be typical. This is particularly likely to occur when the mean is used. With a single subject design, a subject's mean response to an experimental condition may represent behavior that did not occur even once. This has been demonstrated, for example, with the mean response of individual aphasics to aphasia test subjects (Silverman, 1974).

The typical response to an experimental condition also may not be typical when a group design is used. The mean response of the typical group member may not correspond to that of any group member. The mean number of stutterings produced by 25 stutterers during their reading of a 100-word passage, for example, might be 10.5. Since no stutterer could stutter a fraction of a stuttering, this stuttering frequency would not correspond to that produced by any of the 25 stutterers. The lack of "representativeness" of mean data would be of considerable importance for answering some questions since it would lead to incorrect answers.

A second difference between single subject and group designs is the necessity of assuming that subjects do not respond differently to an experimental condition—that is, the necessity of assuming that observed differences in the responses of subjects to an experimental condition result from the effects of extraneous variables or from "chance" (random) fluctuation rather than from real differences in their responses to that condition. While single subject designs do not require such an assumption, group designs implicitly or explicitly do. Without such an assumption, it would not be particularly meaningful to talk about the typical response of a group to an experimental condition. This would be particularly true when an experimental condition had opposite effects on different persons. An example of such a condition would be consecutive readings of a passage. This condition has been shown to result in some stutterers becoming progressively more fluent (adaptation effect) and others becoming progressively more disfluent (Bloom and Silverman, 1973). The only circumstance under which it would probably be meaningful to talk about a typical response to an experimental condition when people differ in their responses to that condition is when the differences are of degree rather than kind—that is, when an experimental condition changes the behavior of all subjects in the same direction but to different degrees. A particular obturator may reduce the hypernasality of all persons with cleft palates who are fitted with it, but not to the same degree. It would be meaningful, therefore, to talk about the effect of this obturator on the speech of the typical person who was fitted with it.

A third difference between single subject and group designs is the minimum number of times it is necessary to run a subject under each experimental condition. With a group design, reliable results are frequently obtainable when a subject is run only once under each such condition. With a single subject design, on the other hand, reliable results would rarely be obtainable if a subject were run only once under each condition. The reason for this difference is that with a group design, factors that reduce reliability (e.g., measurement error, effects of extraneous variables, and random fluctuation) can be kept from biasing the results by using as a measure of performance (criterion measure) the average of the measures from a number of subjects under each condition. Such factors usually would not bias the performance of the majority of subjects in a group under an experimental condition in the same manner.

With a single subject design, the previously mentioned factors that can reduce reliability can be prevented from biasing the results by using as a measure of individual performance (criterion measure) under each condition the average of the measures made under each condition. These factors usually will not bias measures of a subject's performance under a given experimental condition in exactly the same manner. Hence, answers to questions will tend to be more reliable with a single subject design if they are based on a subject's average performance under a condition than on any single performance under it.

A fourth difference between single subject and group designs is what the answers to questions can be used to predict. For research findings to be useful, they must be applicable outside of the experimental situation in which they were generated. With a single subject design, the behavior of a subject under an experimental condition can be used to predict his or her most probable behavior under that condition.

With a group design, the behavior of the mean or median group member under an experimental condition can be used to predict the most probable behavior of the mean or median member of such a group under such a condition. It also can be used to predict the response to an experimental condition of the mean or median member of a population from which a group was selected, if it was randomly selected from that population. A population consists of all individuals who are classified in a particular manner. Thus, the population referred to by the question, "Are adults who have anomia helped by a particular therapy?" consists of all adults who have anomia. If a group were not randomly selected from a population, this type of generalization would be questionable. (The rationale and methodology for random sampling are described in Chapter 9.)

A fifth difference between single subject and group designs is related to the control of order and sequence events. An *order effect* is one that systematically improves or impairs a subject's performance on a series of tasks. An example of an order effect that could impair performance would be fatigue. If an aphasic were to perform a series of 10 tasks one after the other, his performance might systematically worsen as a function of fatigue. This could occur regardless of the ordering of the tasks. An example of an order effect that could enhance a subject's performance on a series of tasks would be learning. A client may score higher on a test following a period of therapy than he did on the same test prior to therapy not because he improved, but because of what he learned during his first exposure to the test.

A *sequence effect* occurs when a subject's performance on a task is enhanced or impaired by his or her doing another task before it. An investigator who sought to determine the effect of a drug on stuttering would have to obtain samples of stutterers' speech both while they were and while they were not under the influence of the drug. If both speech samples were elicited during the same day, it might make a difference whether the "drug" or "no-drug" speech sample was elicited first. If the "drug" speech sample was made first and if the effects of the drug had not worn off completely before the "no-drug" sample was made, this could result in a different stuttering frequency during the "no-drug" condition than probably would have occurred if it had come first. For a sequence effect, then, the ordering of tasks, or experimental conditions, is critical. One ordering may result in sequence effect contamination, while a second ordering may not.

Both order and sequence effects are easier to eliminate in a group design than in a single subject design. In a group design, they can be controlled by administering only one experimental condition to each subject. An investigator who wished to determine the effect of a drug on stuttering could take a group of stutterers and randomly assign them to one or two conditions—i.e., speaking without being under the influence of the drug and speaking while under the influence of the drug. Since each subject would only speak under one condition, there would be no possibility of order or sequence effect contamination.

Order and sequence effect contamination is always a possibility with a single subject design, since subjects are run under more than one condition and often more than once under each condition. These effects can sometimes be prevented by having fairly long intervals between treatments. An investigator who wished to determine the effect of a drug on stuttering with a single subject design could separate drug and no-drug speech samples by 24 hours. This would prevent a sequence effect if the effects of the drug wore off in less than 24 hours. Some order effects, such as fatigue, could probably be eliminated with this same strategy.

A sixth way that single subject and group designs differ is related to statistical procedures for assessing the reliability of research findings. These are less well developed for single subject than for group designs (Kratochwill, 1978).

A seventh way that single subject and group designs differ is in the minimum number of subjects necessary. With a single subject design, research can be done with a single subject (N of 1). Therapy outcome research, for example, can be done with an N of 1 (though a larger N usually would be desirable). "Pure" research also is sometimes possible with an N as small as 1. In some of the research on teaching "language" to chimpanzees, only a single chimpanzee was used. Though research with this type of design can be done with only one subject, many studies that utilize it have more than one (McReynolds and Kearns, 1983; Tawney and Gast, 1984).

The minimum number of subjects necessary when a group design is used almost always exceeds that necessary for a single subject design. Studies that use a group design usually require an N of greater than 10. The minimum N necessary for a particular study is a function of several factors, including how reliable answers to questions have to be. The more reliable they have to be, the larger the N required. An investigator who wished to determine whether a particular therapy resulted in a particular behavioral change would need a larger N if he or she wished to be 99 percent certain of the accuracy of the conclusion than if it were adequate to be 95 percent certain. (Factors that should be considered when estimating the N necessary for a particular study are discussed in Chapter 10.)

The eighth, and final, difference between single subject and group designs to be considered here is the basis on which generalizations are made to the population from which subjects are selected. A group design usually does so on a statistical basis, and a single subject design usually does so on a "logical" basis.

In a group design, if the sample of subjects selected approximates a random sample from the population to which one wishes to generalize, then one could generalize to the population through the use of *inferential statistical procedures.* (These are discussed in Chapter 10.) These procedures permit us to infer characteristics of a population from characteristics of a sample (or samples) from that population. If the population of interest were speech-language pathologists who hold the Certificate of Clinical Competence in Speech-Language Pathology from the American Speech-Language-Hearing Association, and the sample consisted of a group of speech-language pathologists randomly selected from the population (from the American Speech-Language-Hearing Association Membership Directory), the attitudes of speech-language pathologists in the population could probably be inferred reliably from those in the sample through the use of inferential statistics, provided that the sample was large enough (Hsu, 1989).

In a single subject design, generalizations to the population from which subjects are selected usually are made on a "logical" rather than statistical basis. While a single subject from a population cannot be assumed to respond similarly to the majority of persons in the population to an experimental condition, it is unlikely that he or she would be the only person in the population who would respond in this way to the condition. Thus, the behavior of this single subject would represent that of a segment of the population. The size of this segment, however, cannot be specified from the performance of only one subject. After data on the performance of other persons in the population under the experimental condition are gathered, some inferences about the size of this segment can be made. Such data on hundreds of severely communicatively impaired mentally retarded children who were taught American Sign Language (or another manual sign system) suggest that the segment of this population that is likely to benefit from such intervention is quite large (Silverman, 1989).

ADVANTAGES AND DISADVANTAGES OF EACH DESIGN

Advantages and disadvantages of single subject and group designs will be summarized in this section. Much of this discussion is based upon material in Table 6.1.

Single Subject Design

Advantages.   The single subject design has several advantages. First, this design makes it possible to detect individual differences. It does not require an investigator implicitly or explicitly to assume that all persons in a population respond similarly to particular experimental conditions. In fact, it offers a means of testing this assumption. If subjects respond differently to an experimental condition and their responses are adequately reliable, this is evidence that the assumption that all persons in a population respond similarly to an experimental condition is not viable. This characteristic of single subject designs is of particular importance in therapy outcome research since most clinicians are usually not willing to assume *a priori* that particular therapies affect all clients with similar communicative disorders in the same manner.

A second advantage of the single subject design is that it permits generalization to real persons in a population rather than an abstraction—i.e., the "typical" member of a population—who might not exist. A speech-language pathologist may never encounter an aphasic who responds to a particular stimulus as does the "typical" aphasic. This is because of the problem with mean data discussed previously.

A third advantage of the single subject design is that it does not require a large N. The N needed, in fact, may be as few as 1.

Disadvantages. Several characteristics of the single subject design may be disadvantageous under certain circumstances. The first, and perhaps most important, is that the design may be difficult to control for order and sequence effects. The possibility of such effects should be considered when you are planning a study that could be done with either a single subject or group design. If they seem possible and it seems unlikely they can be controlled (e.g., by spacing experimental conditions), you should probably not use a single subject design.

A second possible disadvantage is that statistical procedures may not be available for assessing the reliability of answers. These are available for a wider variety of group designs than single subject ones (Kratochwill, 1978). Before deciding to use a single subject design, you would probably be wise to determine whether an appropriate statistical procedure is available for assessing the reliability of answers, *assuming that you feel it necessary to do so statistically.* In some types of research (e.g., operant conditioning research), this is rarely done (McReynolds and Kearns, 1983; Tawney and Gast, 1984).

A third possible disadvantage is that generalizing to a population may not be "neat" if appropriate statistical procedures are unavailable.

Group Design

Advantages. The main advantages of group designs are that statistical procedures usually are available both for assessing the reliability of answers and for generalizing to the population from which subjects are selected. Also, such designs usually make it possible to control for order and sequence effects and, through randomization, for the effects of extraneous variables. In addition, it is often possible to infer from these data characteristics of the "typical" member of a population or characteristics of the majority of members of a population (statistical procedures for doing both are described in Chapter 10).

Disadvantages. A group design *may* be disadvantageous for several reasons. First, it usually requires an investigator implicitly or explicitly to assume that all members of a population respond similarly to an experimental condition. Observed differences in response should be regarded as a function of extraneous variables, random fluctuation, measurement error, and so on, rather than differences in response to the condition. Without this assumption, it usually would not make sense to average together the responses of individual subjects. The qualifier *usually* was used here because a few group designs, such as analysis of variance, may not require this assumption.

A second possible disadvantage of a group design is that it may require more subjects from a particular population to answer a particular question than are available. A speech-language pathologist who wished to determine the impact of a particular therapy on elementary-school stutterers and had only six such children in his or her caseload would probably have too small an N to use a group design. This N would probably be adequate, however, for a single subject design.

A third possible disadvantage of group designs is that the characteristics of a "typical" subject may not be typical. Mean measures of the characteristics of the subjects in a sample may not be similar to those of most, if not all, subjects in that sample. Suppose we wished to evaluate the effects of an articulation therapy on the speech of 10 children who had multiple articulation errors. As a criterion measure, we might use the number of errors each child made on an articulation test before and after receiving therapy. Suppose the numbers of articulation errors produced by these children before and after therapy were as shown in Table 6.2. It would be reasonable to conclude from these means that the typical child in this group had fewer articulation errors following therapy than before therapy. Actually, the therapy only appeared to influence the articulation of two of the 10 children, and the magnitude of the effect for these children was considerably more than one error. Thus, the mean performance of the children in this group is not representative of the "typical" performance of these children.

A fourth possible disadvantage of the group design pertains to generalizing to the population from which subjects are selected on statistical grounds. If a sample of subjects who were observed did not at least closely approximate a random sample from the population of interest, generalizations to this population on the basis of statistical inference would be of uncertain validity and possibly misleading. If, for example, the children in a kindergarten classroom did not approximate a random sample of kindergarten children in general, attempts to generalize the results of a speech-improvement program con-

TABLE 6.2   Numbers of articulation errors produced by 10 children before and after therapy.

Subject Number	Number of Errors before Therapy	Number of Errors after Therapy
1	3	3
2	11	4
3	4	4
4	1	1
5	3	3
6	9	6
7	2	2
8	2	2
9	4	4
10	1	1
Mean	4	3

ducted in this classroom to the population of kindergarten children through the use of statistical inference would be of uncertain validity and possibly misleading. The children in a particular classroom may not approximate a random sample because the suburbs or the inner city are underrepresented. A speech-improvement program which is effective in the suburbs may not be in the inner city, and vice versa.

CATEGORIES OF SINGLE SUBJECT DESIGNS

Thus far two basic types of designs have been described, differences between them pointed out, and advantages and disadvantages of each summarized. Some of the variations possible within the single subject design will be described in this section and some of those possible within the group design in the next.

The "ABC" notation system is used here for describing single subject design variations. This is the system that appears to be the most accepted by behaviorally oriented psychologists, speech-language pathologists, and others for describing such designs (McReynolds and Kearns, 1983; Tawney and Gast, 1984). The symbols from it that are used in this section are defined below:

A   A baseline condition in which the independent variable is not present—i.e., one in which there is no treatment or intervention.

B   The first treatment or intervention condition.

C   The second treatment or intervention condition that is different from the first.

A–B   A dash is used for separating adjacent conditions.

A_1 The subscript indicates whether this was the first, second, third, etc., time that the baseline was measured.

B_1 The subscript indicates whether this was the first, second, third, etc., time that the treatment was introduced.

Other notation systems that have been used for this purpose include those of Campbell and Stanley (1966) and of Glass, Wilson, and Gottman (1975).

The "A-Only" Design

The A-only design is one in which attributes of behaviors of individual subjects are observed and described as they occur naturally. No attempt is made to manipulate them. Hence, the resulting study is an investigation rather than an experiment. Observations used may have been made by the investigator or communicated to him or her by an informant (or informants). What was observed may be described using words (qualitatively), numbers (quantitatively), or a combination of the two. Those studies in which observations are described mostly using words sometimes are referred to as case studies (Bromley, 1986). The investigator in studies utilizing the A-only design is sometimes referred to as a participant-observer (McCall and Simmons, 1969)—he or she attempts to observe and describe behavior without influencing it (Tawney and Gast, 1984). This type of design has been used for what are referred to as longitudinal diary studies of language acquisition (McReynolds and Kearns, 1983). These are studies in which attributes of a child's language behavior in his or her natural environment are described at periodic intervals. It also has been used for studies of preschoolers' normal speech disfluency (e.g., Silverman, 1972).

The A-only design also has been used for post hoc analyses. It was used, for example, to determine whether there is any reason to believe that the incidence and prevalence of stuttering changed during this century (Van Riper, 1982). This was done by comparing incidence and prevalence figures reported in the literature for various years during this century.

The A-only design is not strictly speaking an experimental one because the identification of functional relationships between dependent and independent variables is not possible. Nothing is manipulated, or varied. Ongoing behavior is merely described. Consequently, it is not possible with this design to reach conclusions about how particular dependent variables are influenced by particular independent ones. For example, it would not be possible using it to identify factors (independent variables) that cause preschoolers to repeat syllables (dependent variable) more frequently in one situation than in another.

The "B-Only" Design

With the B-only design, as with the A-only one, attributes of behaviors of individual subjects are observed and described under a single condition.

While with the A-only design this condition is one in which they occur naturally, with the B-only design it occurs during or soon after an intervention
(treatment, introduction of an independent variable)—not before (which
would be an A-only design). Observations of a target behavior with this design, as with the A-only one, can be made more than once. An audiologist
probably would depend on this type of design to gather data needed for preparing periodic progress reports about how a client is adapting to the use of
a hearing aid. And a speech-language pathologist probably would do so for
assessing how a severely communicatively impaired client is adapting to the
use of an augmentative communication device. With this type of design, a
client's status prior to intervention *would not* be compared systematically to
that during or immediately following it. However, it would be with the design
that is considered next—the A-B one.

The B-only design can be used for assessing therapy outcome, but it
has several limitations when utilized for this purpose. While it can be used
to describe attributes of a client's communication behavior at certain points
during or at termination of therapy, it cannot be used to determine how he
or she has changed as a result of therapy. To do so it would be necessary to
compare these to what they were before therapy began. A second limitation
is that the effects of therapy cannot be differentiated from those due to other
factors that occurred while it was taking place, such as maturation. The need
for a design that allows the effects of a therapy to be differentiated from
those of maturation is particularly important when assessing the impacts of
language intervention strategies on young children (McReynolds and Kearns,
1983).

The "A-B" Design

The A–B design, sometimes referred to as the "simple time series design" (Birnbrauer, Peterson, and Solnick, 1974), combines elements of the A-
only and B-only designs. With it attributes of behaviors are observed and
described both when they occur naturally and during (or immediately following) some intervention. Behavior observed under the intervention (B) condition is compared to that observed under the baseline (A) one to determine if
it had an effect. The design requires that the dependent variable (the target
behavior) be measured and/or described "using words" repeatedly under
both conditions. After doing so several times under the baseline (A) condition, the intervention (B) one is introduced. It is necessary to observe the
target behavior more than once under the baseline condition to ensure that
measurements and/or word descriptions of it will be reliable. The target behavior is repeatedly observed during the intervention condition to monitor
changes in it that occur *over time* (which is why the design is referred to as
a "time series" one). Hence, behavior occurring at a point during the intervention condition can be compared to that occurring at one prior to or following it as well as to that occurring during the baseline condition. In most stud-

ies using this design, changes in the target behavior (dependent variable) are described quantitatively.

This design can be used instead of the B-only one for assessing therapy (intervention) outcome. In fact, it is the one (which has been referred to as the "before and after" design) that speech-language pathologists and audiologists appear to use most often for this purpose clinically (McReynolds and Kearns, 1983). The target behavior would be observed and described prior to therapy as well as during it and when it is terminated. To determine whether the client has improved and, if so, how much, the status of the target behavior would be compared to what it was before therapy. While this design is superior to the B-only one for assessing therapy outcome because it provides baseline (pretherapy) data, it has a limitation when used for this purpose. If the target behavior changes during intervention, it is not possible to tell whether the change was due to intervention or to something else that occurred during this period. This limitation is of particular concern when it appears likely that a target behavior will be affected by something other than intervention such as *maturation* when assessing the effects of a language intervention program on young children or *spontaneous recovery* when assessing the effects of one on adult aphasics.

The A–B design is a "quasi-experimental" one (Campbell and Stanley, 1966; Kratochwill, 1978). Because there is no return to the baseline condition (as there would be in a "true" experimental design) following intervention, it cannot be determined empirically whether the change observed in the target behavior in the B-condition resulted from intervention (i.e., the independent variable that was used) or something else. The A–B design can be transformed into a true experimental one by adding a baseline condition, thereby creating the design discussed next—the A–B–A one.

The "A–B–A" Design

The A–B–A design is the simplest single subject one for demonstrating cause-effect relationships empirically. It is similar to the A–B design in that the target behavior is observed and described periodically under both baseline (A_1) and intervention (B) conditions. However, it differs in that following intervention the baseline condition is reintroduced (A_2) and the target behavior is again periodically observed and described. Descriptions of the target behavior when this design is used are almost always quantitative—i.e., involve measurement.

This design has been classified as a *withdrawal* one (Sidman, 1960). The reason is that it allows you to determine empirically if a target behavior is different in the intervention than it was in the baseline condition and whether the difference was due to the intervention. This is done by withdrawing the intervention—thereby creating the baseline condition a second time—and again observing and describing (measuring) the target behavior. If it returns to approximately what it was during the initial baseline condition, this would be evidence that the change in the target behavior resulted from the intervention. This design is most appropriate for assessing the impacts of interventions that would be expected to affect the target behavior only while they are present. Hence, it would not be appropriate for assessing therapies having impacts that would be expected to persist for a long period of time (hopefully, permanently) following intervention. One type that it usually would be appropriate for assessing is drug therapy (e.g., on stuttering). If A_2 is delayed until the effect of the drug has worn off, it can be inferred whether changes observed in the target behavior (e.g., reduced stuttering) resulted from it.

While this design provides stronger evidence than the A–B one that changes in a target behavior resulted from intervention, the design we will consider next—the A–B–A–B one—can provide even stronger evidence that this is the case.

The "A–B–A–B" Design

The A–B–A–B design is one of the most frequently used single subject ones in behavior modification research (Kratochwill, 1978). There is repeated introduction and withdrawal of an intervention strategy. This design provides stronger evidence that changes in a target behavior result from intervention than does the A–B–A one because it provides for a direct replication (Sidman, 1960) of the effects of the intervention on the target behavior—i.e., the last two conditions (A_2–B_2) replicate the first two (A_1–B_1). Based on these characteristics it has been referred to as the "reversal design" (Baer, Wolf, and Risley, 1968), "withdrawal design" (Leitenberg, 1973), and "equivalent time series design" (Campbell and Stanley, 1966)

While this design is an excellent one for "laboratory demonstrations" of the effects of independent variables (interventions) on dependent ones (target behaviors), there can be ethical concerns about its use clinically for assessing therapy outcome (Tawney and Gast, 1984). The reason is that it requires therapy to be terminated for a period of time after the client has improved so that the target behavior will return to what it was during baseline (A_1)—i.e., so that the client will relapse. In fact, the design requires the client to relapse almost completely—i.e., to have the status of the target behavior in A_2 be approximately what it was in A_1.

The A–B–A–B design, of course, is appropriate only if it is reasonable to assume that the effects of the intervention on the target behavior can be reversed. If intervention resulted in the target behavior being learned *very well*, this probably would not be a reasonable assumption. For example, if as a result of intervention a client learned to produce /r/ correctly in words and had been doing so for a while, it is unlikely that he or she would relapse to baseline (A_1) if therapy was terminated.

The "B–A–B" Design

The B–A–B design is a variation of the A–B–A–B one that can be used when it is not possible to measure the target behavior (i.e., collect baseline data) prior to intervention. It could be used by a speech-language pathologist or audiologist for determining the amount a client is benefiting from an intervention strategy, particularly one that he or she was using when first seen. An audiologist, for example, could use it for determining the amount a client is being helped by the hearing aid he or she is currently using; the client's hearing would first be tested with the aid, then without it, and then with it again. While this design does not provide as strong a demonstration of intervention effectiveness as does the A–B–A–B one, it tends to provide a stronger one than the A–B–A design because it provides two opportunities to demonstrate it.

Multitreatment Designs

The designs discussed thus far are used for assessing the impact of a single intervention strategy (independent variable) on the target behavior (dependent variable). Multitreatment ones are used when it is desired to assess the impact of two or more intervention strategies on it, singly or in combination. They can be particularly useful for determining which of two intervention strategies has the greater impact on it or whether the combination has a greater one than either by itself. An example of a multitreatment design that can be used for determining which of two treatments has the greater impact on a target behavior is the A–B–A–B–C–B–C one. This is an A–B–A–B design to which a second intervention (C) has been added. And an example of a multitreatment design that can be used for determining whether the combination of two treatments has a greater impact than either by itself is the A–B–A–B–BC–B–BC one. This, like the A–B–A–B–C–B–C design, can be viewed as an extension of the A–B–A–B one.

If there are no order or sequence effects, each of the designs mentioned in the preceding paragraph can be used for answering two questions. Those that the A–B–A–B–C–B–C design can be used for answering are the following:

1. Does intervention strategy *B* affect the target behavior?
2. Do intervention strategies *B and C* differ with regard to the amount they affect the target behavior?

And these are the ones that can be answered using the A–B–A–B–BC–B–BC design:

1. Does intervention strategy *B* affect the target behavior?
2. Does the combination of intervention strategies *B and C* affect the target behavior more than *B* by itself?

Abbreviated versions of the multitreatment design have been used in behavioral research. The A–B–A–B–BC–B–BC design, for example, has been abbreviated to A–B–BC–B–BC (Tawney and Gast, 1984).

Multiple Baseline Designs

The designs discussed thus far are single baseline ones because the status of only one target behavior is observed and described. With multiple baseline designs (Baer, Wolf, and Risley, 1968) this is done for two or more target behaviors. One of the most significant advantages of multiple baseline designs is that they can demonstrate the impacts of intervention strategies on target behaviors without it being necessary to withdraw intervention as it is with the A–B–A–B design (Kratochwill, 1978). That is, with these designs it is not necessary to cause a person to "relapse." It should not be surprising, therefore, that these designs have been used clinically for assessing the impacts of intervention strategies.

There are several types of multiple baseline designs. One that can be useful for evaluating intervention strategies has been referred to as the multiple baseline design across behaviors (Tawney and Gast, 1984). With this type of design two or more target behaviors that appear to be functionally independent and should respond to the same intervention strategy are observed and described (measured). The intervention strategy is applied to one but not to the other. If the only target behavior that changes is the one to which it is applied, this is evidence that the strategy is effective. The evidence, of course, would be stronger if this result was replicated on a number of subjects.

An example of the use of this type of multiple baseline design to demonstrate the effectiveness of an intervention strategy is in the study reported by Elbert, Shelton, and Arndt (1967). Two target behaviors were observed and measured periodically: correct production of /r/ and correct production of /s/. The target behavior that the intervention strategy was expected to modify was the articulation error being treated. Thus, when it was produced correctly a higher percentage of the time following intervention and the other was not, this was interpreted as evidence for the effectiveness of the strategy.

The variations of the single subject design discussed in this section should be regarded as representative rather than exhaustive. There are a number of books and papers that describe other variations and further discuss the ones presented here in the reference list (Barlow and Hayes, 1979; Barlow and Hersen, 1973, 1984; Birnbauer, Peterson, and Solnick, 1974; Campbell, 1963; Campbell and Stanley, 1966; Connell and Thompson, 1986; Cook and Campbell, 1979; Cuvo, 1979; Davidson and Costello, 1969; Dukes, 1965; Edgar and Billingsley, 1974; Gottman, 1973; Holtzman, 1963; Horner and Baer, 1978; Jerger, 1964b; Kazdin, 1981, 1982a, 1982b; Kearns, 1986; Kendall, 1981; Kratochwill, 1978; Kratochwill and Brody, 1978; Kratochwill and

Levin, 1980; McReynolds and Kearns, 1983; McReynolds and Thompson, 1986; McCullough, 1984; Merriam, 1988; Pring, 1986; Rickels, Schweizer, and Case, 1988; Rusch and Kazdin, 1981; Sidman, 1960; Stanley, 1985; Strain and Shores, 1979; Tawney and Gast, 1984; Watson and Workman, 1981; Wolery and Harris, 1982; and Yin, 1984).

CATEGORIES OF GROUP DESIGNS

Hundreds of designs have been devised that can be classified as group designs. Many of those that are useful in behavioral research are included in books by Ferguson (1989), Guilford (1978), Hays (1973), Keppel (1982), Lindquist (1953), Siegel (1988), and Winer (1991).

Two general categories of group designs can be identified: (1) those intended to determine whether a *difference* exists, and (2) those intended to determine whether a *relationship* exists. The designs in these categories permit different kinds of questions to be answered. Those in the first category permit the answering of such questions as:

1. Is vocal rest effective in reducing the size of vocal nodules?
2. Does hearing aid A tend to result in better speech discrimination ability for persons with conductive hearing losses than hearing aid B?

Designs in the second category, on the other hand, permit the answering of such questions as:

3. Is auditory discrimination ability positively related to articulation proficiency?
4. Are scores of audiometric test A negatively related to scores on audiometric test B?

The first of these questions can be answered by determining whether there is a *difference* in the average (mean or median) size of the vocal nodules of a group of persons following vocal rest. The second can be answered by determining whether there is a *difference* in the average (mean or median) speech discrimination scores of a group of persons who have conductive hearing losses when hearing aid A and hearing aid B are used. The third can be answered by determining whether there is a *positive relationship* between scores on auditory discrimination tests and scores on tests of articulation proficiency—that is, it would be necessary to determine whether persons who earn high scores on one tend to earn high scores on the other. Finally, the fourth question can be answered by determining whether persons who earn *high* scores on audiometric test A tend to earn *low* scores on audiometric test B, and vice versa.

Designs for Detecting Differences

To answer some questions, it is necessary to determine whether one or more differences exist. These differences can be of several kinds. They can, for example, be differences between percentages (or proportions), as in these questions:

1. Are stutterers more likely to have articulation errors than nonstutterers?
2. Do more children who have hearing losses fail audiometric screening test *A* than audiometric screening test *B*?

The first question can be answered by determining whether a higher percentage (or proportion) of stutterers than nonstutterers have articulation errors; the second, by determining whether the same percentage (or proportion) of children who have hearing losses fail audiometric test *A* as audiometric test *B*.

Other kinds of differences that can be detected by a group design are those between means, or medians, as in these questions.

1. Do kindergarten children tend to have fewer articulation errors after participating in a particular speech-improvement program than before?
2. Does the level of academic achievement of elementary-school stutterers tend to differ from that of their nonstuttering peers?

The first question can be answered by comparing the mean (or median) number of articulation errors of a group of kindergarten children after participating in the program to that before participating in the program; the second, by comparing the mean (or median) academic achievement scores of a group of elementary-school stutterers with that of a matched group of nonstutterers. Note that the first requires a comparison between two measures made on the *same* subjects and the second requires a comparison between single measures made on *different* subjects.

The questions that illustrated group designs for detecting differences involved comparisons between two measures. Such designs also can be used to compare more than two measures. Suppose we wanted to determine whether there were any differences in the percentages of children in kindergarten through sixth grade who had chronic hoarseness. A group design could be used for comparing these seven percentages. Similarly, such a design could be used to compare mean auditory discrimination scores earned by a group of persons who have conductive hearing losses while using five different hearing aid models.

Group designs for detecting differences differ in several dimensions, including: (1) the type of measure for which they are appropriate, (2) the number of measures that can be compared, and (3) their appropriateness for dependent measures, independent measures, or a combination of the two. The type of measure for which a design is appropriate refers to the nature of the criterion measure—whether it is a percentage, a proportion, a frequency count, a mean, a median, a mode, or some other derived measure. A design that is appropriate for detecting differences between percentages may not be appropriate for detecting differences between means.

A third dimension in which these designs differ is their appropriateness for dependent measures, independent measures, and combinations of the two. Dependent measures are measures made on the same subjects or on extremely well-matched groups of subjects (e.g., two groups in which there is one member of a number of pairs of identical twins in each). Independent measures are measures made on unmatched groups of subjects. "Before and after" therapy measures would be examples of dependent measures, since they are made on the same persons. Measures made on unmatched groups such as stutterers and nonstutterers would be examples of independent measures.

Some designs only are appropriate for dependent measures or independent measures, and others are appropriate for combinations of the two. A design appropriate for dependent measures would be necessary to answer this question: "Do dysarthrics who have been fitted with a palatal lift prosthesis tend to be more intelligible with the device than without?" Such a design would be needed because two measures on the same subjects would have to be compared—one with the prosthesis and one without it.

Answering other questions requires a design appropriate for independent measures. Consider the question, "Do dysarthrics who have been fitted with a palatal lift prosthesis tend to be more intelligible than those who have had pharyngeal flap surgery?" A design appropriate for comparing independent measures would be needed here because two groups are being compared, one consisting of dysarthrics who have been treated surgically and the other consisting of dysarthrics who have been fitted with a prosthesis.

To answer some questions, a design appropriate for both dependent and independent measures is necessary. For example, consider the question, "Do palatal lift prostheses tend to increase the intelligibility of the speech of dysarthrics who have inadequate velo-pharyngeal closure more than do pharyngeal flaps?" One design appropriate for answering this question, known as the Type I analysis of variance design (Lindquist, 1953), can be diagrammed as shown in Figure 6.1. If this design were used, measures of the intelligibility of the speech of two groups of dysarthrics would be made before and after physical management. Between-group comparisons would involve independent measures, and "before and after" treatment comparisons would involve dependent measures. Note that this design has an advantage over the one described in the preceding paragraph because it is possible to determine whether the groups differed in degree of intelligibility prior to intervention.

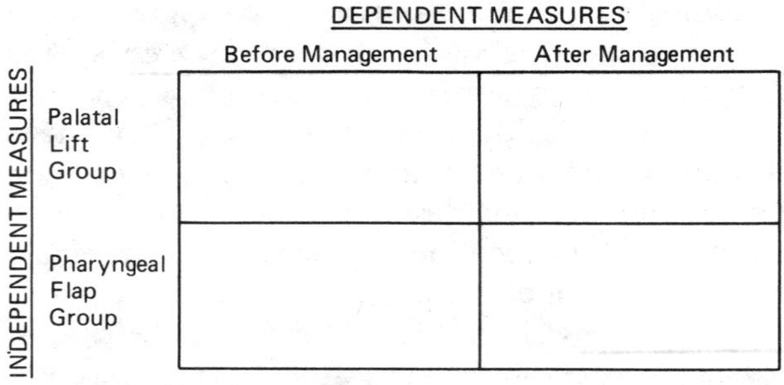

DEPENDENT MEASURES

FIGURE 6.1 Analysis of variance design for assessing the effects of palatal lift prostheses.

Designs for Detecting Relationships

Answering some questions requires a design for detecting relationships rather than differences. There are several kinds of questions about relationships that such designs can help to answer if relationships are found to exist, including those related to: (1) the *direction* of the relationships (positive or negative), (2) the *strength* of the relationships, and (3) the *nature* of the relationships (linear or nonlinear). Suppose you wished to describe the relationship between children's speech disfluency levels in two situations–that is, you wished to determine whether those who tended to be the most disfluent in one situation also tended to be the most disfluent in the other, and vice versa. You might sample the speech of 10 children in the two situations and determine the frequency of speech disfluency per 100 words spoken by each child in each situation. Suppose the disfluency frequencies you obtained were as shown in Table 6.3.

To permit the relationship between the disfluency frequencies in the two situations to be visualized, they were plotted on a two-dimensional graph-

TABLE 6.3   Frequencies of speech disfluency exhibited by 10 children in two situations.

Child	Situation I	Situation II
1	6.3	10.1
2	5.6	9.4
3	4.5	10.1
4	9.0	22.5
5	4.5	8.7
6	3.9	6.1
7	6.8	17.5
8	5.5	10.4
9	12.5	35.4
10	3.4	5.6

ical display known as a *scattergram* (see Figure 6.2). The configuration of this scattergram provides data for answering the following four questions (assuming the answer to the first is yes):

1. Does a relationship exist between these children's disfluency frequencies in the two situations?
2. What is the *direction* of the relationship between the disfluency frequencies in the two situations?
3. Does the relationship appear to be *linear* or *nonlinear*? If nonlinear, what does the *nature* of the relationship appear to be?
4. How *strong* does the relationship between the disfluency frequencies in the two situations appear to be?

What would be the answer to each question based on the configuration of the scattergram in Figure 6.2? The answer to the first question would be yes, since the points are not randomly distributed on the scattergram but are confined to a relatively small segment of it. The configuration of Figure 6.3, incidentally, illustrates what a scattergram might look like if little or no relationship existed between the variables. The points are not confined to a segment of the graph; they are scattered throughout the graph. A child who had a relatively high disfluency frequency in one situation would be about as likely to have a relatively high as a relatively low frequency in the other.

From the configuration of the points in Figure 6.2, it would appear that the *direction* of the relationship between the children's disfluency frequencies in the two situations is "positive." The ordering of the children with

FIGURE 6.2   Scattergram depicting a relatively strong positive relationship between two variables.

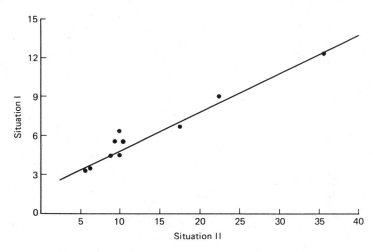

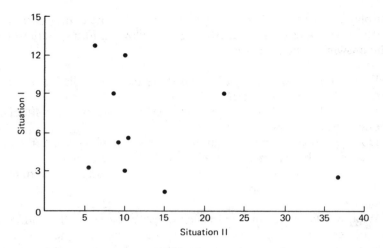

FIGURE 6.3 Scattergram depicting little or no relationship between two variables.

regard to disfluency frequencies is quite similar in the two situations. Children who had relatively high disfluency frequencies in one tended to have relatively high disfluency frequencies in the other, and vice versa. If the direction of the relationship had been "negative," the configuration of the points might have been similar to that in Figure 6.4.

To answer the third question, it would seem reasonable to assume from the configuration of the points in Figure 6.2 that the relationship between the disfluency frequencies in the two situations for these children is *linear*.

FIGURE 6.4 Scattergram depicting a relatively strong negative relationship between two variables.

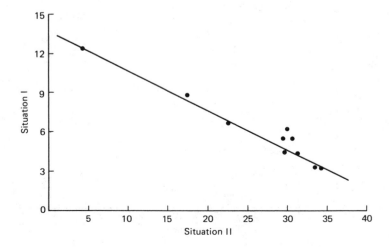

The line that could be drawn on the scattergram from which the points would deviate least and which would be the least complex would be a straight line. When two variables are linearly related, an increase (or decrease) in the magnitude of one is associated with a *proportional* increase (or decrease) in the magnitude of the other. This proportional increase (or decrease) will occur throughout the range of possible values. If two variables are *not linearly related*, on the other hand, an increase (or decrease) in the magnitude of one will not be associated with a proportional increase (or decrease) in the magnitude of the other throughout the range of possible values. Two common nonlinear relationships between variables are depicted in Figures 6.5 and 6.6. The relationship depicted in Figure 6.5, which is *curvilinear,* is the least complex of the possible nonlinear relationships between variables. That depicted in Figure 6.6, which is *cubic,* is one step up in complexity from curvilinear.

To answer the fourth question, it would appear from the configuration of points in Figure 6.2 that the relationship between the relative disfluency frequencies in the two situations for these children is *fairly strong*. The points are not scattered very much; they deviate little from the straight line which best describes the relationship between them. The greater the deviation of the points in a scattergram from the line which best describes the nature of the relationship between two variables, the weaker the relationship between them. The scattergrams in Figure 6.7 illustrate two degrees of linear relationship. The relationship depicted in the scattergram on the top is stronger than that depicted in the scattergram on the bottom.

The discussion thus far has been limited to detecting and describing relationships between two variables. There are group designs for detecting

FIGURE 6.5 Scattergram depicting a relatively strong curvilinear relationship between two variables.

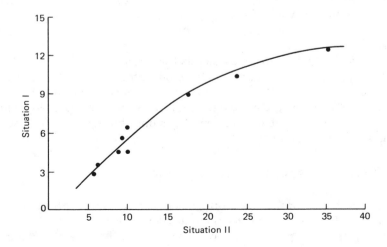

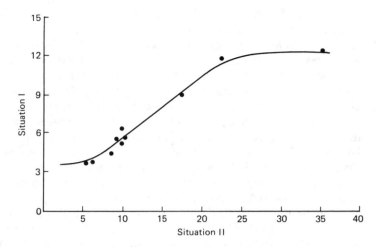

FIGURE 6.6   Scattergram depicting a relatively strong cubic relationship between two variables.

and describing more complex relationships—that is, those involving more than two variables. Such designs could be used for answering such questions as:

1. How well do clinicians agree on how severe stutterers are?
2. What factors influence how severe a stutterer is perceived as being?
3. What factors best differentiate the speech of a child beginning to stutter from that of his peers?

The first question could be answered by determining the extent to which a sample of clinicians would order a group of stutterers in the same manner in the severity of their stuttering. The second could be answered by identifying factors that are related to judgments of stuttering severity. And the third could be answered by identifying factors that are more likely to be related to the speaking behavior of peers who have no history of a stuttering problem. Statistical procedures that could be used to answer these questions (the Kendall coefficient of concordance, multiple regression and correlation, and the discriminant function analysis for questions one through three respectively) are discussed in Chapter 9.

WHICH TYPE OF DESIGN SHOULD YOU USE?

It should be fairly apparent from the discussion in this chapter that usually a number of factors must be considered when you decide whether to use a single subject or group design to answer a question. For some questions, how-

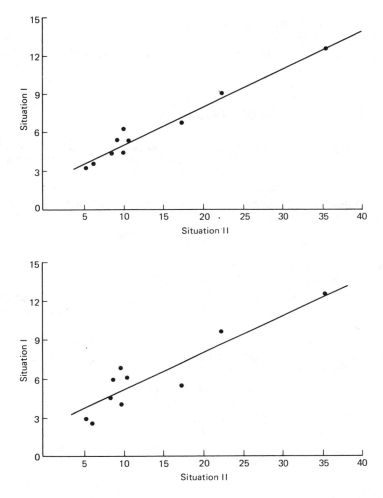

FIGURE 6.7 Scattergrams depicting two degrees of linear relationship. The relationship depicted in the scattergram on the top is stronger than that depicted in the one on the bottom.

ever, only one of these two types would be appropriate because of a single consideration. Such questions include:

1. those that state unequivocally whether they refer to individuals or to typical members of groups,
2. those for which all treatments could not be administered to individual subjects, and
3. those for which an insufficient N would be available for a group design.

For questions where the choice is not clear-cut, you must weigh the advantages and disadvantages of each design and select the one that seems most likely to yield data of adequate validity, reliability, and generality to answer the question. If neither design seems likely to yield data of adequate validity, reliability, and generality to answer a question (or questions), it might be wise to search for some other question (or questions) for which the prospects of collecting such data seem better.

EXERCISES AND DISCUSSION TOPICS

1. Indicate whether you would use a single subject or a group design to answer each of the following questions and state the reasons for your decisions. Also describe the subjects you would observe to answer each question (indicating attributes they would and would not possess) and specify the observations you would make on these subjects and the conditions under which you would make them.

   a. "What impacts does learning to use a communication board have on aphasics?"

   b. "Which of two methods of teaching speechreading tends to produce the best results with hard-of-hearing adults?"

   c. "Do persons who have sensorineural hearing losses tend to respond differently to a particular hearing test than those who have conductive hearing losses?"

2. Using the "ABC" notation, diagram a design you have used during your clinical practicum experience for assessing (auditing) therapy outcome. What limitations does this design have and how could it be improved?

3. Order and sequence effects are discussed in this chapter from the perspective of their possible detrimental impacts on clinical research. How could they also adversely affect the outcome of a diagnosis and/or a therapy session?

7
Types of Data

This chapter will deal with the observations, or data, that serve as the raw material for answering questions. Such observations can be viewed as raw material because they have to be organized in some manner before they can be used for answering questions. (This topic is discussed in Chapters 9 and 10.)

WHAT ARE DATA?

Data can be viewed as an abstraction from the observational process. When you observe an event, you do not attend to, or abstract all aspects of it. You simply attend to a small number (in some cases only one) that are relevant for answering a particular question. If, for example, you wished to determine whether a child had articulation errors, you could administer an articulation test. Most such tests require the child to say a number of words in which the phonemes of the language occur in various positions. The child's production of each word constitutes an event. This event would have a number of attributes, including accuracy of production of each phoneme, voice quality, pitch level, intensity, etc. During a child's production of each word, you would probably attend only to the phoneme (or possibly two phonemes) the word was included in the test to sample. This illustrates what is meant, therefore, by abstracting only those aspects of an event that are relevant for answering a question, which in this case would be: "Is the phoneme (or are the phonemes) which the word was intended to sample produced correctly in the position in which it occurs in the word?" The information abstracted about the accuracy of production of the phoneme could serve as *data* for answering this question.

There may be more than one aspect of an event which, if abstracted, could serve as data for answering a particular question. The accuracy of production of a phoneme in a word, for example, could be described in several ways. First, it could be described on the basis of how it sounds to an observer (or observers). Second, it could be described on the basis of how accurate the postures of the articulators look during production of the phoneme through the use of cineflourography (i.e., X-ray motion pictures). Third, it could be described on the basis of action potentials recorded from the speech musculature during production of the phoneme by means of electromyography. Finally, it might be described on the basis of oral and nasal pressure and flow measurements made during production of the phoneme through the use of appropriate transducers and electronic amplifiers and recording devices. (The use of instrumentation for observing aspects of events is discussed in Chapter 8.)

Strictly speaking, data are symbolic representations of attributes of events. They are not what is abstracted from events but abstractions of what is abstracted from events. As the general semanticists have pointed out (e.g., Johnson, 1946), you cannot express in words or numbers everything you observe. If, for example, the event you were observing was a child telling a story about a picture and the attribute you were attending to was phonological development, the data resulting would be your description of what you observed—in words, or numbers, or both. It would not be what you observed per se.

What relationship should exist, then, between the symbolic representation of what is observed (data) and what is observed? The answer is that the two should be similar in structure. By this we mean that the relationship between data and what is observed should be analogous to that between a *map* and the *territory* it represents. If a map that included Illinois and Wisconsin were similar in structure to the territory represented, Chicago, Illinois, would be north of Champaign, Illinois, and Milwaukee, Wisconsin, would be north of both Champaign and Chicago. If the map indicated that Milwaukee was south of Chicago, the structure of the map would not be similar to the territory. (For further discussion of the man-territory analogy, see Johnson, 1946, pp. 131–133.)

The relationship between map and territory, or between what is observed and its symbolic representation, can be further illustrated by means of the relationship between a pure-tone audiogram and what it depicts. A pure-tone audiogram can be regarded as a *partial* symbolic representation of one aspect of hearing, i.e., threshold for pure tones. It is a partial representation because thresholds are not plotted for all frequencies in the audio range (e.g., they are not plotted for 562 Hz or 1079 Hz). If the configuration of the audiogram is similar in structure to the territory it is supposed to depict—i.e., a person's thresholds for pure tones at selected frequencies—it will accurately indicate the person's thresholds at the frequencies tested. The ordering of these frequencies for threshold would correspond to the person's relative ability to detect the presence of pure tones at the frequencies tested. Not only would the ordering of frequencies for threshold correspond to that in the territory, but the relative degrees of hearing loss at the frequencies tested would also. If a pure tone of one frequency had to be made 10 dB louder than a pure tone of a second frequency to be detected, this would be indicated by the configuration of the audiogram.

A second illustration of the map-territory relationship that is relevant to communicative disorders is the relationship between articulation test results and articulation errors. For articulation test results to be similar in structure to the territory they are supposed to depict—i.e., the articulation errors of the person tested—they have to indicate the speech sounds that are produced incorrectly and how they are produced incorrectly (i.e., omitted, distorted, or substituted for).

The extent to which a data map is similar in structure to the territory it represents determines its validity. The greater the structural similarity, the more valid the data. A description of something is valid if it accurately describes that which it is intended to describe. Aphasia test results are valid to the extent that they accurately describe an aphasic's language deficits. A description of a therapy session would be valid to the extent that it accurately portrayed what occurred during the session. Assessing the validity of data, therefore, involves estimating the degree of structural correspondence between map and territory—between the description of an event and the event itself.

Speech-language pathologists and audiologists use many types of data for answering questions. The following data, for example, were reported in a single issue of the *Journal of Speech and Hearing Disorders:*

1. transcriptions of samples of stuttered speech
2. linguistic analyses of normal speech disfluencies
3. children's scores on the Environmental Language Inventory
4. anecdotal reports of parents functioning as language trainers
5. numbers of syllables spoken per minute
6. judgments of "normalcy" of speech
7. stutterers' self-ratings of reactions to speech situations
8. personality test scores
9. frequency of use of specific syntactic structures
10. scores on the Elicited Language Inventory
11. verbal descriptions of expressive language
12. chronological ages

13. scores on Porch Index of Communicative Ability
14. pure-tone audiometric test results
15. verbal descriptions of apraxics' use of American Indian Sign
16. mean values of temporal integration in dB
17. verbal descriptions of "cocktail party speech" accompanying myelo-meningocele and shunted hydrocephalus
18. auditory localization test scores
19. verbal description of a person with contact granuloma of the vocal cords
20. measures of respiratory function (e.g., tidal volume)
21. measures of speaking pitch level
22. verbal descriptions of X-rays
23. verbal descriptions of the communicative behavior of a young deaf child
24. nasality scores
25. articulation error frequencies

Actually, thousands of different kinds of verbal and numerical descriptions have been used by speech-language pathologists and audiologists to map territories of interest to them.

QUALITATIVE AND QUANTITATIVE DATA

There are two basic types, or classes, of data—qualitative and quantitative. *Qualitative* data are *verbal* descriptions of attributes of events, and *quantitative* data are *numerical* descriptions of attributes of events. Both are used by speech-language pathologists and audiologists to answer questions.

Qualitative Data

Some attributes of events can be more adequately described through words than through numbers. Verbal descriptions of such attributes could be less abstract—that is, could include more information—than numerical ones. Suppose, for example, you wished to describe the response of an aphasic to an aphasia test item. A highly abstract description of such a response would be to assign it a 1 if it were appropriate and a 0 if it were inappropriate. A less abstract description would be to assign it a number that would indicate how close it was to being appropriate, e.g., a number from 0 to 16 as is done with the PICA scoring system (Porch, 1971). The level of abstraction could be reduced even more by describing the aphasic's behavior when the item was presented in as much detail as possible. (Excellent examples of such descriptions of aphasics' response to aphasia test items can be found in Head's classic work, *Aphasia and Kindred Disorders of Speech,* published in 1926.)

Verbal descriptions of attributes of events vary in the degree to which they are similar in structure to the territory they are intended to map. As I indicated earlier in this chapter, this topic has been dealt with in depth by the general semanticists (e.g., Johnson, 1946). They have indicated how the use of language can cause some verbal maps to be more similar in structure to the territory being mapped than others. The following sets of statements illustrate several of the ways in which verbal descriptions of attributes of events can vary in the extent to which they are similar in structure to the territory they are intended to depict. The second statement in each set would probably be judged to be more similar in structure than the first.

1a. John said his first word when he was 10 months old.
1b. John's parents first remembered hearing him produce sounds which they interpreted as a meaningful word when he was 10 months old.
2a. John is a moderately severe stutterer.
2b. John's stuttering was judged moderately severe in the situation in which he was observed.
3a. John's study was rejected by the *Journal of Speech and Hearing Research* because it was poorly designed.
3b. An associate editor for the *Journal of Speech and Hearing Research* felt that John's study was poorly designed and rejected it.
4a. John is a good clinician.
4b. John behaves in a manner that is consistent with my internal standard regarding what constitutes a good clinician.
5a. Stutterers do not stutter when they are alone.
5b. Some stutterers report they do not stutter when they are alone.
6a. The articulation test results indicated that John had a relatively severe articulation problem.
6b. Based on the articulation test results, I felt that John had a relatively severe articulation problem.

Qualitative data (i.e., verbal descriptions of attributes of events) vary with regard to level of validity, reliability, and generality. The greater the structural similarity between the description of an attribute of an event and what occurred, the more valid the description. The "b" descriptions in the preceding paragraph, therefore, would probably be regarded as more valid than the "a" descriptions.

The level of reliability of qualitative data is a function of the interaction between the observer and the observed. Some persons tend to be more reliable observers than others. They are more likely to *consistently* abstract the relevant aspects of an event. They have fewer biases that would tend to distort their observations.

The level of generality of qualitative data is a function of the representativeness of the sample of events observed. Samples selected by a random procedure (i.e., table of random numbers) that are relatively large usually are the most representative. They permit relatively accurate inferences to be made regarding the class of events of which they are representative. If you wished to determine the distribution of attitudes of ASHA certified speech-language pathologists and audiologists toward a piece of legislation before the Congress, you could select a random sample of such individuals from the most recent *American Speech-Language-Hearing Association Directory* and ask each to complete a questionnaire. Assuming your sample was adequately large, the distribution of attitudes in the sample would probably correspond closely to that in the population (i.e., the total group of ASHA certified speech-language pathologists and audiologists). The distribution of attitudes in the sample would serve, therefore, as a fairly accurate "map" of the distribution of attitudes in the population. The data in the sample thus would have some generality.

Is qualitative data inferior to, or less scientific than, quantitative data? While there is no reason for regarding one form of data as intrinsically inferior or superior to the other, the answer to this question would depend on the territory being described. Verbal descriptions would be more similar in structure to some territories than numerical descriptions would be. For such territories, verbal descriptions would be superior to numerical ones. On the other hand, some territories can probably be described more precisely through numbers than through words. For such territories, qualitative data would be inferior to quantitative data. An investigator's choice would be expected to depend on which he or she feels provides the most accurate map for the territory.

Quantitative Data

Some attributes of events can be described and communicated more adequately through numbers than through words. This is particularly likely to be true for those attributes which involve quantities, or magnitudes. The following statements concern the frequency of occurrence of an articulation error:

1. During the session John produced /s/ correctly most of the time.
2. During the session John produced /s/ correctly 80 percent of the time.

The second would probably be regarded as more adequately describing John's production of /s/ during the session than the first, since the meaning of "80 percent" is less ambiguous than that of "most." Hence, the second would be a more adequate map of the territory than the first.

The defining characteristic of quantitative data is that they consist of number symbols, or numerals. Numerals function semantically in the same manner as words—i.e., they have *assigned* meanings. Meanings are assigned to both classes of symbols; they do not exist in nature. To identify the meanings that have been assigned to a given word, you can look it up in a dictionary. If it has more than one meaning, its meaning in a particular situation has to be inferred from context. Numerals function similarly in that each can be assigned several meanings; to determine their meaning in a given situation you have to know the context in which they are being used. The numerals 10, 20, and 30, for example, would have different meanings in the following five contexts:

1. They could be used to designate types of communicative disorders.
2. They could be used to designate positions in a rank ordering for hypernasality.
3. They could be used to designate points on an equal-appearing interval scale of articulation defectiveness.
4. They could be used to designate frequencies of occurrence of stuttering.
5. They could be used to designate degrees of hearing loss in dB.

The first context illustrates the *nominal* meaning of numerals, or number symbols. In this context they are used merely to designate, or label, categories. Letters of the alphabet, words, or other symbols could be substituted for them. The numeral 10, for example, could be used to designate spastic dysphonia, 20 to designate Broca's aphasia, and 30 to designate conductive hearing loss. The numerals on the backs of football players' jerseys also have this meaning.

The second context illustrates the *ordinal* meaning of numerals. In this context they are used to designate locations in rank order. They indicate the relative amount of an attribute each individual possesses relative to that possessed by the other individuals ranked. The numeral 10, for example, could be used to designate the individual in a group of three who was most hypernasal and 30 the one in the group who was least hypernasal.

The third context illustrates the *interval* meaning of numerals. In this context they designate points on a continuum which have equal amounts of the attribute being measured between them. If the numerals 10, 20, and 30 had interval meaning, the amount of increase in articulation defectiveness between a speech sample assigned the numeral 10 and one assigned the numeral 20, for example, would be equal in magnitude to the amount of increase in articulation defectiveness between a sample assigned the numeral 20 and one assigned the numeral 30. If these numerals had ordinal rather than interval meaning, the amount of increase in articulation defectiveness between them would not be assumed equal.

The fourth context illustrates the *ratio* meaning of numerals. In this context they designate points on a continuum which both have equal amounts of an attribute between them and are related to an *absolute* zero. Because of the presence of an absolute zero, the magnitudes between points, as well as those represented by the points themselves, have meaning. A speech sample assigned the numeral 20, for example, would contain articulation that is twice as defective as one assigned the numeral 10. And one assigned the numeral 10 only would be one-third as defective in articulation as one assigned the numeral 30. These relationships would not hold for numerals with ordinal or interval meanings, since such numerals are not related to an absolute zero.

The fifth context illustrates the *logarithmic* meaning of numerals. In this context numerals designate points on a continuum which have *unequal*, but known, mathematically defined amounts of an attribute between them. Since the numerals on the decibel scale have logarithmic meanings, a person who had a 30 dB hearing loss would hear less well than a person who had either a 20 dB or 10 db one, and the magnitudes of the differences between these amounts of hearing loss could be estimated.

These five meanings for numerals (nominal, ordinal, interval, ratio, and logarithmic) are ones that are most often encountered by speech-language pathologists and audiologists. They will be further discussed in the final section of this chapter, which is concerned with measurement.

Quantitative data, like qualitative data, vary in validity, reliability, and generality. The factors that influence these are the same for quantitative data as for qualitative data.

The validity of quantitative data is a function of the degree of structural similarity, or isomorphism, between the meanings of the numerals used to describe, or quantify, an attribute of an event and the attribute being described. The more valid the data, the greater the degree of similarity, or isomorphism. If ordinal numerals are used to describe the ordering of a group of individuals on the basis of a particular attribute and the individuals are orderable on the basis of that attribute in the manner designated by the numerals, then the numerals are isomorphic to the attribute being described and hence validly describe that attribute. Suppose you had five stutterers who varied considerably in severity in relation to the others, with 1 designating mildest stuttering and 5 most severe stuttering. The numerals would be isomorphic to the territory and hence valid if, for example: (1) the stutterer assigned the numeral 2 was more severe than the stutterer assigned the numeral 1 and less severe than the stutterers assigned the numerals 3, 4, and 5; (2) the stutterer assigned the numeral 5 was more severe than any of the others; and (3) the stutterer assigned the numeral 1 was less severe than any of the others. For the numerals to be a valid map of the territory, therefore, they would have to rank order the stutterers in a manner that would be consistent with the relative severities of their stuttering.

The reliability level of quantitative data, like that of qualitative data, is a function of the interaction between the observer and the observed. The factors mentioned as influencing this interaction in the discussion of qualitative data also apply here. The main difference between the two is that the level of reliability of quantitative data can usually be estimated more precisely than that of qualitative data.

The factors mentioned as influencing the generality of qualitative data also influence the generality of quantitative data. Random sampling and a sufficiently large N maximize the probability of adequate generality for both types of data. The main difference between the two for generality is similar to that for reliability—i.e., the generality of quantitative data usually can be estimated more precisely than that of qualitative data. Statistical inference, which is the approach used to estimate the generality of quantitative data, is discussed in Chapter 10.

MEASUREMENT-RELATED PROPERTIES
OF QUANTITATIVE DATA

The measurement-related properties of the five most frequently encountered types of quantitative data in speech-language pathology and audiology research—nominal, ordinal, interval, ratio, and logarithmic—were summarized briefly in the preceding section. These properties will be discussed here in greater depth. It is essential for speech-language pathologists and audiologists to develop as good an intuitive understanding of them as they can. Without such an understanding, quantitative data cannot be accurately interpreted or applied.

The Nature of Measurement

Measurement can be defined as *the assignment of numerals to attributes of (objects and) events according to rules.* This definition is a slightly modified version of one formulated by the late S. S. Stevens (1951, p. 1), who was a pioneer in psychological and psychophysical measurement. There are several terms in this definition to which particular attention should be paid. The first is the term *numeral*. Numerals, as was indicated earlier in this chapter, are number symbols. Their meanings are determined by the rules used to assign them. Numerals on nominal, ordinal, interval, ratio, and logarithmic scales have different meanings because they are assigned by different rules. Therefore, it is necessary to know the rules by which a particular set of numerals was assigned to grasp their meaning.

The second important aspect of this definition is that numerals are assigned to *attributes* of objects and events rather than to objects and events themselves. When you describe an object or event, you only describe certain attributes of it, not all possible ones. Objects and events possess infinite numbers of attributes (Johnson, 1946).

The third important point of this definition is that the term *objects* is in parentheses, to indicate that it could be deleted from the definition. Objects can be classified as events. What you abstract as an object on the macroscopic (observable) level would be classified as an event on the submicrocopic (molecular) level since its configuration would be constantly changing (Johnson, 1946). The eventness, or process nature, of objects is apparent even if they are observed on the macroscopic level over a relatively long period of time (Johnson, 1946). The author's 1982 Toyota did not have the same attributes in 1992 that it had when it was new. The attributes (or characteristics) of a hearing aid after two years of use are unlikely to be identical to what they were when it left the factory. Since the attributes of phenomena classified as objects vary as a function of time on both macroscopic and submicroscopic levels, they are not sharply differentiable from phenomena classified as events. It would appear justifiable, therefore, to classify them as events rather than to place them in a separate category.

The rules used for assigning numerals to attributes of events on nominal, ordinal, interval, ratio, and logarithmic scales are presented and discussed in the following sections.

Nominal Scales

Numerals on a nominal scale are assigned to categories, or subclasses, of attributes of events by means of the rule that states "do not assign the same numeral to different classes or different numerals to the same class" (Stevens, 1951, p. 26). They merely label, or identify, such categories or subclasses. The particular numeral assigned to a particular category or subclass is *arbitrary*. It is desirable, however, that the categories of subclasses be *mutually exclusive* and *exhaustive* with regard to the attribute being scaled. That is, all events that possess the attribute being scaled should be (1) assignable to only one category or subclass, and (2) assignable to a category or subclass. Suppose the attribute you wished to scale was articulation errors. The following three categories, or subclasses, could be used for this purpose, and a numeral could be assigned arbitrarily to identify each:

1. sound substitutions
2. sound omissions, additions, and inversions
3. sound distortions

These categories would probably be regarded as both mutually exclusive and exhaustive, since individual articulation errors would be assignable to only one category and all such errors could be assigned to a category. The specific ordering of the numerals that is used to label the three categories is completely arbitrary. Any of the six—i.e., $(N)(N-1)$—possible permutations of these three numerals (see Figure 7.1) would serve equally well.

The events assigned to any one category must be equivalent with regard to the attribute being scaled, or fall within the defined domain of that category. They do not have to be equivalent, however, with regard to any other attributes. The relation between such events for the attribute scaled is referred to as *equivalence* and is symbolized by the familiar sign $=$. The

123
321
132
231
213
312

FIGURE 7.1   Permutations of numerals on a nominal scale.

equivalence relation is defined logically as being *reflexive, symmetrical,* and *transitive* ($x = x$ for all values of x; if $x = y$, then $y = x$; and if $x = y$ and $y = z$, then $x = z$). These qualities are further defined in the section on ordinal scales.

Nominal scales have been constructed for a variety of attributes of interest to speech-language pathologists and audiologists. Some such scales are an end in themselves and others are a means to an end. Several examples of the first type would be Angle's (1907) three classes of malocclusion—i.e., Class I (Neutrocclusion), Class II (Distocclusion), and Class III (Mesiocclusion); Jerger's four types of Bekesy audiogram tracings (Jerger, 1960); and Schuell's five major diagnostic categories of aphasia (Schuell, Jenkins, and Jimenez-Pabon, 1964). The second type would include instances where qualitatively defined categories, or subclasses, are arbitrarily assigned numerals to facilitate computer analysis. The category "male," for example, might be assigned the numeral 1, and "female" the numeral 2. Or the numeral 1 might be assigned to conductive hearing loss, 2 to sensori-neural hearing loss, and 3 to mixed hearing loss. Various statistical analyses can be performed on observations that have been categorized in this way, including determining the number and percentage of total observations that fall into each category.

Ordinal Scales

Numerals on an ordinal scale are assigned to N categories, or subclasses, or events to designate a *rank order.* The categories, or subclasses, ordered may contain only a single event (e.g., a person). While the ordering of the N numerals designates the ordering of the N categories with regard to the amount of the target attribute they possess, it is arbitrary whether 1 or N is used to designate the greatest amount of the attribute. Thus, if 10 events (e.g., speech samples) were rank ordered, the one with the greatest amount of the target attribute (e.g., hypernasality) could be assigned either the numeral 1 or the numeral 10.

With an ordinal scale, the differences in the amount of the target attribute between the categories ranked are not necessarily the same. There are not necessarily equal intervals between scale points. This is illustrated in Figure 7.2. The difference in the amount of the target attribute between the category assigned the numeral 1 and the category assigned the numeral 2 in

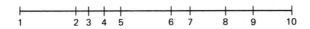

FIGURE 7.2 An ordinal scale.

this figure is greater than the difference between the category assigned the numeral 2 and that assigned the numeral 3. If the 10 numerals on this scale had been assigned to 10 samples of speech to designate an ordering on the basis of articulation defectiveness, the difference in degree of articulation defectiveness between the sample assigned the numeral 1 and that assigned the numeral 2 would be greater than the difference in degree of articulation defectiveness between the sample assigned the numeral 2 and that assigned the numeral 3.

Categories on an ordinal scale can be labeled by words and certain other symbols rather than (or in addition to) numerals. The labels "mild," "moderate," and "severe" can be attached to categories on an ordinal scale, as can the labels "poor," "fair," "good," "very good," and "excellent"; and A, B, C, D, E. The labels "correct" and "incorrect"; "+" and "−"; and "+", "±", and "−" also can be attached to categories to define ordinal scales.

For a scale to have ordinal properties, the numerals have to be assigned by rules that result in a specific relationship between the categories ranked. This relationship, according to Hempel (1952, pp. 58–62), is based on the relations of *coincidence* (sharing the same place or being equal to another) and *precedence* (being less than or greater than another). For the relationship between categories on a scale to be ordinal, Hempel states that the two relations have to meet the following conditions.

1. Coincidence must be *transitive*; i.e., whenever x stands in coincidence to (or in the same category as) y and y stands in coincidence to (or in the same category as) z, then x stands in coincidence to (or is included in the same category as) z. In other words, if John lives in the same state as Jim and Jim lives in the same state as Joe, then John lives in the same state as Joe.
2. Coincidence must be *symmetric*; i.e., whenever x stands in coincidence to (or is included in the same category as) y, then y stands in coincidence to (or is included in the same category as) x. In other words, if John lives in the same state as Jim, then Jim lives in the same state as John.
3. Concidence must be *reflexive*; i.e., any event x stands in coincidence to (is includable in the same category as) itself with regard to the attribute being measured. Another way of stating the same thing is that $x = x$ for all values of x. In other words, all events included in a category are equivalent with regard to the attribute on the basis of which they were assigned to the category. Thus, all individuals classified as having a conductive hearing loss would have pathology in the outer and/or middle ear.

4. Precedence must be *transitive*; i.e., if x stands in coincidence to y and y stands in precedence to z, then x stands in precedence to z. In other words, if Bloodstein's (1987) Phase II stuttering is more severe than his Phase I stuttering, and his Phase III stuttering is more severe than his Phase II stuttering, then his Phase III stuttering should be more severe than his Phase I stuttering.

5. Precedence must be *coincidence-irreflexive*; i.e., if x stands in coincidence to (or is equal to) y, then x does not stand in precedence to y. In other words, if John has the same threshold for a 1000 Hz tone as Jim, then John does not have a higher threshold or lower threshold for this tone than Jim.

6. Precedence must be *coincidence-connected*; i.e., if x does not stand in coincidence to (or is not equal to) y, then x stands in precedence to y or y stands in precedence to x. In other words, if John does not have the same threshold for a 1000 Hz tone as Jim, then John either has a higher threshold or a lower threshold for this tone than Jim.

There are six conditions, then, that Hempel indicates need to be satisfied for numerals to have ordinal properties. The first three, incidentally, also must be satisfied for numerals to have nominal properties (see section on nominal scales).

Ordinal scales are the type that has probably been used most frequently to measure, or quantify, attributes of events of interest to speech-language pathologists and audiologists. There are at least three reasons for the frequent use of this type of scale. First, ordinal scales are simpler to construct than other types which indicate magnitudes, or quantities (i.e., interval, ratio, and logarithmic scales). The reason for this is that the other types require the six conditions for ordinal measurement to be satisfied in addition to some others. (These additional conditions are indicated in the sections in which the three types are discussed.)

A second reason for the frequent use of ordinal scales is that ordinal level measurement is all that is required for answering many questions. Such questions often are similar in form to one of the following:

1. Does Person A (or Group A) *have more of (or less of) an attribute* than Person B (or Group B)? Other phrases that could occur instead of the italicized one include: (a) have a higher (or lower) score on a task, (b) have a longer (or shorter) response time, and (c) exhibit a higher frequency (or lower frequency) of a behavior.

2. Do persons who exhibit a relatively high level (or relatively low level) of an attribute under one condition (or on one task) also tend to exhibit a similar level under one or more other conditions (or on one or more other tasks)? Another way of phrasing this question would be: Does

Condition A (or Task A) tend to rank order persons in the same manner as Condition B, etc. (or Task B, etc.)?

A third probable reason for the frequent use of ordinal scales is that some attributes, or dimensions, do not lend themselves to higher than ordinal level measurement—i.e., they do not lend themselves to interval or ratio level measurement. An example would be a scale in which the categories, or points, include several dimensions, such as Bloodstein's (1987) four-phase scale for describing the development of stuttering. It would be extremely difficult, if not impossible, to construct such a scale so there would be equal intervals between points for all dimensions included.

Interval Scales

Numerals on interval scales are assigned by the same rules as those on ordinal scales, *plus* one additional rule: they must be assigned in such a manner that the interval widths between successive numerals are equal in magnitude with respect to the attribute being scaled. This requirement is graphically portrayed in Figure 7.3 for the attribute "distance." The distance between the numerals 1 and 2 in this figure is equal to that between the numerals 2 and 3, 3 and 4, 4 and 5, 5 and 6, 6 and 7, 7 and 8, 8 and 9, and 9 and 10. The equality of these interval widths can be checked with a ruler.

Interval scales can be constructed for psychological attributes as well as physical ones. In addition to equal physical distances between points, there can be *equal-appearing* perceptual distances between points—distances that appear approximately equal based on observer judgments. The Lewis-Sherman Scale of Stuttering Severity (Lewis and Sherman, 1951) represents an attempt to develop a scale on which the perceptual distances between points are equal appearing. This scale consists of nine sets of speech segments, each of which has been assigned a numeral between 1 and 9. The segments assigned the numeral 1 contain the mildest stuttering and those assigned the numeral 9 the most severe. The segments were selected from a larger group that were rated by the method of equal-appearing intervals for "degree of stuttering severity." This method, which is described in Chapter 8, is thought to result in measurement that approximates interval level. Theoretically, differences in stuttering severity between speech segments assigned the numeral 1 and those assigned the numeral 2 would be approximately equal to those between speech segments assigned the numerals 2 and 3, 3 and 4, 4 and 5, 5 and 6, 6 and 7, 7 and 8, and 8 and 9. The interval widths on this scale, incidentally, were estimated by means of a rating procedure and

FIGURE 7.3   An interval scale.

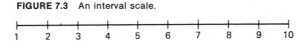

with a few exceptions were found to be fairly equal (Berry and Silverman, 1972).

Because of the equality of interval widths, the *differences* between numerals on interval scales can be manipulated arithmetically. That is, they can be added, subtracted, multiplied, and divided. The difference in the amount of an attribute between events designated by the numerals 1 and 3 would be twice that between events designated by the numerals 1 and 2 and half that between events designated by the numerals 1 and 5. If these numerals were points on an interval scale of stuttering severity, the difference in severity of stuttering between a speech segment designated by the numeral 1 and one designated by the numeral 3 would be twice that between speech segments designated by the numerals 1 and 2 and half that between speech segments designated by the numerals 1 and 5.

While the differences between numerals on an interval scale can be manipulated arithmetically, this cannot be done with the numerals themselves. The reason for this restriction is that the numerals on such a scale are not related to an absolute, or "true," zero. Thus, a speech segment that was assigned the numeral 2 would not necessarily contain stuttering that was twice as severe as that in a segment assigned the numeral 1 nor half as severe as that in a segment assigned the numeral 4.

Scales that have been regarded either implicitly or explicitly as having interval properties have been developed for a number of attributes of interest to speech-language pathologists and audiologists. Such scales would include those which were constructed by the method of equal-appearing intervals, e.g., the Lewis-Sherman Scale of Stuttering Severity (Lewis and Sherman, 1951). They also might include scales based on age ratios such as IQ (i.e., MA/CA × 100). Numerals on IQ scales could be regarded as having either ordinal or interval properties. The interpretation would depend on whether you were willing to assume, for example, that the increase in "intelligence" from an IQ of 60 to an IQ of 70 is equivalent to the increase from an IQ of 95 to one of 105. If you were willing to assume that the intervals between points on the IQ scale are approximately equal throughout the *entire* range of possible IQs, then you would be justified in regarding numerals on this scale as having interval properties. On the other hand, if you would not be willing to make this assumption, it would be safest to regard such numerals as having ordinal properties.

Scales that are claimed to have interval properties should probably be regarded as having ordinal properties unless it has been demonstrated unequivocally that the equal interval assumption is viable. Regarding them as such in most instances would probably not cause any problems.

Ratio Scales

Numerals are assigned by the same rules on ratio scales as on interval scales with the exception that they are required to be related to an absolute, or true, zero. This requirement is portrayed graphically for the attribute "distance" in Figure 7.4. Because ratio scales have as their origin a true zero point, the numerals on such scales, as well as the intervals between them, are isomorphic to the structure of arithmetic and can be manipulated arithmetically. A speech segment assigned the numeral 4 on a ratio scale of stuttering severity would contain stuttering that is twice as severe as that in a speech segment assigned the numeral 2 on this scale. A ratio scale theoretically could be constructed for the attribute stuttering because it would be possible to have a speech segment which contained zero stuttering. It might not be possible, on the other hand, to construct a ratio scale for the attribute "intelligence" because it would be difficult to define zero intelligence.

The decision on whether a scale has ratio properties may not be unequivocal. Frequency of articulation errors would probably be regarded as a scale with ratio properties if it were viewed as a *frequency* scale, since the numeral 4, for example, would indicate twice as many articulation errors as the numeral 2. On the other hand, it would probably not be regarded as a ratio scale of *articulation defectiveness*, since four errors would not necessarily be judged to represent twice the degree of articulation defectiveness as two errors. It would probably not be regarded even as an interval scale of articulation defectiveness since interval widths between successive numerals are unlikely to be judged equal. The change from one to two articulation errors, for example, would probably be judged to represent a greater increase in articulation defectiveness than would the change from 15 to 16 such errors. Hence, a scale of articulation defectiveness based on frequency of articulation errors would probably be regarded as having ordinal properties.

While one measure of a particular attribute might not result in a scale that has ratio properties, another such measure might result in a scale with these properties. It might be possible, for example, to construct a ratio scale of articulation defectiveness by using a psychological scaling procedure such as *direct magnitude-estimation* (see Chapter 8) rather than frequency counts of articulation errors. With this approach, each of a group of speech segments that contained a wide variety of frequencies and types of articulation errors would be assigned a number by a panel of listeners that would be instructed to indicate how defective the articulation was in it as compared to the articulation in a "standard" speech segment. The standard speech segment would be arbitrarily assigned a point value, e.g., 100. Each listener would be instructed to assign a point value to each speech segment that would indicate how defective he or she considers the articulation in it to be as compared to that in the standard speech segment. A listener who felt, for example, that

FIGURE 7.4 A ratio scale.

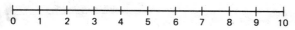

0   1   2   3   4   5   6   7   8   9   10

the articulation in a particular speech segment was twice as defective as that in the standard segment would assign that segment 200 points. On the other hand, a listener who felt the articulation in a particular speech segment was half as defective as that in the standard segment would assign it 50 points. The listener could assign any number of points desired to a speech segment as long as it reflected a judgment on how defective the articulation was in it as compared to that in the standard segment. The mean of the point values assigned to each segment could be computed and used as its *scale value*— i.e., the point, or value, on the scale to which it is assigned. Assuming the listeners *rated the speech segments as instructed*, the resulting scale should at least come close to having ratio properties. A segment with a mean point value of 100, for example, would be approximately twice as defective in articulation as one with a mean point value of 50, and approximately half as defective in articulation as one with a mean point value of 200.

The unit of measurement of a ratio scale is arbitrary. For the attribute "length," for example, you can convert from inches to feet (or from feet to inches) by multiplying (or dividing) all numerals by the *positive constant* 12. The conversion, or transformation, from one unit of measurement to another by *multiplying* or *dividing* all numerals by a positive constant does not influence the ratio properties of a scale.

Ratio scales for attributes of interest to speech-language pathologists and audiologists have been developed from several types of measures including the following:

1. Frequency counts. One attribute that has been scaled by this measure is frequency of moments of stuttering.
2. Temporal (time) measures. One attribute that has been scaled by this type of measure is duration of moments of stuttering.
3. Length (distance) measures. The amount of opening between the poste-

TABLE 7.1 Relationships between ratio scale values and logarithmic scale values for the base numbers 2 and 10.

Ratio Scale Value	Logarithmic Scale Value (Base 2)	Logarithmic Scale Value (Base 10)
0	(2^0) 1	(10^0) 1
1	(2^1) 2	(10^1) 10
2	(2^2) 4	(10^2) 100
3	(2^3) 8	(10^3) 1000
4	(2^4) 16	(10^4) 10000
5	(2^5) 32	(10^5) 100000
6	(2^6) 64	(10^6) 1000000
7	(2^7) 128	(10^7) 10000000
8	(2^8) 256	(10^8) 100000000
9	(2^9) 512	(10^9) 1000000000

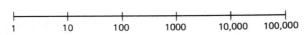

FIGURE 7.5   A logarithmic scale.

rior surface of the velum and the anterior surface of the posterior pharyngeal wall during the production of /a/ has been measured in millimeters from lateral headplates (X-rays) to assess velopharyngeal closure.
4. Voltage measurements. Output voltages from some types of electro-
acoustical instrumentation used in audiology have been recorded and
measured.
5. Observer judgments. Scales for attributes of communicative behavior
which at least approximate ratio measurement have been constructed through the use of psychological scaling methods such as direct
magnitude-estimation. (Several such scales are described in Chapter 8.)

Logarithmic Scales

Logarithmic scales, like ratio scales, are constructed from numerals that
meet the conditions for ratio level measurement. To construct a logarithmic
scale from such numerals you multiply each by a particular *base* number.
(Only numerals with ratio properties can be used to construct logarithmic
scales because numerals with nominal, ordinal, and interval properties cannot
be manipulated arithmetically.) The base numbers used most often for scaling attributes of communicative behavior are 2 to 10. Relationships between
ratio scale values and logarithmic scale values for the base numbers 2 and 10
are illustrated in Table 7.1.

These relationships demonstrate one of the main advantages of logarithmic over ratio scales. A logarithmic scale can present data more compactly
than a ratio scale. Scale values up to 10,000 are included in the logarithmic
scale depicted in Figure 7.5 in the same space as for scale values up to 10 in
the ratio scale depicted in Figure 7.4. The compactness of logarithmic scales
in comparison to ratio scales is illustrated further in Figure 7.6.

Because logarithmic scales are derived from numerals with ratio scale
properties, the numerals on such scales can be manipulated arithmetically.
Logarithmic scales can be transformed into ratio scales for the same reason.

Logarithmic scales have been used to quantify a number of attributes
of interest to speech-language pathologists and audiologists, including the in-

FIGURE 7.6   Comparison between ratio and logarithmic scales.

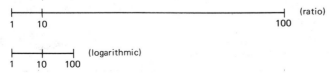

tensities and fundamental frequencies of voices. They also have been used to record the effects of speech therapies on articulation errors over time (e.g., Mower, 1969).

EXERCISES AND DISCUSSION TOPICS

1. How does a clinical evaluation report serve as a "map" of a "territory"?

2. Specify two types of qualitative and two types of quantitative data that an audiologists might gather during a hearing aid evaluation.

3. Indicate what *attribute* or what *event* you would attempt to describe verbally or numerically to answer the following questions. For each, specify two ways you could describe this attribute of this event that probably would be sufficiently reliable and valid for answering the question.

    a. "How much does production of /s/ tend to improve after 10 weeks of daily therapy using a particular program?"

    b. "How much better does a particular hard-of-hearing child tend to understand speech while he or she is using a hearing aid than while he or she is not using it?"

    c. "How intelligible is the esophageal speech of a person who has had a total laryngectomy?"

4. You are to evaluate the numerical properties of the scores yielded by three diagnostic tests. Indicate what measurement scale you feel the scores from each are on and give your reasons.

8

Approaches
to Generating Data

This chapter describes some approaches (or strategies) for generating the types of data necessary to answer questions of relevance to speech-language pathology and audiology—specifically, approaches that have proved useful for describing attributes of communicative behavior. It will attempt to develop in the reader an intuitive understanding of these approaches and of the types of questions they can answer, as well as factors to be considered when designing and evaluating the results of studies utilizing these approaches.

ROLE OF THE OBSERVER
IN THE DATA-GENERATING PROCESS

Before beginning our discussion of approaches for describing attributes of events of interest to speech-language pathologists and audiologists, we will consider the data-generating process itself, particularly the role of the observer in this process. The observer is a component of all schemes for generating data, since all of them rely on observer judgment to some extent. With psychological scaling (rating) procedures, which are discussed elsewhere in this chapter, the importance of the observer in the process is obvious because the data are observer judgments. It may not be as obvious, however, for physical measurement, i.e., measurement of physical attributes of events that utilizes electronic or other types of instrumentation. Examples of such instruments would be rulers and dial voltmeters. Both may appear to result in "objective" measurement, i.e., measurement not influenced by observer judgment; distances may appear to be indicated by the marks on rulers and voltages by the position of the pointer on voltmeter dials. Rulers and voltmeters do not read themselves, however. Someone has to decide which mark on a ruler corresponds to the distance being measured and which number on the voltmeter dial the indicator is pointing at. Also, the accuracy of the calibration of such devices obviously influences the accuracy of the measurement it is possible to obtain from them. And the accuracy of their calibration is partially a function of observer judgment, since they are calibrated by some human agent. For these reasons, observer judgment is an unavoidable component of any data-generating process or scheme.

The presence of an observer (or observers) in the process introduces error into it. A group of observers who measure the same thing, for example, may not record the same measurement. This can be demonstrated by means of a relatively simple task such as measuring the length of a line with a ruler. How long is this line?

———————————————

To answer this question, 10 students at Marquette University were handed a card on which a line of this length had been drawn and a foot ruler graduated in sixteenths of an inch. All measured the line with the same ruler. They were told to measure the line and record their measurement on a blank card which they had been given. Their length estimates ranged from 2.00 inches to 2.25 inches, with a mean of 2.07 inches. While the differences between estimates are relatively small, they could be large enough in some instances to make a difference that would result in a difference in an answer to a question.

The presence of an observer in the process can introduce two types of error: random and systematic. Both were described in Chapter 7. *Random error*, as indicated previously, is present to some degree in all data-generating processes. It can arise from several sources, including insufficient accuracy in making and in recording (writing down) observations. If, for example, you were measuring distances with a ruler, random error could result occasionally from not placing the ruler at the exact point from which you wished to begin to measure, or from reading distances from the ruler incorrectly, or from writing down distances inaccurately after you had read them. The nature of random error is such that if you were to describe again an aspect of an event (or object) after you had made an error (or errors), you would be unlikely to make the same error (or errors). Because random error does not replicate itself— i.e., does not occur whenever a data-generating process is repeated—it does not bias the resulting data. It does not, for example, cause numbers from a measurement process to be consistently larger or smaller than they should be. While random error can be reduced by such means as making all measurements twice, it is doubtful whether it ever can be completely eliminated.

The second type of error, *systematic error*, is usually of more concern to investigators than the first because it *biases* the resulting data. For example, it causes the numerals generated by a measurement process to be consistently larger or smaller than they should be. In the case of measuring distances with a ruler, systematic error could result from consistently placing the end of the ruler at a point that was not the one from which you wished to begin to measure, or consistently misreading the ruler in the same manner (e.g., interpreting the gradations as occurring every $\frac{1}{16}$ inch rather than every $\frac{1}{8}$ inch), or consistently recording distances incorrectly after reading them (e.g., indicating inches rather than millimeters after numerals).

Observer-related systematic error can be introduced from several sources, including:

1. A measuring "instrument" or process being improperly administered or conducted. An investigator, for example, may not administer an educational or psychological test in the manner in which it was supposed to be administered. An investigator who deviated from the instructions in the test manual for administering the test might obtain scores that are biased—i.e., consistently higher or lower than they should be.

2. Subjects not performing a task as instructed. They may, for example, not make the judgement they were instructed to make. Suppose a group of subjects were told to rate a series of speech segments from cleft palate speakers for degree of nasality, thus requiring them to ignore articulation errors and other deviations of speech, voice, and language usage. They may not be able to keep the other deviations present in the speech segments from influencing their nasality ratings, which would cause these ratings to be biased.

3. Experimenter bias. An experimenter's outcome expectations or hypotheses can bias the measurements he or she makes (Rosenthal, 1976). For example, a speech-language pathologist who expected a particular treatment to be effective in reducing stuttering severity might rate stutterers as less severe after the administration of the treatment than before more often than the effects of the treatment would justify. Such errors would not represent deliberate, or conscious, attempts to deceive but "wishful thinking." (This topic is further discussed in Chapter 11.)

4. Subject bias. This phenomenon is closely related to, and is sometimes the result of, experimenter bias. Subjects may respond to experimental conditions in the manner which they feel the experimenter either would like them to respond or expects them to respond. That is, they have thoughts about an experiment that can influence their performance on an experimental task. As Orne has pointed out:

> Insofar as the subject cares about the outcome, his perception of his role and of the hypothesis being tested will become a significant determinant of his behavior. The cues which govern his perceptions—which communicate what is

expected of him and what the experimenter hopes to find—can therefore be crucial variables. . . . They include the scuttlebutt about the experiment, its setting, implicit and explicit instructions, the person of the experimenter, subtle cues provided by him, and of particular importance, the experimental procedure itself. All of these cues are interpreted in the light of the subject's past learning and experience. (Orne, 1969, p. 146)

If clients were asked, for example, to describe the effects a particular therapy had on them as part of a study of the effectiveness of that therapy, and if they surmised that the person who was conducting the study either expected (or hoped) to find it effective in certain ways, they might be more likely to indicate that it had at least "a little" effect in these ways than they would if they had had no information concerning the expected (or hoped for) outcome. Hence at least some of their statements could be biased.

Data-generating schemes used by speech-language pathologists and audiologists can be divided into two groups. The first includes those that use an "instrument" to supplement observer judgment. The instrument helps the observer to "abstract" the attribute he or she wishes to describe. A speech-language pathologist who wished to describe the extent of increase in sympathetic nervous system activity in response to a feared stimulus as part of a desensitization procedure could use a psychogalvanometer to assist in observing and measuring this activity. Or an audiologist who wished to describe thresholds for pure tones could use a pure-tone audiometer to help abstract this phenomenon.

An instrument used to supplement observer judgment need not be electronic. Most, if not all, educational and psychological tests could probably be used for this purpose. So also could tests of communicative ability such as articulation tests, aphasia tests, language development scales, auditory discrimination tests, and tests of speechreading ability. Other "instruments" that could be used for this purpose include questionnaires and structured interviews.

The second group of data-generating schemes includes those that rely primarily upon observer judgement. The observer is the most important component of such schemes. Psychological scaling techniques, which have been used a great deal by speech-language pathologists and audiologists for quantifying attributes of communicative behavior, are representative of the schemes in this group. These techniques require the observer to make various kinds of judgments, including the following:

1. deciding to which of a group of categories an event should be assigned
2. deciding which member of each of a series of pairs of events possesses the greater amount of an attribute
3. rank ordering a group, or series, of events on the basis of the amount of an attribute they possess
4. assigning numerals between 1 and a specified upper limit (usually 7 or

9) to events on the basis of the amount of some attribute they possess, so that the intervals between successive numerals will be equal-appearing with respect to an attribute

5. assigning numerals between 1 and a specified upper limit (usually 7 or 9) to events on the basis of the amount of some attribute they possess, so that each event is assigned the numeral of the category on the scale that comes closest to indicating the amount of the attribute it possesses (the amount of the attribute possessed by each category on the scale would be specified either verbally or nonverbally)

6. assigning points to each of two events which sum, or add up, to a particular constant (e.g., 100) so that the points assigned to each of the two correspond to the relative amount of the attribute being measured that it possesses in relation to that possessed by the other (e.g., if one member of a pair were judged to possess twice the amount of an attribute as the other, it would be assigned 66.67 points and the other would be assigned 33.33 points)

7. assigning points to events on the basis of the amount of an attribute they possess as compared to that possessed by a "standard" event, or stimulus

Each of these tasks is associated with a psychological scaling technique that is described elsewhere in the chapter.

Several data-generating schemes of each type are described in this chapter. While these are not the only ones that have been used in speech and hearing research, they include those that have been used most often.

SCHEMES THAT UTILIZE AN INSTRUMENT TO SUPPLEMENT OBSERVER JUDGMENT

Schemes that utilize an instrument to supplement observer judgment can be divided into two groups. The first consists of those that utilize electronic or other instruments for physical measurement; and the second, those that do not utilize such instruments—e.g., those that utilize tests, structured tasks, and questionnaires.

Schemes That Utilize Electronic or Other Physical Measurement Instrumentation

Various types of instruments are used by speech-language pathologists and audiologists to measure physical attributes of communicative behavior. Information about such instruments can be found in the chapter by Borden and Harris in *Speech Science Primer* (1980) as well as the books by Code and Ball (1984), Cudahy (1988), Curtis and Schultz (1986), Decker (1989), and McPherson and Thatcher (1977).

Most instrumentation schemes for measuring attributes of events that are electrical signals or can be transduced (i.e., converted) into electrical signals contain certain components. These components, which are diagrammed in Figure 8.1, can be regarded as defining a series of stages for the process of measuring such signals.

The first stage in the process is *detection*. Its purpose is to detect the presence (and absence) and possibly the magnitude of the signal of interest. If the phenomenon is not an electrical signal, it is transduced into an electrical signal.

The detection stage for measuring speech and other acoustical signals consists of a microphone and possibly a preamplifier. The microphone transduces acoustical signals into electrical signals. The function of the preamplifier is to amplify the electrical signals (i.e., voltages) generated by the microphone, with very little distortion, to the point where their magnitude is within the sensitivity range of the "amplifier" stage.

The detection stage for measuring biological electrical signals—such as those resulting from muscle action potentials, brain waves, and changes in skin resistance—consists of electrodes which either would be attached to the surface of the skin (i.e., surface electrodes) or inserted into muscle fibers or other tissue (i.e., needle electrodes) and an appropriate preamplifier. The function of the preamplifier here would be to increase the magnitudes of the electrical signals detected by the electrodes, with very little distortion, to the point where their magnitude is within the sensitivity range of the "amplifier" stage.

While these two types of detection stages are probably the ones that have been used most frequently in speech and hearing research, several other types have also been used. These would include: (1) strain gages that trans-

FIGURE 8.1   Instrumentation scheme for measurement.

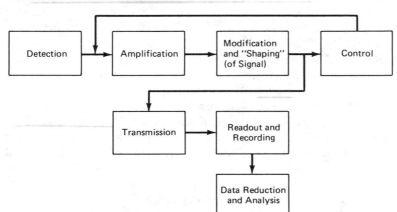

duce mechanical pressures, or stresses, into electrical signals, (2) pneumotac-tographs that transduce rates of air flow into electrical signals, and (3) photoelectric cells that transduce light intensities into electrical signals. An appropriate preamplifier would be fitted to each such transducer.

The second stage in instrumentation schemes for measuring electrical signals is *amplification.* The function of this stage is to increase the magnitude of the electrical signal from the detection stage to the point where it is within the sensitivity range of the readout and recording device being used. The electrical signal from the detection stage may have to be passed through a series of amplifiers, rather than a single amplifier, to increase its magnitude to the point where it is within the sensitivity range of this device. It may also modify the output of the detection stage in such a way that the "noise" (i.e., extraneous signals) in the system will be reduced.

A third stage that may be included in instrumentation schemes for measuring electrical signals is the *modification and shaping* of the signals outputed by the amplifier stage. One of the primary functions of such a stage would be to remove "noise" (extraneous information to what is being measured) from these signals—i.e., to make the figure, or what the investigator wishes to observe, stand out better from the background (other information in the signal).

A modification and shaping stage may consist of a filter network. There are three basic types of filter networks—high pass, low pass, and band pass. Their function is to emphasize or deemphasize specific frequency components of a signal. A *low pass* filter network is used to reduce or eliminate from a signal frequency components *above a specified frequen*cy. A low pass filter network thus would emphasize the low frequency components of a signal. A *high pass* filter network is used to eliminate from a signal frequency components *below a specified frequen*cy. A high pass filter network thus would emphasize the high frequency components of a signal. A *band pass* filter network is used to reduce or eliminate from a signal *both* frequency components above a specified frequency and below a specified frequency; it consists of a high pass and a low pass filter network. A band pass filter network thus would emphasize a particular "band" of the frequency components of a signal—those between specified upper and lower frequency limits.

The next stage usually included in instrumentation schemes for measuring electrical signals is *control.* Its function is to keep the amplitude or some other attribute of the electrical signal outputed by the amplification stage (or modification and shaping stage, if one is used) *within certain limits.* This is a feedback component that functions in much the same manner as a thermostat on a furnace and an automatic record level on a tape recorder. It measures the average amplitude (or other attribute) of the output signal from the amplification stage (or possibly that of the shaping stage if one is used). If the amplitude (or value of some other attribute of the signal) is too great, it adjusts the amplification stage to attenuate, or weaken, it. If, on the other hand, the magnitude is insufficient, it adjusts the amplification stage to increase it. This process keeps the amplitude (or other attribute) of the signal within the sensitivity range of the device used to record the signal. A microcomputer, or microcomputer circuitry in the amplifier, ordinarily is used for this purpose.

The next stage consists of a device for *transmitting* the signals outputed by the amplification stage (or shaping stage if one is used) to a readout and recording device. The simplest such device would be an electrical cable (i.e., jumpcord) that would connect the output of the amplification stage (or a modification and shaping stage if one were used) to the input of a readout and recording device. Radio telemetry instrumentation also could be used for this purpose. The output signals from the amplification stage (or modification and shaping stage if one were used) would be fed into a radio transmitter and beamed to a radio receiver that could be anywhere from a few feet to hundreds of thousands of miles (e.g., astronauts in space) away. The radio receiver would be connected to a readout and recording device.

The next, and possibly last, stage in such instrumentation schemes consists of a device for *recording and reading out,* or displaying, the output signals from the transmission stage. Without such a device, these signals could not be measured.

Several types of readout and recording devices can be used in instrumentation schemes for measuring electrical signals. The simplest type consists of a *meter,* which indicates the value of the attribute of the signal being measured at given moments in time. This value may be indicated by a pointer (Figure 8.2) or a digital display (Figure 8.3).

FIGURE 8.2   A typical meter that indicates values of the attribute being measured by a pointer.

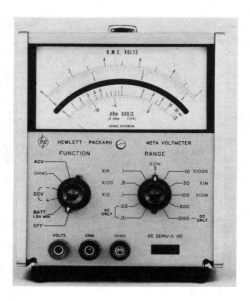

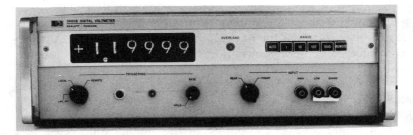

FIGURE 8.3 A typical meter that indicates values of the attribute being measured by a digital display.

Another class of readout and recording devices that can be used in such schemes include *oscillographic recorders* (see Figure 8.4) and *strip chart recorders* (Figure 8.5). Both will indicate changes in the configuration of a signal during a specified period of time by means of a continuous line drawn on a strip of paper. The primary difference between them is that an oscillographic recorder can handle a wider range of rates of change in the configuration of a signal than a strip chart recorder can. Strip chart recorders are most useful when the rate of change in the configuration of a signal is relatively slow. The line may be drawn in ink by a pen, by a light on photosensitive paper, or by a heated stylus on heat-sensitive paper. The strip of paper may be in a roll or in a Z-fold pack (i.e., folded in a fanlike manner similar to computer

FIGURE 8.4 A typical multi-channel oscillographic recorder.

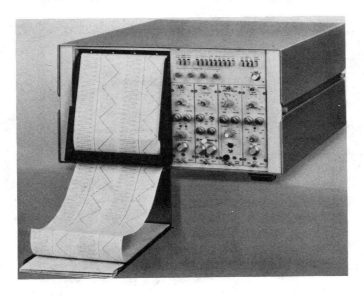

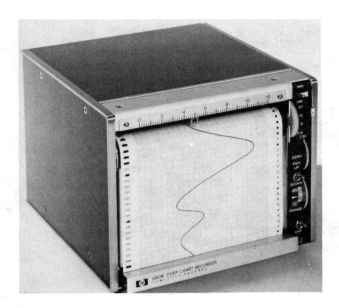

FIGURE 8.5   A typical single-channel strip chart recorder.

readout paper). Some such recorders have more than one channel—that is, they can indicate changes in the configurations of several signals simultaneously on the same strip of paper.

A third class of devices for displaying changes in the configurations of electrical signals are *oscilloscopes* (Figure 8.6). The oscilloscope display is similar to an oscillographic recorder display. The only real difference is that the signal is "painted" with light on a glass televisionlike screen, not inscribed on a strip of paper. A signal displayed on an oscilloscope screen can be photographed if a permanent record of it is desired. Microcomputers can be programmed to function as oscilloscopes—changes in the configurations of electrical signals would be displayed on the monitor screen.

A fourth class of devices used for this purpose are ones that *record changes in the configurations of electrical signals on a magnetic medium.* There are two types of magnetic media that are used for this purpose. The first is magnetic tape. The type of device that is used most often for recording on such tape is referred to as an *instrumentation tape recorder* (Figure 8.7). These can be used to record both biological electrical signals and electrical signals from transducers (e.g., strain gages). They usually have more than one channel (i.e., most can record signals from several sources simultaneously).

A second type of magnetic medium that is used for the purpose is a computer disk, either a "floppy" or "hard" one (Silverman, 1987). A microcomputer (e.g., an IBM compatible, a Macintosh, or an Apple II) would be

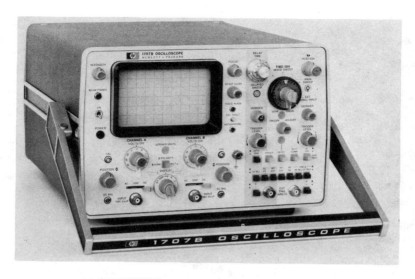

FIGURE 8.6   A typical oscilloscope.

FIGURE 8.7   A typical instrumentation magnetic tape recorder.

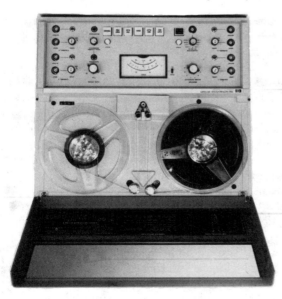

used for recording (and hence storing) the electrical signal data on the disk. Signals recorded in this manner can be displayed graphically (in whole or part) on a monitor screen and/or printed using a dot-matrix or laser printer. They also can be subjected to various statistical analyses, with the results displayed on a monitor screen and/or printed.

The final class of devices that will be mentioned here for displaying changes in the configurations of electrical signals are *X-Y recorders* (Figure 8.8). These recorders automatically plot the value of an independent variable versus a dependent variable directly on sheets of graph paper. Electrical signals from two transmission stages are inputed into the recorder. Plots produced by X-Y recorders can provide information concerning the *nature of* the *relationship* (e.g., linear or nonlinear), *the direction* of the relationship (i.e., positive or negative), and the *strength of the relationship* (i.e., degree of correlation) between the two signals, or variables, being measured. A plot from such a recorder could, for example, provide information on how thresholds for pure tones (X) vary as a function of their frequency (Y). A microcomputer, with appropriate hardware and software, can simulate the type of display produced by an X-Y recorder.

FIGURE 8.8 A typical X-Y recorder.

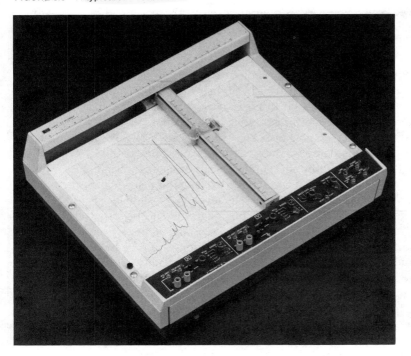

The readout and recording devices mentioned here are not the only such devices that have been used in instrumentation schemes for measuring attributes of events relevant to speech-language pathology and audiology. However they are probably the ones that have been used most often for this purpose.

The readout and recording stage is the final stage of some instrumentation schemes for measuring electrical signals. The signals plotted by an oscilloscope, X–Y recorder, strip chart recorder, or oscillographic recorder are measured by an observer (or observers). Other such schemes possess an additional stage that is concerned with *data reduction and analysis.* The output of the "readout and recording" stage, for example, could be fed into a computer for organization, measurement, and statistical analysis. Computer data reduction and analysis is particularly likely to be incorporated into an instrumentation measurement scheme that produces too many signals to be measured by an observer in a relatively short period of time, or when the statistical analyses to be made of the data are relatively complex. Signals that have been recorded on a magnetic medium (tape or disk) usually are the simplest to analyze in this manner.

Now that the functions of individual components of instrumentation schemes for measuring electrical signals have been described, we can indicate how such a scheme might be used to measure an attribute of communicative behavior. Suppose we wished to measure a stutterer's anxiety level in certain situations outside the clinic. One measure of this that could be used would be the galvanic skin response (GSR). To *detect* changes in skin resistance (associated with changes in anxiety level) electrodes could be attached to the stutterer's skin in an inconspicuous place. The electrical signals from the electrodes could be fed into a miniature *preamplifier, amplifier*, and from there into a miniature *radio transmitter*. The preamplifier, amplifier, and radio transmitter circuitry could be fitted into a very small case and attached to the stutterer's body or clothing so that it would not be visible. The signals from the transmitter could be picked up by a *radio receiver* located at the clinic (providing the clinic was not too far away). They could be fed into an *amplifier* (or series of amplifiers) to increase their magnitude to the point where they would be within the sensitivity range of a strip chart recorder. A *control* device could be used to keep the level of the signals within the sensitivity range of the device. If the baseline magnitude of the signals transmitted became weaker because the stutterer moved farther away from the location of the radio receiver, the degree of amplification would be increased. On the other hand, if the baseline magnitude of these signals became stronger because the stutterer moved closer to the location of the radio receiver, the degree of amplification would be reduced. The signals from the amplifier might be fed through a *filter* before being transmitted by means of an electrical cable to the *strip chart recorder*. The function of the filter would be to remove extraneous signals, or "noise," from the output of the amplifier stage.

This would be likely to "simplify" the strip recorder plot, thereby making it easier to interpret.

This instrumentation scheme, of course, is not the only one that could be used for measuring changes in skin resistance that occur outside a clinic setting. It is merely intended to illustrate how such a scheme might function.

Measuring Readouts from Instrumentation Schemes. This section will describe how quantitative data are abstracted from meter dials, oscilloscope screens, and the displays from such devices as strip chart recorders, oscillographic recorders, and X-Y recorders or of computers that have been programmed to simulate these.

The quantification of electrical signals involves the assignment of numerals to one or more of their attributes (i.e., their amplitudes, frequencies, phase relationships, etc.). The numerals assigned usually have *ratio* properties and for this reason can be manipulated arithmetically. The process by which numerals are assigned may be relatively simple. This is usually the case when the readout device is some sort of meter, e.g., a VU meter. VU meters are used by both speech-language pathologists and audiologists to measure the loudness levels of auditory signals, including speech. Some have a dial with numerals around its perimeter ranging from -20 to $+3$ and a pointer. The position of the pointer indicates the numeral that corresponds to the loudness level of the signal. This numeral is used to designate its loudness level at that moment in time. Since the loudness level of a signal may vary considerably during a relatively short period of time, the pointer may be moving almost continuously. The fact that the loudness level of a signal may not remain constant can create problems when it is necessary to assign a single number to designate it for a particular period of time. One approach that could be used to generate such a value would be to average the numerals indicated by the pointer at specified intervals during this period of time. If this time interval were 60 seconds, for example, the dial might be read every five seconds and the mean of these values computed.

The measurement of electrical signals displayed by strip chart recorders, oscillographic recorders, X-Y recorders, oscilloscopes, or computers ~~DISTANCE MEASURE~~ that have been programmed to simulate one of these devices usually involves ~~MEASURE~~ a *distance measuring*, or *frequency counting*, or *both* a distance measuring and ~~DURATION~~ frequency counting operation. ~~MEASURE~~

A *distance measuring operation* involves determining how far (in inches or millimeters) a particular point in a display deviates from a baseline. The numeral assigned to that point is this value. The *baseline* could be the magnitude, or level, of the phenomenon being measured prior to the administration of an experimental treatment. The baseline for measuring the degree of reaction to a feared stimulus through changes in skin resistance, for example, could be the level of skin resistance immediately prior to the presentation of this stimulus. The deviation from a baseline can be estimated in several ways.

It can be measured with a ruler, or by counting the number of squares in the grid printed on the readout paper between the baseline and the point on the display you wish to measure. The amount of deviation from a baseline following administration of a treatment is apt to vary to some extent. If it is necessary to assign a single number to designate the amount of deviation from a baseline during a specific period of time, the mean of a series of deviation measures made during this period of time could be used. The amount of change in skin resistance during a one-minute period following the presentation of a feared stimulus could be designated by the mean amount of deviation from the baseline measured at five-second intervals. It would be necessary to attach + and − signs to the deviation measures if they occurred in both directions from the baseline (i.e., + if the signal were above the baseline and − if it were below the baseline). For the point on the section of strip chart in Figure 8.9 marked with an arrow, the deviation from the baseline would be approximately 13 millimeters. The direction of the deviation would be "negative" since the signal falls below the baseline. (Note that the readout has a one-millimeter grid printed on it).

The measurement of displays could involve a *frequency counting operation*. This involves determining the number of times a particular attribute, or configuration, of a signal occurs. Frequency of occurrence usually is specified with relation to a particular time interval. Thus, a frequency counting operation may also require a distance measuring operation. The frequency of occurrence of an attribute may be related to a particular time interval that would correspond to a particular distance on the readout paper strip—i.e., the number of inches (or millimeters) of the readout marked by the pen or stylus during the time interval to which the frequency count is related. The frequency of a tone could be determined from an oscillographic recorder readout by counting the number of cycles that were inscribed by the stylus during a one-second time interval. The number of inches of paper that pass under the stylus during a given time interval is estimated from information supplied by the manufacturer of the readout device concerning the speed at which the paper is moving. If six inches of paper passed under the stylus each second, the frequency of a tone would correspond to the number of cycles that were inscribed on a six-inch strip of the paper.

The measurement procedures for oscilloscope screen tracing are essentially the same as those for oscillographic recorder readouts. The attributes of signals that can be measured from oscilloscope screen tracings include frequency and amplitude. Frequency can be estimated by counting the number of cycles displayed on the screen with the oscilloscope set to display a particular time interval. If the interval were 50 milliseconds (i.e., $^{50}/_{1000}$ second) and 10 cycles were displayed on the screen, the frequency of the signal (e.g., tone) would be 200 cycles per second. Amplitude can be estimated by a grid inscribed on the oscilloscope screen. It can be measured in millimeter deviation from a baseline, as with an oscillographic recorder, or in volts (a measure

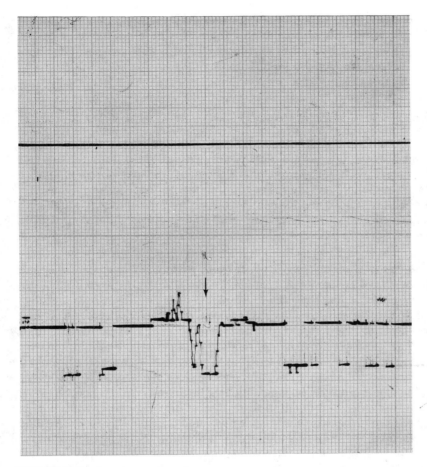

FIGURE 8.9   Section of a "readout" from a two-channel strip chart recorder.

of the electrical magnitude of a signal). Measurements can be made directly from the screen display or from printouts or photographs of the screen display.

Measurements of attributes of speech and other auditory signals from magnetic tape recordings are made in a variety of ways. In some cases, such signals are fed into an instrumentation measurement scheme before being measured. They are passed through an amplifier stage and a modification and shaping stage and then are transmitted to a readout and recording device such as a strip chart recorder, X-Y recorder, oscillographic recorder, oscilloscope, meter, or computer programmed to function as such a device. The instrumentation scheme helps to abstract the target attribute from the taped signal and thus facilitates the measurement process. A taped speech signal might be fed into a sound spectrograph (e.g., Sonograph) to analyze and display its spectral characteristics—i.e., the amount of energy present at specific frequencies during given moments in time. Several characteristics of the speech spectra could be measured from the resulting spectrogram, or Sonogram (e.g., vowel formant frequencies).

It sometimes is possible to program a computer to make the various types of distance and frequency measurements described in the preceding paragraphs (Silverman, 1987). Whether using a computer for this purpose would save time is a function of how long it would take to set up the computer to make them. If, for example, only a few measurements had to be made and it would take several days to set up a computer to make them, it probably would be faster to make them "by hand" instead of by computer.

Measurements of attributes of communicative behavior from magnetic tape recordings also are made by means of rating procedures. A number of such procedures, classified as *psychological scaling methods*, are described in the final section of this chapter.

Sources of Error in Measurements from "Readout" Devices. There are several sources of random and systematic error that can influence the accuracy of quantitative data derived from meter dials and from strip chart recorders, X-Y recorders, oscillographic recorders, oscilloscopes, and similar types of displays. These can be grouped under three main headings: (1) gross errors, (2) systematic errors, and (3) random errors (Stout, 1962, pp. 21–26).

Gross errors consist of mistakes in reading meters and other readout displays and in recording numbers resulting from measurement processes. Misreading a meter would be an example of such an error. The pointer on a VU meter indicates −2 but is read as indicating −3. Perhaps the person misread the meter because the signals measured previously were −3 and he or she expected further −3 readings. It is well known that your expectations can influence your perceptions (Johnson, 1946). Gross errors also include mistakes in recording (e.g., writing down or typing) the numbers that result from a measurement process. One of the most common errors of this type is transposition. The person making and recording the measurements from a meter may read 35.2 but write down 32.5. Gross errors can be reduced by making each measurement several times, preferably with one measurement not immediately following the next. These errors usually do not bias the measurement process in any meaningful way because they occur infrequently and tend to be random.

Systematic errors can be grouped under three main headings: (1) instrumental errors, (2) environmental errors, and (3) observational errors. Instrumental errors include those that result from shortcomings of the instrument, or misuse, or loading effects of the equipment. The performances of all components of instrumentation measurement schemes probably deviate to some degree from their nominal values (i.e., those specified by their manufacturers) even when they are new. If the instruments included in such schemes are not recalibrated periodically, this deviation is likely to increase because of use and age. If the deviation is fairly small, it may not bias the measurement process in any meaningful way.

The problem of instrumental errors resulting from *shortcomings of equipment* can be illustrated by means of the pure-tone audiometer. All such audiometers, even when they are new, would not measure exactly the same thresholds at given frequencies, because of factory calibration error. Differences in threshold measurements arising from factory calibration error are likely to be too small to be significant clinically. However, if pure-tone audiometers are not recalibrated periodically, error due to use and age may increase to the point where threshold measurements will not be sufficiently accurate for at least some clinical purposes.

Instrument calibration errors can be handled in two ways. The best, but usually the most expensive, is to have the instrument recalibrated. The second is to determine the extent of the calibration error and apply a *correction factor.* If you knew, for example, that the amount of hearing loss indicated by a pure-tone audiometer at 1000Hz was 5 dB too great, you could subtract 5 dB from the degree of hearing loss indicated by this audiometer at this frequency.

Instrumental error also can result from *misuse* of components of instrumentation measurement schemes. Failure to use or maintain an instrument according to the manufacturer's instructions can cause instrumental error. Failure to use the recommended type of earphones on an audiometer, for example, could result in an impedance mismatch that would probably cause the loudness levels of the pure tones generated by that audiometer to deviate from their nominal values. Such errors can be reduced or eliminated by following manufacturers' recommendations regarding the use of instruments.

The *loading effects* of components of instrumentation measurement schemes is another source of instrumental error. What sometimes happens is that the measurement process influences what is being measured. The circuitry of a measuring instrument (e.g., a voltmeter) can interact with that of the instrument producing the signal being measured (e.g., a pure-tone audiometer), altering this signal and hence producing inaccurate measurements. To avoid this source of error, it is essential to "isolate" the circuitry of measurement instruments from the circuitry of the instruments producing the signals being measured.

The second subclass of systematic errors is *environmental errors.* These result from factors external to a measuring device (i.e., in the environment in which it is being used) which can influence the functioning of one or more of the components within it and thus influence the accuracy of measurements made with it. Environmental factors that can influence the functioning of the components of such schemes include temperature, humidity, barometric pressure, and stray electrical and magnetic fields. The accuracy of the calibration of many electronic instruments is dependent on their being used

INSTRUMENTAL ERRORS

ENVIRONMENTAL ERRORS

in an environment in which the temperature is maintained within a specified range. If such an instrument is used in a room in which the temperature is either above or below this range, measurements may be biased. It may be possible to use this instrument in such an environment if the effect of the temperature in the room where the measurements are being made on the resulting measurements is known. A correction factor can be applied to measurements made in this environment. If they are too high, a constant can be subtracted from them; and if they are too low, a constant can be added to them. The most direct way to control for the effects of environmental factors is to use instrumentation measurement schemes in environments that conform to manufacturers' recommendations.

The third subclass of systematic errors are *observational errors*. Different persons measuring the same phenomenon with the same instrumentation under identical environmental conditions will not necessarily produce duplicate results. An observer may consistently record values from a VU meter that are higher or lower than they should be because of the angle at which he or she views the meter. For these values to be accurate, the meter must be read from directly in front. If it is viewed at an angle, the indicator may appear to be pointing to a different number on the scale than that which it would appear to be pointing to if it were viewed from in front. This source of error can be reduced or eliminated by having measurements made by more than one observer and by using the average of the measurements made of a particular phenomenon as the measure of that phenomenon.

The third, and final, classification of measurement error based on Stout's scheme is *random error*. The sources of this type of error were described at the beginning of this chapter and in Chapter 6.

Schemes That Utilize Instruments That Are Not Electronic or Intended for Physical Measurement

Measurement schemes which utilize instruments that are not electronic or intended for physical measurement are described in this section. These instruments include tests, structured tasks, semantic differentials, Likert-type scales, questionnaires, and structured interviews.

Schemes Utilizing Tests and Structured Tasks. Speech-language pathologists and audiologists have used many types of tests and structured tasks to facilitate the observation and description of attributes of communicative behavior. The performance of such a task permits the target attribute either to stand out sufficiently from other behavioral attributes or to occur at an appropriate time for it to be observed and described. If, for example, the target attribute were "accuracy of articulation of certain consonant phonemes in initial, medial, and final positions in words," having a child respond to the stimulus items on a picture articulation test would make it possible for the production of these phonemes in the desired contexts to be observed at an "appropriate" time and their accuracy assessed.

The numerals (i.e., scores) assigned to target behavioral attributes by tests may be on any level of measurement. However, while such scores could have nominal, ordinal, interval, ratio, or logarithmic properties, they rarely exceed those for ordinal measurement. The intervals between them (with regard to the attribute being measured) are usually not equal *throughout the range of possible scores*, and they are usually not related to an absolute zero. Interpretations of the magnitudes of the differences between test scores, therefore, have to be made with considerable caution. Because one child's performance on an articulation test improved by four points while a second child's performance on the same test improved by two points does not necessarily mean that the first child's articulation improved twice as much as the second child's. In fact, it may not even be true that the first child's articulation improved more than the second child's. The first child's four-point increase may have resulted from learning to produce /s/ blends in the initial positions in words, while the second child's two-point increase may have resulted from learning to produce /s/ and /r/ correctly in the initial positions of words. Regardless of the score differences, many speech-language pathologists would look upon the second child as having improved more than the first. If this were the case, it probably would be most appropriate to interpret scores on the test as having nominal rather than ordinal properties.

The data generated by schemes utilizing tests and structured tasks will consist of scores and/or verbal descriptions. The former, like all numerals assigned to attributes of events, are subject both to random and to systematic measurement error. The sources of random and systematic error which influence test scores are the same as those indicated for instrumentation measurement schemes, i.e., gross errors, systematic errors, and random errors.

Gross errors include mistakes in reading test and subtest scores and in recording such scores. Recording subtest scores incorrectly on a test profile summary sheet or a data sheet would be an example of such an error. Scores could be recorded incorrectly either because they are misread or because they are written down incorrectly (e.g., numbers are transposed).

Systematic errors, as previously indicated, are of three types: instrumental errors, environmental errors, and observational errors. *Instrumental errors* include those that result from shortcomings of the test instrument. Age norms developed for interpreting test scores, for example, may not be accurate. If the normative group used to standardize a language development scale was not representative of the population of which it was supposed to have been representative, scores from this scale may be consistently interpreted as indicating higher (or lower) language ages than would be the case. Hence language age estimates based on this scale would be biased.

Instrumental errors also include those resulting from *misuse* of test instruments. If an educational or psychological test is not administered according to the instructions in the test manual, the scores obtained may be systematically higher (or lower) than they should be.

Environmental errors include those due to factors external to the device which influence the accuracy of measurements made with it. If a test were administered in an environment that caused the testee to become "anxious," this could cause his or her score to be lower than it would have been in a relatively "relaxed" environment.

Observational errors include those which result from differences in internal standards among test administrators. All testers would not necessarily evaluate a given test performance in the same manner. A response that one tester would consider to be "within normal limits" another may regard as "not within normal limits." One tester may classify a slightly lateralized /s/ production on an articulation test as "within normal limits," and another may classify it as "not within normal limits." Thus, one tester may consistently identify higher percentages of children as having a lateral lisp than would another.

The third, and final, source of error that can influence test scores is *random error*. While this type of error, as previously indicated, will not bias measurements (i.e., cause them to be consistently higher or lower than they should be), it will reduce their reliability. One source of random error in a test situation may be inconsistency of response by the testee to the test stimuli. It *sometimes* is possible to reduce this source of error by administering test items more than once.

These types of errors, of course, can also influence the accuracy of data generated by tests and structured tasks which consist of verbal descriptions.

The Semantic Differential Technique. The semantic differential technique (Osgood, Suci, and Tannenbaum, 1957; Snider and Osgood, 1968) was developed by Professor Charles Osgood and his associates at the University of Illinois in the 1940s. With this approach, subjects are provided with a set of seven-step, bipolar adjectival scales and instructed to indicate for each scale the direction and intensity of its association to the stimulus being rated. If, for example, we wished to determine a client's attitude toward a hearing aid, one scale that might be included in the semantic differential for this purpose would be:

acceptable ___ : ___ : ___ : ___ : ___ : ___ : ___ unacceptable

If a client's attitude toward the hearing aid was *very closely related* to one or the other of these adjectives, he or she would mark the scale in the following manner:

acceptable _x_ : ___ : ___ : ___ : ___ : ___ : ___ unacceptable

or

acceptable ___ : ___ : ___ : ___ : ___ : ___ : _x_ unacceptable

If a client's attitude toward the hearing aid was *quite closely* (but not extremely) *related* to one or the other of these adjectives, he or she would mark the scale in the following manner:

acceptable ___ : _x_ : ___ : ___ : ___ : ___ : ___ unacceptable

or

acceptable ___ : ___ : ___ : ___ : ___ : _x_ : ___ unacceptable

If a client's attitude was *only slightly related* to one or the other of these adjectives, he or she would mark the scale in the following manner:

acceptable ___ : ___ : _x_ : ___ : ___ : ___ : ___ unacceptable

or

acceptable ___ : ___ : ___ : ___ : _x_ : ___ : ___ unacceptable

Finally, a client who felt that his or her attitude toward the hearing aid was either *neutral* on the scale or that both adjectives were *completely irrelevant* would mark in the following manner:

acceptable ___ : ___ : ___ : _x_ : ___ : ___ : ___ unacceptable

A semantic differential that can be used, with minor modification, for assessing attitudes toward persons who have almost any type of communicative disorder is reproduced in Figure 8.10.

Both the construction and administration of semantic differentials have been described in considerable detail (Osgood, Suci, and Tannenbaum, 1957; Snider and Osgood, 1968). This section will therefore be devoted primarily to a discussion of specific considerations in constructing and analyzing semantic differentials to measure attitudes toward therapies.

Constructing a Semantic Differential. One of the first considerations in constructing a semantic differential is generating the set of bipolar adjectival scales. The specific scales selected will be determined by the stimulus to which reactions are desired. The stimulus, incidentally, does not have to be a word or words—any observable object or event (e.g., a tape recording) could serve as the stimulus.

Three approaches, singly or in combination, are useful for generating a set of scales for a semantic differential. The first is to consult the thesaurus sample of bipolar adjectival scales that Osgood and his associates included in *The Measurement of Meaning* (pp. 53–61). The second is to conduct a brainstorming session in which the members of a group are asked to suggest scales relevant to their reactions to the stimulus. The third is to solicit responses from a number of persons to a statement such as this: "Please list all the adjectives you can think of that describe (the stimulus)." Bipolar scales are constructed from adjectives used by two or more persons.

FIGURE 8.10 A representative semantic differential task.

THE PERSON WHO IS SPEAKING

afraid	___:___:___:___:___:___:___	not afraid
mature	___:___:___:___:___:___:___	immature
unlovable	___:___:___:___:___:___:___	lovable
speech intelligible	___:___:___:___:___:___:___	speech unintelligible
intelligent	___:___:___:___:___:___:___	unintelligent
secure	___:___:___:___:___:___:___	insecure
natural	___:___:___:___:___:___:___	unnatural
no sense of humor	___:___:___:___:___:___:___	sense of humor
speaks rapidly	___:___:___:___:___:___:___	speaks slowly
unselfish	___:___:___:___:___:___:___	selfish
dishonest	___:___:___:___:___:___:___	honest
fluent	___:___:___:___:___:___:___	disfluent
cautious	___:___:___:___:___:___:___	rash
witty	___:___:___:___:___:___:___	dull
speech monotonous	___:___:___:___:___:___:___	speech not monotonous
stable	___:___:___:___:___:___:___	unstable
employable	___:___:___:___:___:___:___	unemployable
unsociable	___:___:___:___:___:___:___	sociable
loud	___:___:___:___:___:___:___	soft
old	___:___:___:___:___:___:___	young
coordinated	___:___:___:___:___:___:___	uncoordinated
dominant	___:___:___:___:___:___:___	submissive
speech dysrhythmic	___:___:___:___:___:___:___	speech rhythmic
speech unpleasant	___:___:___:___:___:___:___	speech pleasant
hesitant	___:___:___:___:___:___:___	not hesitant
boring	___:___:___:___:___:___:___	interesting
unfriendly	___:___:___:___:___:___:___	friendly
cowardly	___:___:___:___:___:___:___	brave
confused	___:___:___:___:___:___:___	orientated
superior	___:___:___:___:___:___:___	inferior
speech slow	___:___:___:___:___:___:___	speech fast
reputable	___:___:___:___:___:___:___	disreputable
optimistic	___:___:___:___:___:___:___	pessimistic
excitable	___:___:___:___:___:___:___	calm
handicapped	___:___:___:___:___:___:___	not handicapped
untrustworthy	___:___:___:___:___:___:___	trustworthy
relaxed	___:___:___:___:___:___:___	tense
contrary	___:___:___:___:___:___:___	agreeable
reliable	___:___:___:___:___:___:___	unreliable
extrovert	___:___:___:___:___:___:___	introvert
rich	___:___:___:___:___:___:___	poor
insane	___:___:___:___:___:___:___	sane
contented	___:___:___:___:___:___:___	discontented
soothing	___:___:___:___:___:___:___	aggravating
not frightened	___:___:___:___:___:___:___	frightened
not frustrating	___:___:___:___:___:___:___	frustrating
alert	___:___:___:___:___:___:___	not alert

FIGURE 8.10 Continued

THE PERSON WHO IS SPEAKING

speaks poorly	___:___:___:___:___:___:___	speaks well
discourteous	___:___:___:___:___:___:___	courteous
quarrelsome	___:___:___:___:___:___:___	congenial
lazy	___:___:___:___:___:___:___	industrious
deaf	___:___:___:___:___:___:___	not deaf
emotional	___:___:___:___:___:___:___	unemotional
realistic	___:___:___:___:___:___:___	idealistic
approachable	___:___:___:___:___:___:___	unapproachable
not talkative	___:___:___:___:___:___:___	talkative
not aggressive	___:___:___:___:___:___:___	aggressive
weak	___:___:___:___:___:___:___	strong
positive self concept	___:___:___:___:___:___:___	negative self concept
uneducated	___:___:___:___:___:___:___	educated
deliberate	___:___:___:___:___:___:___	impulsive
nervous	___:___:___:___:___:___:___	calm
sensitive	___:___:___:___:___:___:___	insensitive
able to carry on conversation	___:___:___:___:___:___:___	unable to carry on conversation
scrupulous	___:___:___:___:___:___:___	unscrupulous
independent	___:___:___:___:___:___:___	dependent
masculine	___:___:___:___:___:___:___	feminine
confident	___:___:___:___:___:___:___	not confident
frustrated	___:___:___:___:___:___:___	not frustrated
competent	___:___:___:___:___:___:___	incompetent
inhibited	___:___:___:___:___:___:___	uninhibited
depressed	___:___:___:___:___:___:___	happy
organized	___:___:___:___:___:___:___	unorganized
accept	___:___:___:___:___:___:___	reject
isolated	___:___:___:___:___:___:___	not isolated
comfortable	___:___:___:___:___:___:___	uncomfortable
insincere	___:___:___:___:___:___:___	sincere
enthusiastic	___:___:___:___:___:___:___	unenthusiastic
soothing	___:___:___:___:___:___:___	aggravating
kind	___:___:___:___:___:___:___	cruel
naive	___:___:___:___:___:___:___	sophisticated

After they have been selected, the scales are ordered by means of a table of random numbers. Whether the positive or negative adjective in each pair appears on the left is also randomly determined. Ordering the scales for the response sheet (see Figure 8.10) can be facilitated by writing or typing each pair of adjectives on a separate card.

Administering a Semantic Differential. To administer a semantic differential, present a response sheet to each subject along with a set of instructions. The author has found the set included in *The Measurement of Meaning* (pp. 82–84) quite satisfactory. To maximize the probability that a subject will understand what is required, it is advisable to read the instructions aloud while the subject follows along on his or her copy.

Analyzing Semantic Differential Ratings.   To facilitate analysis of semantic differential ratings, the seven points between pairs of adjectives are each assigned a numeral. The set usually assigned is either

$$1, 2, 3, 4, 5, 6, 7$$
$$\text{or}$$
$$-3, -2, -1, 0, +1, +2, +3$$

If the first set is used, the numeral 4 would be assigned to the center of the scale, 1 to the lower end, and 7 to the upper end. The lower end of the scale could be associated with the negative adjective and the upper end with the positive.

The numerals in the second set are more descriptive of the bipolar nature of the adjectives than those in the first. However, they are more difficult to manipulate arithmetically because some have negative values. Since both sets lead to the same result, and since the numerals in the 1 to 7 set are easier to manipulate arithmetically than those in the -3 to $+3$ set, the 1 to 7 set is usually used.

Data concerning attitudes toward an event (e.g., a therapy program) can be abstracted from semantic differential ratings. Obviously, the ratings assigned to individual scales by persons doing the task can provide information about their reactions to, or attitude toward, the stimulus. Comparable information for the "typical" member of a group can be derived by computing the mean or median of the ratings assigned to each scale. The closer an individual or average rating is to the center of a scale, the less likely the adjectives defining that scale are to be relevant to reactions to the stimulus.

Data generated by the semantic differential technique, of course, are subject to the same sources of error as mentioned in the preceding section for tests and structured tasks.

The Likert Methodology.   Likert-type scales can be used to generate data for attitude assessment. They consist of a series of statements about a subject, each of which reflects either a favorable or an unfavorable attitude toward it. The number of statements reflecting each usually is approximately equal. Printed below each statement is a response line, similar to the following:

Strongly Agree   Agree   Undecided   Disagree   Strongly Disagree

Respondents are told to circle, or place a checkmark over, the response that best describes their reaction to the statement. Responses can be analyzed in several ways. The simplest is to indicate percentages for each individual statement. Because three responses—agree, undecided, and disagree—usually are easier to interpret than five, the two "agree" categories and the two "disagree" categories may be combined. If this is done, statements can be made similar to the following: 70 percent of hearing-impaired clients six months after being fitted with a particular type of hearing aid agreed with the statement, "The benefits I gained from using the aid have exceeded my expectations."

It sometimes is desirable to describe the overall reaction of respondents to the subject to which the statements refer. This can be done by assigning the scale value indicated below to each of their responses to each statement reflecting a favorable attitude:

Strongly agree	5
Agree	4
Undecided	3
Disagree	2
Strongly Disagree	1

For each statement reflecting an unfavorable attitude, the scale would be reversed (e.g., the scale value assigned for "strongly agree" would be 1). The average (mean or median) of the ratings assigned by a respondent to the various statements would indicate the degree to which his or her attitude toward the subject was favorable.

Likert-type scales have been used a great deal by speech-language pathologists and audiologists. They have been used, for example, to assess individual clients' attitudes toward their communicative disorder—e.g., the *Iowa Scale of Attitude toward Stuttering* (Johnson, Darley, and Spriestersbach, 1963).

Likert-type scales are subject to the same sources of error as the other data-generating schemes discussed in this chapter. For further information about such scales, see Best and Kahn (1989, pp. 195–198) and Henerson, Morris, and Fitz-Gibbon (1987, Chapter 6).

Schemes That Utilize Questionnaires or Structured Interviews. Questionnaires and structured interviews are among the most frequently used tools for generating data in speech and hearing research. They are used for this purpose in almost every study (e.g., for finding out the ages of subjects). Both require subjects to answer questions and/or respond to statements. Structured interviews can be looked upon as oral questionnaires—i.e., instead of writing responses, subjects give information orally and face-to-face.

Structured interviews, of course, are always administered personally and usually individually. Answers to questions and responses to statements are either written down by the interviewer (sometimes on a printed form) or are tape recorded and transcribed later. Interviews for generating research data are conducted in a manner similar to those used by clinicians for gathering case-history data. Hence, a case-history interview would be an example of a structured interview!

Questionnaires can either be administered personally or by mail. While the former is usually preferable, individuals who have the desired information cannot always be contacted personally without the expenditure of a great deal of time and money in travel. One problem that can be encountered when using mailed questionnaires is that the rate of return may be too low. This is particularly likely to occur if the questionnaire is relatively long (would take more than five minutes to complete) and/or those who are asked to complete it see no advantage to themselves in doing so. A questionnaire administered in this manner, therefore, should be kept as short as possible, and a strong case should be built in the letter accompanying the questionnaire for why it would be advantageous to recipients to complete and return it.

There are two types of response forms that can be used in questionnaires and structured interviews: closed-form and open-form. With the closed-form, or restricted, type you usually are asked to check items from a list of suggested responses. The following example illustrates the closed-form item:

> Why did you choose to do graduate work at this university? Kindly indicate three reasons in order of importance, using the number 1 for the most important, 2 for the second most important, and 3 for the third most important.
>
> RANK
>
> (a) ASHA accreditation _____
> (b) Advice of someone _____
> (c) Reputation of institution _____
> (d) Expense factor _____
> (e) Financial aid _____
> (f) Location _____
> (g) Other _____ _____
>   (kindly indicate)

When using the closed-form type, it is a good idea to provide for unanticipated responses by including an "other" category.

The open-form, or unrestricted, type calls for a free response in your own words. The following item seeks the same type of information as in the previous example:

> Why did you choose to do graduate work at this university?

While this type provides the possibility for greater depth of response than the closed-form one, the data it generates tend to be more difficult to interpret and summarize than those from the other. Both types, of course, can be used in the same questionnaire or structured interview.

Questionnaires and structured interviews are subject to the same sources of error as the other data-generating schemes discussed in this chapter.

Both questionnaires and structured interviews are used a great deal in educational and social science research. A number of books and articles have been written by investigators in these fields that can be helpful when designing a study in which they will be used. Three that I have found particularly helpful were written by Best and Kahn (1989), Chadwick, Bahr, and Albrecht (1984), and Henerson, Morris, and Fitz-Gibbon (1987).

SCHEMES THAT RELY PRIMARILY ON OBSERVER JUDGMENT: PSYCHOLOGICAL SCALING METHODS

The use of psychological scaling methods for quantifying observable aspects of communicative behavior is considered in this section. Further information needed both to interpret the results of experiments in which scaling methods are used and to design such experiments is provided in Appendix C.

Need for Psychological Scaling Techniques in Speech, Language, and Hearing Research

We will attempt to indicate the need for psychological scaling techniques in speech, language, and hearing research through answers to the following questions:

1. What are the *purposes* of scaling techniques?
2. What can scaling techniques *do* for a researcher interested in speech, language, and hearing?
3. In what ways have scaling techniques been used in speech, language, and hearing research?

Psychological scaling techniques provide a methodology for quantifying a variety of attributes of events of interest to speech-language pathologists and audiologists with levels of validity and reliability that are sufficiently high for most purposes. An *event* is a phenomenon that occurs in a certain place during a particular interval of time. All events have attributes, or measurable properties. Speech can be classified as an event, since it is a "phenomenon that occurs in a certain place during a particular interval of time." Since all events have attributes, or measurable properties, what are the attributes of the event "speech" and how are they defined? Literally hundreds of attributes of speech have been delineated. (To prove this to yourself, examine the indexes of representative speech-language pathology and speech science texts.) Many have been defined on the basis of observer judgment. In fact, they *are* observer judgments. The observer is the "instrument" by which such attributes are abstracted from the speech signal. After an attribute of this type has been identified, investigators may attempt to identify the physical attributes of the speech signal that results in observers detecting it. They may even attempt to synthesize the configuration of physical attributes they identify (through the use of a computer) and have observers listen to the synthesized signal to determine whether they detect the target attribute. An example of an attribute that has been studied in this manner is hypernasality. This attribute was initially detected in the speech signal by observers and hence was an observer judgment. Later, investigators attempted to identify the physical aspects of the speech signal that cause observers to hear hypernasality and to generate a synthesized signal based on the aspects identified. The taped synthesized signal was then played for groups of observers to determine whether it sounded hypernasal to them. Since hypernasality is an observer judgment, it follows that the most valid indicator of its presence would be observer judgment.

If you are willing to accept the assumption that at least some attributes of speech events are observer judgments—i.e., are the result of the interaction between the observer and the speech event—then for an instrumentation scheme for measuring, or quantifying, such attributes to have *at least face validity* (or appear intuitively to be valid), it would have to involve observer judgment. It would have to require one or more observers to indicate in some manner the amount of the target attribute present in each speech stimulus. Thus, the observer (or panel of observers) would function as a "measuring instrument" with his or her (their) judgments being the "readout." This readout can be of any type that reflects the relative amount of the target attribute present in the stimuli, including words, numbers, and marks on a line.

Psychological scaling techniques are methodologies that can be used for "measuring" the relative amounts of target attributes present in speech events through the use of observer judgments. With these methodologies, an observer (or panel of observers) is instructed to indicate in some manner the relative amount of a target attribute present in each of a group of stimuli (e.g., speech segments). Since they provide instrumentation measurement schemes in which the readout is an observer judgment, these methodologies have *at least face validity* for measuring attributes of speech events which are observer judgments.

Thus in response to the first two questions presented at the beginning of this section, the purpose of psychological scaling techniques is to provide methodologies for measuring, or quantifying, attributes of events which are observer judgments. Such techniques can do a great deal for investigators in speech, language, and hearing since many attributes of events of interest to speech-language pathologists and audiologists are observer judgments.

How have psychological scaling techniques been used in speech, language, and hearing research? What attributes have they been used to measure, or quantify? Due in large part to the pioneering methodological research of Professor Dorothy Sherman of the University of Iowa, psychological scaling methods have been used for quantifying numerous attributes of speech events. A partial list of such attributes is presented in Table 8.1. This list was compiled from a search of the first 13 volumes of the *Journal of Speech and Hearing Research* for papers in which psychological scaling methods had been used. It includes most of the attributes that were scaled in the studies reported in these papers. The studies cited in Table 8.1, in addition to indicating applications that have been made of psychological scaling methods in speech, language, and hearing research, provide information that could be useful to investigators who wish to rate a set of stimuli for one or more of the attributes listed. Aspects of the scaling methodologies used by the investigators in the studies cited may be utilized by other investigators who wish to quantify these same attributes.

Psychological Scaling Methods as Measuring Instruments

Psychological scaling methods are measuring instruments in the same sense that rulers and thermometers are, because they result in numerals being assigned to attributes of events which have certain characteristics (see Chapter 7). They have these characteristics because of the rules that are used to assign them. As indicated in Chapter 7, the rules used to assign numerals to attributes of events determine the meaning of the numerals—i.e., the "level of measurement" of the scale which they define. A *scale* consists of a succession or progression of steps or degrees, or a graduated series of categories. The "rules" used for assigning numerals with psychological scaling methods *theoretically* result in one of three types of scales: ordinal, interval, or ratio (the characteristics of each are described in Chapter 7). We emphasize "theoretically" to highlight the fact that psychological scaling methods do not always result in numerals, or ratings, that possess the characteristics they are supposed to possess (i.e., achieve the level of measurement they are supposed to achieve). There are several reasons why this may be the case. One of the most common is the inability of observers to assign numerals, or rate the stimuli, in the manner in which they are instructed.

To illustrate how psychological scaling methods are used to assign numerals to attributes of events, we will discuss the following six, which are representative, from this frame of reference: paired, or pair, comparisons (Edwards, 1957); rank order, or order of merit (Guilford, 1954); equal-appearing intervals, or category scaling (Edwards, 1957); successive intervals, or successive categories, or graded dichotomies (Edwards, 1957); constant sums (Guilford, 1954); and direct magnitude-estimation (Prather, 1960). These methods,

TABLE 8.1   Representative attributes of events of interest to speech-language pathologists and audiologists that have been quantified by means of psychological scaling methods.

Attribute	References
Abstraction of words, level of	II, 161
Articulation defectiveness, severity of	III, 191; III, 303
Articulation proficiency, degree of	VI, 49
Bizarreness, degree of	XII, 246
Breathiness, severity of	XII, 246; XII, 747
Difficulty of listening to compressed speech, degree of	XI, 875
Effeminant voice quality, degree of	IX, 590
Esophageal speech, acceptability of	X, 417
Favorability of description, degree of	X, 339
Force or strain while speaking, degree of	IV, 281
Foreign dialect, degree of	VIII, 43
General merit of speech sample, degree of	IX, 248; IX, 323
Harshness, severity of	I, 155; I, 344; XII, 246
Hoarseness, severity of	XII, 246
Intelligibility, degree of	XII, 246; XXIV, 441
Language development, level of	X, 41; X, 828
Language usage, intricacy of	XI, 837
Lipreading ability, level of	II, 340
Loudness, level of	XII, 103; XII, 246
Moment of nonfluency, severity of	I, 132
Nasal emission, severity of	XII, 246
Nasality, degree of	I, 383; II, 40; II, 113; IV, 381; V, 103; X, 549; XI, 553; XII, 246
Preference, degree of	I, 86; V, 370
Pitch, level of	XII, 246; XII, 747
Pitch variability, degree of	XII, 747
Quality of EDR audiometric records, level of	IV, 41
Representativeness to intended vowel, degree of	IV, 203
Rhythm pattern, normality of	IV, 281
Roughness, degree of	XII, 330
Sibilant intensity, level of	XII, 747
Similarity, degree of	VI, 239; VII, 310; VIII, 23; X, 225
Social adequacy, degree of	V, 79
Speaking rate, normality of	IV, 281; XII, 246; XII, 747
Stress, normality of	XII, 246
Stuttering severity, degree of	I, 40; I, 61; V, 256; V, 332; VI, 91; VIII, 263; VIII, 401; XIII, 360
Vowel imitation, abruptness of	I, 344

(Roman numerals refer to volumes of the *Journal of Speech and Hearing Research;* Arabic numbers, to the first pages of papers in which the attributes were scaled.)

incidentally, are the ones that have been used most frequently in speech, language, and hearing research.

Paired (Pair) Comparisons.   With this method, which theoretically results in an ordinal scale, all possible pairs of stimuli are compared to an *internally generated standard* (or scale) for the attribute being rated, or scaled, and the stimuli in each pair are ordered on the basis of the amount of the attribute which each is judged to possess. The task is performed by a group, or panel, of observers. Each observer is presented with all possible ordered pairings (i.e., permutations) of the stimuli to be scaled. The number of such pairings that will result from a set of stimuli of a given size (N) can be determined by multiplying the number of stimuli by the number of stimuli minus one, or

$$N (N - 1)$$

For a set of 10 stimuli, the number of pairs rated would be

$$N (N - 1) = 10 (10 - 1) = 90$$

and for a set of 100 stimuli it would be

$$N (N - 1) = 100 (100 - 1) = 9900$$

Note how the number of pairs increases dramatically as the number of stimuli increases.

Observers are told to indicate the stimulus in each pair which possesses the greater amount of the attribute being scaled, or rated. They perform this task by comparing the amount of the target attribute they observe in each of the two stimuli in a pair to their internal standard, or scale, for that attribute. For example, an observer who was presented with speech segments from two persons who have hypernasal speech and was asked to indicate which was the most hypernasal would perform this task by comparing the level of hypernasality he or she perceived in the two segments to his or her internal standard, or scale, for degree of hypernasality and, on the basis of these comparisons, would indicate which is the most hypernasal.

Rank Order (Order of Merit).   With this method, which theoretically results in an ordinal scale, sets of stimuli are compared to an internally generated standard, or scale, for the attribute being rated, and the stimuli in the set are ordered on the basis of the amount of the target attribute they are judged to possess. The task is performed by a group, or panel, of observers. Each observer is presented with the set of stimuli and is told to rank order them on the basis of the amounts of the target attribute which they possess. He or she is instructed to indicate the ordering of the stimuli by assigning the numeral to each stimulus which designates its position. The highest numeral assigned (N) is equal to the number of stimuli being ordered.

Observers may be instructed to assign either 1 or N to the stimulus possessing the greatest amount of the target attribute. They rank order the stimuli by comparing the amount of the target attribute they perceive in each to their internal standard, or scale, for that attribute. For example, an observer who was presented with speech segments from five persons who have hypernasal speech and was told to order them on the basis of the amount of hypernasality they possess (with 1 designating least hypernasality and 5 designating most) would perform this task by comparing the level of hypernasality he or she perceived in the five segments to his or her internal standard, or scale, for degree of hypernasality and on the basis of these comparisons indicate the ordering of the stimuli.

This method can be viewed as an extension of the method of paired comparisons. The only real difference in the judging task is that observers are required to order N rather than two stimuli.

Equal-Appearing Intervals (Category Scaling). With this method, which theoretically results in an interval scale, each of a set of stimuli is compared to an internally generated scale, or continuum, for the attribute being rated, which is divided into a specified number of equal-size segments (usually 5, 7, or 9), and the numeral is assigned to it that designates the segment of the internally generated continuum which corresponds to the amount of the attribute it is judged to possess. The task is performed by a group, or panel, of observers. Stimuli are presented to observers one at a time. Observers are instructed to assign the numeral between 1 and the number that corresponds to the number of points on the scale (e.g., 7) to each stimulus that indicates the amount of the target attribute it possesses. They are informed that the scale is one of equal intervals—from 1 to 7 (or some other value)—with 1 representing the least possible amount of the target and 7 (or some other value) representing the greatest possible amount; 4 (or some other medial value) represents the midpoint between 1 and 7 with respect to the attribute, with the other numbers falling at *equal distances* along the scale. For example, an observer who was presented with speech segments from five persons who have hypernasal speech and was told to assign a numeral to each on the basis of the amount of hypernasality present (with 1 designating least possible hypernasality, 7 designating most possible hypernasality, and the numbers between falling at equal distances along the scale) would perform this task by comparing the amount of hypernasality he or she perceived in each speech segment to each of the seven segments of his or her internal scale for degree of hypernasality and on the basis of these comparisons assign each a numeral between 1 and 7. Observers may assign the same numeral to two or more speech segments. They would rate in such a manner if they felt the degree of hypernasality present in the segments fell within the same segment of their internal scales for hypernasality.

Successive Intervals (Successive Categories; Graded Dichotomies).
With this method, which theoretically results in an interval scale, each of a
set of stimuli is compared to an internally generated scale, or continuum, for
the attribute being rated, which is divided into a specified number of segments (usually 5, 7, or 9) that are not necessarily of equal size, and the numeral is assigned to it that designates the segment of the internally generated
continuum that corresponds to the amount of the attribute it is judged to
possess. The task is performed by a group, or panel, of observers. Stimuli are
presented to observers one at a time. Observers are instructed to assign the
numeral between 1 and the number which corresponds to the number of
points on the scale (e.g., 7) to each stimulus which indicates the amount of
the target attribute it possesses. They are informed that the scale contains a
specified number of points which range from 1 to 7 (or some other value). In
some instances, each point on the scale is *anchored,* or defined, and in others
only the extremes are anchored. A seven-point scale (that could be used for
assessing attitudes toward statements with Likert methodology) on which
each point is anchored is illustrated by the following:

_____	:	_____	:	_____	:	_____	:	_____	:	_____	:	_____
Completely		Mostly		Slightly		Undecided		Slightly		Mostly		Completely
Disagree		Disagree		Disagree				Agree		Agree		Agree
(1)		(2)		(3)		(4)		(5)		(6)		(7)

On the other hand, such a scale may have only the extremes anchored:

Strongly
Disagree ____ : ____ : ____ : ____ : ____ : ____ : ____ Strongly Agree
        1   2   3   4   5   6   7

For example, an observer who was presented with speech segments from
five persons who have hypernasal speech and was asked to assign a numeral
between 1 and 7 to each on the basis of the amount of hypernasality exhibited by the speaker with the points on the scale defined as (1) no hypernasality, (2) extremely mild hypernasality, (3) mild hypernasality, (4) moderate
hypernasality, (5) moderately severe hypernasality, (6) severe hypernasality,
and (7) extremely severe hypernasality would perform this task by comparing
the amount of hypernasality he or she perceived in each speech segment to
that designated by each of the seven modifiers on his or her internal scale of
hypernasality and on the basis of these comparisons would assign each a numeral between 1 and 7. The observer may assign the same numeral to two
or more speech segments if he or she feels the amount of hypernasality present in them is designated by the same modifier.

    The primary difference between the methods of equal-appearing inter-
vals and successive intervals is the assumption made regarding the sizes of
the segments of the internally generated scale for the attribute. With the

method of equal-appearing intervals, these segments are assumed to be of equal size. With the method of successive intervals, no assumption is made regarding the relative sizes of segment widths; the segment widths are estimated from the data.

Constant Sums. With this method, which theoretically results in a ratio scale, *all possible pairs* of stimuli are compared to an internally generated scale for the attribute being rated, and a judgment is made regarding the relative amount of the attribute possessed by each member of each pair. The proportion of 100 points is then assigned to each of the stimuli in each pair which reflects the relative amount of the attribute possessed by each member of each pair. The points assigned to the stimuli in each pair always total 100. To illustrate this method, suppose that one of the stimuli in a pair was judged to possess twice as much of a target attribute (e.g., nasality) as the other. The former would be assigned 67 points and the latter 33 points.

The task is performed by a group, or panel, of observers. Each observer is presented with all possible ordered pairings (i.e., permutations) of the stimuli to be scaled. The number of such pairings which will result from a set of stimuli of a given size (N) can be determined by multiplying the number of stimuli by the number of stimuli minus one, or

$$N (N - 1)$$

Note that the manner of presentation of stimuli to observers is the same as for the method of pair comparisons.

Observers are told to indicate for each pair of stimuli both the stimulus that possesses the greater amount of the target attribute and the *ratio* of the amount of the attribute this stimulus possesses in relation to that possessed by the other stimulus through proportional point assignments to the two stimuli. They perform this task by comparing the amount of the target attribute they observe in each of the two stimuli in a pair to their internal scale for that attribute. For example, an observer who was presented with speech segments from two persons who have hypernasal speech and was asked to indicate how much more hypernasal the most hypernasal speaker was than the least hypernasal speaker (through a proportional assignment of 100 points) would perform this task by comparing the levels of hypernasality he or she perceived in the two segments to his or her internal scale for degree of hypernasality and on the basis of these comparisons would make the point assignments. Observers could make any point assignments they wished as long as the points totaled 100 and portrayed the ratio of degree of hypernasality exhibited by the two speakers.

Direct Magnitude-Estimation. With this method, which theoretically results in a ratio scale, each of a set of stimuli is compared to a point on an internally generated scale, or continuum, for the attribute being rated, and a numeral is assigned to each stimulus which designates the relative amount of the attribute that it possesses as compared to the amount of the attribute at that point on the internally generated scale. If the point on the internally generated scale that is serving as the standard were assigned a value of 100 points, and a stimulus to be rated were judged to possess three times the amount of the attribute as the standard, it would be assigned 300 points. If a stimulus, on the other hand, were judged to possess one-half as much of the attribute as the standard, it would be assigned 50 points.

The rating task is performed by a group, or panel, of observers. Stimuli are presented one at a time. The observers are presented with a stimulus of the type they will be rating to use as a standard, prior to beginning the rating task. The amount of the target attribute present in this stimulus is assigned a value of 100 points. The observers are instructed to assign the number of points to each stimulus which represents the relative amount of the target attribute it possesses with reference to that possessed by the standard stimulus. If, for example, the observers felt a stimulus possessed twice the amount of the target attribute as the standard stimulus, they would assign it 200 points. If, on the other hand, they felt it possessed only half the amount of the target attribute as the standard, they would assign it 50 points. They can use any point assignment they feel appropriate. They need not limit themselves to even fractions and even multiples of the 100 points assigned to the standard. They can use any point assignment they choose as long as it represents their judgment of the amount of the target attribute possessed by a stimulus in relation to that possessed by the standard. If, for example, observers were presented with speech segments from five persons who have hypernasal speech and were told to assign points to each on the basis of the amount of hypernasality each possesses in relation to that present in the speech segment of a sixth person (standard) which is assigned 100 points, they would perform this task by comparing the amount of hypernasality they perceived in each speech segment they were asked to rate and in the standard segment to their internal scale for degree of hypernasality, and on the basis of these comparisons they would assign each stimulus a number of points. The standard would serve as an *anchor* to align their internal scales of hypernasality. They can assign the same number of points to two or more speech segments if they feel the speakers in these segments exhibit the same amounts of hypernasality.

Considerations in the Choice of a Scaling Method

Six scaling methods were described in the previous section. How do you decide which to use for quantifying a particular attribute of a particular set of stimuli? A number of factors should be considered when making such a decision, including: (1) minimum level of measurement required, (2) number of stimuli to be rated, (3) maximum number of judges available, (4) age and intelligence level of the judges, (5) computational ease, (6) maximum length of judging session, (7) necessity that ratings for stimuli scaled at differ-ent times be comparable, (8) statistical sophistication of the audience to whom the results are to be reported, (9) duration of individual stimuli, and (10) judges' reactions to the scaling task. We will discuss each as it relates to the choice among the six scaling methods that have been described.

   Minimum Level of Measurement Required.   The question of concern here is whether the minimum acceptable level of measurement for judges' ratings is ordinal, interval, or ratio. This level usually can be inferred from the *kinds of statements* you want to be able to make about the ratings or the *kinds of questions* you want to be able to answer using them. If, for example, you decided to rate "before and after" therapy speech samples for degree of articulation defectiveness and you wanted to make a judgment from these ratings on whether the clients' articulation was *less defective* after therapy than before it, only *ordinal* measurement would be required. On the other hand, if you wanted to be able to make a judgment regarding the *amount of reduction* in articulation defectiveness following therapy (assuming there was such a reduction), *ratio* measurement would be required.

   Any of the six scaling methods can be used if *only ordinal* measurement is required. They have been empirically demonstrated to order sets of stimuli in the same manner.

   If the minimum level of measurement required is *interval*, then equal-appearing intervals, successive intervals, constant sums, or direct magnitude-estimation could be used. If observers perform the rating tasks *as instructed,* these methods should result in ratings that have properties which *approxi-mate* (or come close to achieving) interval level measurement.

   If *ratio* measurement is required, either constant sums or direct magni-tude-estimation can be used. Both methods should result in ratings with prop-erties approximating those for ratio level measurement *if* the observers per-form the rating tasks as instructed.

   Number of Stimuli to Be Rated.   If the number of stimuli to be rated were fewer than 10, this probably would not be an important consideration. However, if this number exceeds 10, three of the scaling methods (i.e., pair comparisons, rank order, and constant sums) may not be practical. The rea-son for pair comparisons and constant sums is that too many stimulus pairs may have to be rated. As I have already indicated, the number of stimulus pairs that have to be rated when these methods are used is the product of the number of stimuli times this number minus one, or $N = 10$

$$N(N - 1)$$

$$\frac{10(10-1)}{10(9)}$$
$$90$$

For 20 stimuli, the number of stimulus pairs would be

$$20(20 - 1)$$

or 380. Obtaining 380 ratings would probably be too time-consuming in most instances. Pair comparisons and constant sums would rarely be practical when the number of stimuli to be scaled exceeded 50.

The method of rank order may not be practical to use when the number of stimuli to be scaled exceeds 10, because it may be quite difficult for an observer to keep in mind the amount of the target attribute possessed by each stimulus while ordering them. This is particularly likely to be the case when the stimuli, or events, to be ordered are auditory (e.g., speech segments).

Maximum Number of Judges Available. Some scaling methods require larger panels than others to achieve scale values that possess a given level of reliability. Equal-appearing intervals, for example, tends to require fewer judges to achieve scale values that have a given level of reliability than does direct magnitude-estimation. Also, a variation of direct magnitude-estimation in which an interval rather than a point standard is used (referred to as direct interval-estimation) appears to require fewer raters than direct magnitude-estimation to achieve scale values which have a given level of reliability (Silverman and Johnston, 1975).

Age and Intelligence Level of the Judges. Some rating tasks are more difficult than others. The task associated with the method of pair comparisons probably would be easier for children and for adults with below-normal intelligence than those associated with the other scaling methods.

Computational Ease. Some scaling methods require less computation than others to derive scale values. Equal-appearing interval scale values, for example, require less computation than successive interval scale values. While computational ease probably would not be one of the first considerations in selecting a scaling method, it nevertheless would probably make sense if two or more methods would serve *equally well* to select the one which requires the least amount of computation.

Maximum Length of Judging Session. The number of stimuli that can be rated in a given amount of time is different for different methods. Fewer stimuli can be rated in a given amount of time with pair comparisons and constant sums than with the other methods. Equal-appearing intervals, successive intervals, and direct magnitude-estimation would probably require approximately the same amount of time to rate a given number of stimuli. The time required for rank order is apt to be longer than for equal-appearing intervals, successive intervals, or direct magnitude-estimation, particularly if the number of stimuli to be ranked is relatively large or the differences in the amounts of the target attribute they possess are relatively small.

Necessity That Ratings for Stimuli Scaled at Different Times Be Compa-
rable.   With some scaling methods, the rating assigned to a stimulus to indicate the amount of the target attribute it possesses is apt to be influenced by
the amount of that attribute present in the other stimuli with which it is
rated. This is almost certain to be a problem when the methods of pair comparison, constant sums, and rank order are used. If it is necessary for ratings
for stimuli scaled at different times to be comparable, the safest method to
use probably would be direct magnitude-estimation (assuming the same standard stimulus is used for rating all stimuli).

Statistical Sophistication of the Audience to Whom the Results Are to
Be Reported.   Some scaling methods require a better statistical background
to understand intuitively than do others. Equal-appearing intervals, for example, would not require as much statistical sophistication to understand as
would successive intervals. While this would not usually be one of the main
considerations in the choice of a scaling method, if two or more methods
would be equally appropriate for a particular purpose, it would probably make
sense to choose the one requiring the least statistical sophistication to understand, or interpret.

Duration of Individual Stimuli.   The duration of individual stimuli may
be a relevant consideration in the choice of a scaling method, particularly
with regard to the practicality of pair comparisons and constant sums. If their
duration is relatively long, the judges may not be able to remember both
members of a pair well enough to make a pair comparison or constant sum
rating that is adequately reliable. Also, if their duration is relatively long, the
number of stimuli that could be rated in a given period of time by these
methods may be too few to be practical.

Judges' Reactions to the Scaling Task.   Observers' "levels of belief" in
their abilities to perform rating tasks are apt not to be a constant. They would
probably be more confident of their ability to make pair comparison judgments than direct magnitude-estimation judgments. If they do not believe
they can perform the rating task they are asked to perform, they may not try
too hard and their ratings may not be adequately reliable.

For further information about methodological considerations when designing scaling experiments, see Appendix C.

SCHEMES THAT RELY PRIMARILY ON OBSERVER JUDGMENT:
OBSERVATION WITH SYSTEMATIC CLASSIFICATION

Observation with systematic classification has been one of the main strategies used for generating data to answer questions in all research areas. It has
been utilized by speech-language pathologists and audiologists for clinical as

well as research purposes. A clinician, for example, who *classifies* a client's voice as "breathy" based on *observation* of his or her speech during an evaluation session is using it. So also is one who on the basis of a phonological analysis on a sample of a child's speech describes him or her as evincing certain sound substitutions and/or omissions.

Data generated in this manner usually consists of "words," though the data can have a numerical component. It involves assigning attributes of an event you have observed to categories. "Stuttering severity," for example, would be an attribute of the event "speaking behavior." The category to which this attribute would be assigned would be either "mild," "moderate," or "severe." Other labels or sets of categories, of course, could be substituted—e.g., the set of seven categories that define the *Iowa Scale of Stuttering Severity* (Johnson, Darley, and Spriestersbach, 1963). If this scale were used, each category would be designated by a numeral between 1 and 7. These numerals would possess the attributes of those on a nominal scale and possibly also those on an ordinal one (see Chapter 7).

The process used here is quite similar to that described in the preceding section. Both psychological scaling techniques and those utilizing observation with systematic classification involve assigning attributes of events to categories. With the former, the categories are designated by numerals that possess ordinal, interval, or ratio scale characteristics (see Chapter 7). With the latter, on the other hand, the categories are either designated by words (or phrases) or by numerals that have nominal scale (and possibly also ordinal scale) characteristics. The mental processes involved are the same—the only difference is the manner in which categories are designated and defined.

Data derived from observation with systematic classification are subject to the same types of error as are those derived from psychological scaling techniques and the other strategies described in this chapter. They are neither more nor less likely than the others to yield "incorrect" answers!

For further information about the use of observation with systematic classification for generating data in behavioral research, see Best and Kahn (1989).

EXERCISES AND DISCUSSION TOPICS

1. You are to rate each of five utterances for "degree of syntactic complexity" by means of six psychological scaling methods: pair comparisons, rank order, equal-appearing intervals, successive intervals, constant sums, and direct magnitude-estimation. The utterances are:

   a. "David is tired."

   b. "Yes."

   c. "She ate a lot of candy."

   d. "My father really wanted to help us, but he didn't have time."

e. "Fortunately, Ted has plenty of money."

A. *Pair Comparisons*

Instructions. Printed below are five pairs of utterances in a random order. Indicate whether you feel the first or second utterance in each pair is most *complex* syntactically.

a. "Fortunately, Ted has plenty of money."
"My father really wanted to help us, but he didn't have time."

b. "David is tired."
"Yes."

c. "Fortunately, Ted has plenty of money."
"David is tired."

d. "My father really wanted to help us, but he didn't have time."
"Yes."

e. "She ate a lot of candy."
"My father really wanted to help us, but he didn't have time."

B. *Rank Order*

Instructions. Printed below are five utterances in a random order. Assign a number between 1 and 5 to each which indicates its relative degree of syntactic complexity as compared to the other four utterances. Assign 1 to the utterance you feel is *most* complex syntactically and 5 to the utterance you feel is *least* complex syntactically. Do not assign the same number (or rank) to more than one utterance.

a. "David is tired."

b. "Yes."

c. "My father really wanted to help us, but he didn't have time."

d. "She ate a lot of candy."

e. "Fortunately, Ted had plenty of money."

C. *Equal-Appearing Intervals*

Instructions. Printed below are five utterances in a random order. Assign a number to each which designates its location on a seven-point scale of "syntactic complexity." The scale is one of equal intervals—from 1 to 7—with 1 representing *least* possible syntactic complexity and 7 representing *most* possible syntactic complexity; 4 represents the midpoint between 1 and 7 with respect to complexity, with the other numbers falling at equal distances along the scale. Do not attempt to place utterances between any two of the seven points, but only at these points. You, of course, can assign the same number to two or more utterances if you feel they are equivalent with regard to syntactic complexity.

a. "David is tired."

b. "Yes."

c. "My father really wanted to help us, but he didn't have time."

d. "She ate a lot of candy."

e. "Fortunately, Ted has plenty of money."

D. *Successive Intervals*

Instructions. Printed below are five utterances in a random order. Assign a number to each which designates its location on a seven-point scale of "syntactic complexity." On the scale 1 represents *least* possible syntactic complexity and 7 represents *most* possible syntactic complexity; 4 represents the midpoint between 1 and 7 with respect to complexity. Do not attempt to place utterances between any two of the seven points, but only at these points. You, of course, can assign the same number to two or more utterances if you feel they are equivalent with regard to syntactic complexity.

a. "David is tired."

b. "Yes."

c. "My father really wanted to help us, but he didn't have time."

d. "She ate a lot of candy."

e. "Fortunately, Ted has plenty of money."

E. *Constant Sums*

Instructions. Printed below are five pairs of utterances in a random order. Assign points to the two utterances in each pair so that the total number of points assigned to the utterances in a pair is 100. The proportion of 100 points assigned to each of the utterances in a pair should reflect the relative amount of syntactic complexity possessed by each member of the pair. If, for example, you felt that one utterance in a pair was twice as complex syntactically as was the other, you would assign it 67 points and the other 33 points.

a. "Fortunately, Ted has plenty of money."
   "My father really wanted to help us, but he didn't have time."

b. "David is tired."
   "Yes."

c. "Fortunately, Ted has plenty of money."
   "David is tired."

d. "Fortunately, Ted has plenty of money."
   "Yes."

e. "She ate a lot of candy."
   "David is tired."

F. *Direct Magnitude-Estimation*

Instructions. Printed below are five utterances in a random order. Assign the number of points to each utterance that you believe represents its relative degree of syntactic complexity with reference to the following *standard* utterance that has been assigned a value of 100 points.

   "She works hard."

The point assignment you make to each utterance should represent, with reference to the standard, its relative syntactic complexity. For example, if you feel that an utterance is *twice* as complex syntactically as the standard, you assign it *200 points.* On the other hand, if you feel that an utterance is *half* as complex syntactically as the standard, you assign it *50 points.* You may, of course, use any point assignment you wish to represent your judgment of an utterance's syntactic complexity so long as it represents your judgment of the syntactic complexity of the utterance in relation to the standard utterance.

a. "David is tired."

b. "Yes."

c. "My father really wanted to help us, but he didn't have time."

d. "She ate a lot of candy."

e. "Fortunately, Ted has plenty of money."

2. Three speech-language pathologists rated a videotaped sample of stuttered speech on a seven-point equal-appearing interval scale of stuttering severity. The first assigned it a 2 (mild); the second a 4 (moderate); and the third a 6 (severe). What factors might account for the differences in their ratings?

3. How might psychological scaling techniques be used clinically (e.g., for assessing therapy outcome)?

4. Describe an instrumentation scheme for measurement (see Figure 8.1) that is used clinically by either speech-language pathologists or audiologists.

9

Organizing Data for Answering Questions: Descriptive Techniques

Once the data have been gathered—whether qualitative or quantitative— they have to be organized, or structured, in a manner that will permit the question or questions posed by the investigator to be answered. Without such organization, the answers derived for the data are less likely to be accurate. You can easily be deceived if you attempt to answer questions merely by skimming through, or eyeballing, the available data. You may, for example, inadvertently give too much weight or too little weight to certain aspects of your data, possibly as a function of experimenter bias (see Chapter 8). Suppose a question you were attempting to answer concerned the effectiveness of a particular therapy, and to answer it you recorded a number of observations (both qualitative and quantitative) before and after administration of the therapy to 20 persons who had a certain communicative disorder. If you skim the available data, you might tend to pay more attention to aspects of it that suggest the treatment was effective than to those that suggest it had little or no effect. Another clinician whose theoretical orientation would give him or her a set not to find the therapy effective might tend to pay more attention to aspects of the data that suggest the treatment had little or no effect. Thus, two persons skimming the same data could arrive at different answers to a question if they had different expectations, or sets (biases).

Another reason why you can be easily deceived if you attempt to answer questions merely by skimming data is that the data needed to answer a particular question may not stand out sufficiently from the other data in the set in

which it is included to provide an accurate answer to the question. The problem here can be viewed as one of inadequate separation between figure and
background, or between signal and noise. To illustrate this problem, suppose
you wished to answer the following question: "How was the communicative
behavior of a group of aphasics different following therapy?" If you merely
skimmed the pre- and posttherapy observations you had recorded in their
folders rather than systematically abstracting, organizing, and summarizing
these observations, you might not be able to get a sufficiently good impression of how this behavior was different to answer the question accurately. It
would be difficult, if not impossible, to remember all the relevant observations recorded in the folders.

A third reason (which is related to the second) why skimming the data
is deceptive is that several observations are likely to be relevant to a particular
question. It may not be possible to integrate them sufficiently to arrive at an
accurate answer without first organizing and summarizing them.

Several approaches can be used for organizing and summarizing sets
of data for answering questions. These include statistical analysis, graphical
display, tabular presentation, and narrative description. The first three approaches are the ones customarily used for organizing and summarizing
quantitative data. The last two are customarily used for organizing and summarizing qualitative data. This chapter will discuss organizing qualitative and
quantitative data through these approaches.

STRATEGIES FOR ORGANIZING QUALITATIVE *(verbal descriptive)*
DATA FOR ANSWERING QUESTIONS

The primary emphasis of this section will be on the organization of qualitative (i.e., verbal descriptive) data for clinical case studies. Such data have been
used most frequently by speech-language pathologists and audiologists in this
context.

Observations should be summarized and organized so that they can be
used for answering the questions posed by the investigator. This involves
several processes, the first of which is *abstracting* from the available data
those relevant for answering each question. Suppose you administered three
articulation tests to a child both before and after she received a particular
program of therapy and had transcribed her responses to the test stimuli pho-
nemically. These transcriptions, of course, would be qualitative data. If one
of your questions was whether her production of /s/ at the beginnings of
words was any different after the period of therapy than preceding it, to answer it you would have to abstract the data on the production of /s/ in the
initial position from the remaining articulation test data.

Once the data relevant for answering a question are abstracted, they
are summarized and organized. A child's production of /s/ in the initial position in words as sampled before and after a period of therapy by three articu-

lation tests can be summarized and organized by means of a table such as that shown in Table 9.1.

After the data have been summarized and organized, they can be used to answer the question. The data in the table indicate that the production of /s/ was different following therapy on all three articulation tests. Specifically, they indicate that /s/ was produced correctly in the initial positions of words following therapy (at least in the words sampled by these articulation tests and in the situation in which they were administered).

Abstracting Relevant Data

It is necessary to abstract from the available observations, or data, those that *may* be relevant for answering each of the questions posed. We emphasize "may" to highlight the fact that it is not always possible to determine at this stage of the process exactly which data of those available will be relevant for answering a particular question. If there is any reason to believe that an observation may be relevant for doing so, it should be abstracted.

One strategy that may assist the abstraction process is recording each observation on a card. For answering a question, you would select those cards from the pile on which you have recorded observations that may be relevant. In most instances this would be a better strategy than reading through the available data and attempting to remember those that may be relevant for answering a particular question.

An alternative strategy to the one described in the preceding paragraph is entering each observation as a record in a computer database file. Each such record would be the computer equivalent of a card. To identify those relevant for answering a particular question, you could BROWSE through the records ("cards") in the database file and/or use the program's FIND function to locate those containing certain words. The information contained in some or all of these records could be printed "as is" or transferred electronically to a word-processing program for inclusion in a report or other document.

Organizing and Summarizing Relevant Data

After the observations that may be relevant have been abstracted, they are organized and summarized in a manner which permits the answer to the

TABLE 9.1   A child's production of /s/ in the initial position in words as sampled before and after therapy by three articulation tests.

Articulation Test	Before-Therapy Production	After-Therapy Production
I	/θ/	/s/
II	/θ/	/s/
III	/θ/	/s/

question to be as evident as the available data allow. Several approaches can be used here. First, the data can be organized in tabular form—i.e., summarized in a table. To illustrate the possibilities for organizing and summarizing qualitative data in tabular form, Table 9.2 presents references to representative tables containing qualitative data from articles published in the *Journal of Speech and Hearing Disorders.*

A second approach for organizing and summarizing is to set down the qualitative observations in narrative form. Speech-language pathologists and audiologists typically use this approach in evaluation reports for summarizing relevant observations (both formal and informal) made on clients. They also typically use this approach for daily logs of therapy sessions.

This approach is employed in most clinical case studies for summarizing and organizing qualitative observations. The following two paragraphs from case studies published in the *Journal of Speech and Hearing Disorders* illustrate this application:

Subject 1 in Condition A usually produced touch velopharyngeal closure and his port configuration was oval. . . . . Openings lateral to midline palate-posterior pharyngeal wall contact often were observed in this subject. The subject elevated his palate so it usually contacted the posterior pharyngeal wall. The uvula contracted during two trials. Only one lateral pharyngeal wall or palatopharyngeus muscle could be seen at one time, and it moved toward midline only on one trial and then gag was involved. The subject reported gag on three trials. The subject frequently produced a Passavant's ridge. The ridge varied across trials from slight to marked displacement. No other forward movement of the posterior wall of the pharynx was observed. Laryngeal click was usually heard at the end of trials. (Shelton, Paesani, McClelland, and Bradfield, 1975, p. 238)

TABLE 9.2   References to representative tables that have been used to organize and summarize qualitative data in the *Journal of Speech and Hearing Disorders.*

Data Tabulated	Reference		
	Volume	Year	Pages
Phonetic transcriptions of children's utterances	39	1974	24, 27
Survey of earmold manufacturers' nomenclature	38	1973	459–460
Comparison of three children's phonemic errors	37	1972	454
Child's pattern of phonemic change	37	1972	457–460
Summary of speech, language, and hearing findings in three cases of Laurence-Moon-Biedl syndrome	37	1972	411
Description of parent-child interactions	37	1972	224–225
Samples of the utterances of three children	37	1972	70–71
Examples of the sentence repetitions of four children	36	1971	32
Patterns and generalizations found in the articulatory and auditory discrimination behavior of two groups of subjects	35	1970	138–139
Clinical impression vs. cineradiographic evaluation for eight cases of idiopathic hypernasality	35	1970	48
Summary of voice symptoms and associated factors in psychogenic and neurogenic dysphonias	33	1968	229

Once the desired pitch had been obtained, we directed Craig to continue produc-ing phrases. He progressed quickly and by the third therapy session was able to converse using his new voice, which tended to confirm the nonorganic basis of the voice problem. Occasional pitch breaks occurred, however, and the somewhat hoarse quality persisted. Samples of conversational speech and reading were then tape-recorded so he could identify and tabulate instances when he reverted to the old pitch. At that stage both Craig and his mother were pleased with the results of therapy and encouraged. Others had also commented on his improve-ment. The stabilization phase of therapy continued in the speech clinic and then in various other places where Craig was often accompanied by the clinician. Dur-ing the last few sessions we observed consistently low pitch and a voice quality that was almost clear of roughness. To evaluate Craig's voice in more stressful situations, one clinician attended his English class; the voice was clear, of natural pitch, and audible to those sitting in the back of the room. With the great satisfac-tion of Craig and his mother and with our confidence, it was mutually agreed to terminate therapy six weeks after its initiation. An interview two months later revealed that Craig's voice had remained consistently normal. (Yairi, 1974, p. 375)

Note the degree of similarity between (1) the first paragraph and an excerpt from an evaluation report, and (2) the second paragraph and an excerpt from a progress note regarding the impact of therapy on a client.

Summarizing and organizing qualitative data involves the assignment of observations to *categories* (see Chapter 8). This is true regardless of whether the data are to be summarized and organized in tabular or in narra-tive form.

The categories to which observations are assigned can be categorized in various ways. Some, for example, can be viewed as spatial, some as tempo-ral, some as combinations of these two, and some as neither of these two. An example of a set of *spatial* categories that might be used by a speech-language pathologist or audiologist to organize qualitative observations would be "right ear" and "left ear." An example of a set of *temporal* categories would be "sta-tus prior to receiving therapy" and "status following therapy." An example of a corresponding set of *spatial-temporal* categories would be "status of left ear prior to therapy" and "status of left ear following therapy." And, finally, an example of a set of categories that could be regarded as *neither temporal nor spatial* would be "receptive language" and "expressive language."

The categories to which observations are assigned are determined by, or a function of, the question or questions asked. If you wished to determine, for example, whether a child's speech articulation were any different after a period of therapy than before it, two categories to which you would assign your observations would undoubtedly be "speech articulation prior to thera-py" and "speech articulation following therapy." On the other hand, if your question concerned the current status of a child's communication behavior, several of the categories you might use would be "hearing acuity," "speech fluency," "language usage," and "voice quality."

A given observation may be assigned to more than one category and used to answer more than one question. Suppose a speech-language patholo-gist showed a pencil to a person who had had a stroke and asked this person to name and describe it. Further suppose that the speech-language pathologist regarded the response as appropriate and all phonemes as correctly articulated. This observation, or judgment, could be assigned to more than one category and could be used to answer more than one question. For example, it could be assigned to the category of "receptive language functioning" and could be used to answer the question: "Does the person exhibit a disturbance in receptive language functioning?" It could also be assigned to the category "dysarthria" and could be used to answer the question: "Does the person exhibit any disturbances in the functioning of the articulators for speech?" Other categories to which this observation could be assigned include "auditory acuity," "auditory perceptual functioning," "conceptual functioning," and "word-finding ability."

The discussion in this section provides only a very general introduction to the organization and analysis of qualitative data. If you wish to pursue this topic further, you may find information in the sociology literature about participant observation in field research useful. You may also find useful the paper by Hinds, Scandrett-Hibden, and McAulay (1990) and the book by Bromley (1986) which deals with this topic in the context of individual case studies.

STRATEGIES FOR ORGANIZING QUANTITATIVE DATA FOR ANSWERING QUESTIONS

The remainder of this chapter is devoted to a discussion of strategies for organizing quantitative data through the use of descriptive statistics and graphical displays. For statistics, the discussion emphasizes when it is appropriate to use each and how each is interpreted, rather than the mathematical model which underlies it. To develop an intuitive understanding of what statistics are and what they can do, it is necessary to have at least a little experience computing them. A computational appendix has been included to provide such experience for descriptive as well as inferential statistics (see Appendix A). The latter are discussed in Chapter 10. This appendix contains computational formulas, "worked" examples, Minitab commands, and exercises (including answers).

The statistical methods included in the computational appendix should be regarded as representative rather than exhaustive. This is particularly true of the inferential statistical methods, which are discussed in Chapter 10. While this appendix contains a test of statistical significance appropriate for almost any set of data, these tests constitute only a small sample of those that have been developed. The tests included were selected because they are among the ones that have been used most frequently by speech-language pathologists and audiologists judging by research reports published in the journals of the American Speech-Language-Hearing Association.

All statistics in the computational appendix are computed from a single set of data, which consists of frequencies per 100 words spoken of four types of speech disfluency (i.e., interjection of sounds and syllables, part-word repetition, word repetition, and revision-incomplete phrase) for each of 56 elementary-school children. This set of data was selected for inclusion in the appendix because it can be segmented in ways that make it possible to compute the various statistics included therein. The fact that the frequencies relate to speech disfluencies rather than to some other event of interest to speech-language pathologists and audiologists, of course, is irrelevant to the statistical analyses made of them. What the frequencies represent has no effect on such analyses—i.e., on the computational procedures used. It does, of course, affect the interpretation of the results of such analyses.

Descriptive Statistics

Descriptive statistics describe an aspect, or attribute, of a set of measures—i.e., of a set of quantitative data. They provide indices for specific attributes of the distribution of the data in such a set. The data tabulated in the table at the beginning of Appendix A illustrate this concept. The frequencies of interjection, part-word repetition, word repetition, and revision-incomplete phrase presented in this table for 56 children (a total of 224 measures) constitute a set of quantitative data.

If you were to skim the 224 measures in this table *without looking at the column headings,* they probably would provide little information about the disfluency production of these children. About the only question they would permit you to answer reliably about the children's disfluency production would be: "Were the children homogeneous with regard to the amount of disfluency they produced?" Merely skimming these data would be sufficient to establish that they were not homogeneous with regard to this aspect of their disfluency because their frequencies were different—e.g., 4.83 is not the same as 0.00.

Before these data could be used for answering other questions about these children's disfluency production, they would have to be organized and summarized. The organization and summarization of quantitative data, like qualitative data, involves the assignment of observations to *categories.* Some such categories have nominal scale characteristics. Others have ordinal, interval, ratio, or logarithmic scale ones (see Chapter 7 for a description of these measurement scales). The assignment of measures to a set of categories results in a *distribution.* To illustrate the concept of distribution, let us again refer to the data table in Appendix A. The categories "interjection," "part-word repetition," "word repetition," and "revision-incomplete phrase" define a nominal scale; the 56 measures that are assigned to each constitute a distribution. Furthermore, the categories "second grade," "third grade," "fourth grade," "fifth grade," and "sixth grade" define an ordinal scale and the measures that are assigned to each also constitute a distribution.

Thus far we have only considered what are referred to as *univariate* distributions. The characteristic of such distributions is that observations are assigned to categories on the basis of only a single attribute of the data. With respect to our illustration, this attribute would be either type of disfluency or grade level of the child producing the disfluency.

In some instances it may be advantageous to categorize observations on the basis of more than one attribute. The resulting distribution would be *multivariate*. The type of multivariate distribution encountered most frequently in speech and hearing research is the *bivariate*. In such distributions, observations are assigned to categories on the basis of two of their attributes. The data table in Appendix A can be viewed as a bivariate distribution. Each of the 224 measures can be regarded as having been assigned to one of the 20 joint categories, or cells. The resulting distribution, or matrix, is illustrated in Table 9.3. The number in each cell indicates how many of the 224 measures were assigned to it.

The data table in Appendix A provides some information about the disfluency production of the children whose speech was sampled. Merely skimming these data as categorized provides the information necessary to answer at least one question: "Did the children tend to produce more revisions and incomplete phrases than interjections?" A casual inspection of these data suggests that the frequencies for revision-incomplete phrase tend to be higher than those for interjection. On the other hand, merely skimming these data would probably not be sufficient to answer the question: "How much more frequently did the children tend to produce revisions and incomplete phrases than they did interjections?" To answer this question and most others these data would be appropriate for answering, further organizing and summarizing of the data are necessary. *Descriptive statistics* can be used for this purpose.

TABLE 9.3   Data table from Appendix A viewed as a bivariate distribution.

	I	PW	W	R-IP
Second Grade	15	15	15	15
Third Grade	11	11	11	11
Fourth Grade	9	9	9	9
Fifth Grade	11	11	11	11
Sixth Grade	10	10	10	10

What do descriptive statistics describe? What sorts of questions are they helpful in answering? These questions will be considered in the three sections which follow. The first deals with measures of *central tendency*; the second, measures of *variability*; and the third, measures of *association*.

Measures of Central Tendency. These indices designate the "average," "typical," or most frequently occurring number in a set of numbers. A number provided by such an index is regarded as *representative* (in some respect) of the numbers in the set from which it was computed.

When the numbers in the set from which indices of central tendency are computed are measures of attributes of persons or of behaviors, they provide information concerning the average, typical, or most frequently occurring amount of an attribute. They designate an amount, or magnitude, of an attribute that in some respect can be regarded as "representative" of that present in the set. If the numbers in a set were scores on a test of language proficiency that had been administered to a class of kindergarten children, it would be possible to designate through the use of indices of central tendency: (1) the average score earned by these children, (2) the score earned by the "typical" member of the class, and (3) the score earned most often by the children in the class. Similarly, if the numbers in a set were a particular stutterer's stuttering frequencies in 15 situations, you could designate through the use of these indices: (1) the average rate at which he or she stuttered in these situations, (2) the rate at which he or she stuttered that was most typical, and (3) the rate at which he or she stuttered most often. The values yielded for these three types of "representativeness" will be quite similar in some instances and quite dissimilar in others.

There are three commonly used measures of central tendency: the *mean*, the *median*, and the *mode*. Each describes one of the types of representativeness referred to in the preceding paragraph. Computational formulas and worked examples for all three are in Appendix A.

The *mean* is probably the most commonly used measure of central tendency, in part because it is usually the easiest to compute. It is merely an arithmetic average: you add together the scores (or other numbers) you wish to average and divide the total by the number of them that were added.

The mean can be used to answer questions such as these:

1. How many hours of therapy did the average child receive?
2. How long, on the average, was a particular cerebral palsied child able to sustain the vowel /a/ during a series of 10 trials?
3. Did the children tend to be less "nasal" following a particular type of cleft palate surgery than before?

Note that answering the first question requires averaging a single measure (i.e., time) from a number of persons; the second, a number of measures from a single person. The mean can be used as a measure of central tendency for both intersubject and intrasubject measures. The third question was included to indicate that the mean sometimes is used to describe the performance of persons *as a group*. Other measures of central tendency also may be used for this purpose.

⊬ Strictly speaking, measures from which a mean is computed must have interval or ratio properties (see Chapter 7). If the properties of such measures do not include equal intervals between scale points, their mean may not be readily interpretable with regard to the magnitude, or amount, of an attribute it represents. Suppose you administered a language test to a group of children on three occasions—i.e., before, halfway through, and after completing a program of therapy—and the means of their scores at these three points were 80, 110, and 120, respectively. If these scores could be assumed to have interval or ratio properties and be *reliable*, the following conclusions would be possible:

1. The children performed better after participating in the therapy program.
2. They exhibited some improvement halfway through the program.
3. The amount of improvement they exhibited tended to be greater during the first than the second half of the program.

If, on the other hand, the scores could only be assumed to have ordinal properties (see Chapter 7), the third conclusion would not be possible. Without being able to assume equal intervals between scale points, you would have no way of knowing whether greater improvement occurred during the first or second half of the therapy program. That is, if the scores on this test lacked the equal interval property, a child could conceivably have to modify his or her language behavior less to go from 80 to 110 than to go from 110 to 120.

Means, as well as other statistics that require measures to have interval or ratio properties, have been used in speech, language, and hearing research (and in other behavioral science areas) with measures that have been demonstrated to have only *ordinal* properties. The argument against using such statistics with ordinal data can be summarized as follows:

> In developing procedures, mathematical statisticians have assumed that techniques involving numerical orderings, or categorization, are to be applied when these numbers or classes are appropriate and meaningful within the experimenter's problem. If the statistical method involves the procedures of arithmetic used on numerical scores, then the numerical answer is formally correct. Even if the numbers are the purest nonsense, having no relation to real magnitudes or the properties of real things, the answers are still right *as numbers*. The difficulty comes with the *interpretation of these numbers back into statements about the real world* [italics added]. If nonsense is put into a mathematical system, nonsense is sure to come out. (Hays, 1973, p. 74)

Thus, while means and other statistics that are appropriate for measures having interval or ratio properties can be computed with numbers having the properties of any measurement scale—even those with nominal properties such as numerals on the backs of football players—they may not lead to accurate answers because of the difficulty of translating them back into statements about the real world.

While the mean is an appropriate measure of central tendency for data having interval or ratio scale properties, it is not necessarily a good index of representativeness for such data. A mean value may not designate the number most representative of a set. In fact, it may designate a number that *never occurs* in the set of which it is supposed to be representative. An example would be the statement that in 1973 the average household contained 3.48 persons (Golenpaul, 1973). This, of course, would not indicate the size of any household. In instances such as this (i.e., one in which the mean is not representative because fractional amounts cannot occur), it probably would make most sense to round the mean to a whole number.

A more serious problem can exist when a set of data contains one or more extreme scores. The mean of such a set often is not representative. Suppose the language ages shown in Table 9.4 were earned by two groups, each consisting of five children. The only difference between the groups is the language age earned by the fifth child in each. The language age earned by the fifth child in Group II is considerably higher than that earned by any of the other children in this group. While the mean language age computed for the children in Group I would appear to be representative of those earned by the children in this group, this would not appear to be the case for Group II. The mean language age for this group is higher than that earned by four of the five children.

Another artifact that can occur when means are used is that the relationship between the means of sets of scores for a group of persons may not be representative of those between the scores in such sets for the majority of individuals in the group. Table 9.5, for example, shows two sets of scores and their means. While it would appear from these means that the stutterers tended to be more fluent following therapy, actually *only one of the five* was more fluent following therapy.

TABLE 9.4   Language Ages earned by two groups, each consisting of five children.

Mean Artifact

Group I	Group II
3.5 years	3.5 years
5.0 years	5.0 years
6.0 years	6.0 years
6.5 years	6.5 years
7.0 years	14.0 years
Mean = 5.6 years	Mean = 7.0 years

TABLE 9.5 Percentages of words stuttered by five clients before and after a period of therapy.

Stutterer	Percent before Therapy	Percent after Therapy
1	5.2	5.3
2	3.4	3.6
3	7.0	7.0
4	1.1	1.2
5	30.0	12.5
Mean	9.3	5.9

In summary, the mean is a very useful measure of central tendency, but it does have several limitations that you should be aware of both as a user and a consumer of statistics.

The next measure of central tendency that we will consider is the *median*. Except for the mean, it is probably the most frequently used such measure.

The median of a set is that measure which occurs at the midpoint of the set when they are ordered from lowest to highest (or from highest to lowest). The median, for example, of the following set of five measures would be 50.0:

25 26 50 60 200

If a set contains an *odd* number of measures, the computation of the median is straightforward. You merely identify the measure that occurs at the midpoint of the ordering. If a set contains an *even* number of measures, the determination of the median is a little more complex, since it involves an interpolation process. To illustrate this process, let us use the following set, which consists of six measures:

10 20 30 40 43 43

The median of this set would be 35, i.e., half the distance between the third and fourth measures.

The median can be used to answer such questions as those listed in the previous section that would be appropriate to answer through the use of the mean. It can also be used to answer questions similar to the following:

1. How many hours of therapy did the "typical" child receive?
2. What score falls at the 50th percentile for six-year-olds on a particular language test?

Note that to answer the first question it is necessary to identify the measure of the child at the center of the distribution, i.e., the child whose time in therapy is exceeded by that of 50 percent of the children. The second question was included to point out that *the median is the 50th percentile* and, therefore, the appropriate statistic for answering such questions.

The median can be computed from measures having ordinal, interval, or ratio properties. Thus, one difference between the mean and median is that the latter is appropriate for ordinal data.

The main disadvantage of the median as compared to the mean in instances where both would be appropriate concerns ease of computation. The mean is almost always less time-consuming than the median to compute.

Another variable on which mean and median differ is degree of stability. The mean tends to be a more stable (hence, more reliable) measure of central tendency than the median. A sample mean typically provides a more reliable estimate of a population mean than a sample median does of a population median. Partially for this reason, significance tests for differences between means tend to be more *powerful* than comparable tests between medians, and confidence intervals for means tend to be *narrower* than those for medians (significance tests and confidence intervals are discussed in Chapter 10).

One other possible limitation of the median in comparison to the mean is that it is relatively insensitive to extreme measures. Note that the median of all three of the following sets of measures is the same, i.e., 50:

5 19 50 75 80

15 40 50 55 60

15 25 50 75 1000

If for some reason you want your index of central tendency to be influenced by extreme measures, the mean probably would be a better choice than the median.

The final measure of central tendency we will consider is the *mode*. The mode of a set, or distribution, is the measure that occurs most frequently. The mode of the following set of 10 measures would be 7 since this is the value which occurs most often:

7 7 7 8 9 10 11 11 12 13

The mode can be used to answer such questions as the following:

1. What was the most typical (i.e., most frequently occurring) response of a person (or group) to a particular test task?
2. Is a stutterer's speech fluency most likely to improve, become worse, or stay the same after receiving a particular therapy?

While the reason the mode would be appropriate for answering the first question should be obvious, it may be less so for the second. The mode is appropriate for answering such questions as the second—i.e., "probability" questions—because the category most stutterers fall into (the modal category) designates the most probable outcome.

The mode is appropriate for measures having nominal, ordinal, interval, or ratio properties. It is the only measure of central tendency that can be used with nominal data.

The mode is generally regarded as a less stable (hence, less reliable) measure of central tendency than either the median or the mean. Partially for this reason, significance tests for data treated as nominal tend to be less powerful than those for data treated as ordinal, interval, or ratio (this concept is discussed in Chapter 10).

While the mean, median, and mode are the most frequently used measures of central tendency in speech and hearing research, they are not the only such measures. Two others are the geometric mean and the harmonic mean (Campbell, 1974, pp. 73–74). Since these measures have rarely been used in speech and hearing research (or for that matter in research in any behavioral science), they will not be described here.

Measures of Variability.   These indices designate the spread, dispersion, homegeneity, or variability of a set of numbers. They indicate how far the numbers in a set deviate from an index of central tendency computed for the set. The more they deviate, the larger the value of the index.

When the numbers in a set are measures of attributes of persons or behaviors, they provide information about the degree of variability of such attributes. In a sense, they provide information about the degree of representativeness of indices of central tendency. The less variable the measures in a set, the more representative would be any index of central tendency. Suppose five children who had a rare neuromuscular disorder and were approximately the same age earned the following scores on a test of articulation proficiency:

75 77 78 78 80

The median score would be 78. Since the other scores deviate little from the median, it would be quite representative of them. If, however, the scores earned by these children had been the following:

25 40 78 90 150

the median (which again is 78) would have deviated considerably from several of the scores and hence would not have been particularly representative of them.

There are three commonly used indices of variability: the range, the interquartile (or semi-interquartile) range, and the standard deviation. Computational formulas and worked examples for all are in Appendix A.

The *range* is a frequently used measure of variability. It is relatively simple to compute, since it is merely the difference between the highest and lowest measures in a set. In some instances, the highest and lowest measures are reported rather than the difference between them. In the example above, the articulation test scores could be reported as *ranging* from 25 to 150, rather than the *range* being reported as being 125 (i.e., $150 - 25 = 125$).

The range can be used to answer such questions as the following:

1. What was the age range of the clients receiving a particular therapy?
2. How variable was a client's stuttering frequency during a series of 10 telephone calls?

Note that the range can be used as an index of both intrasubject and intersubject variability.

The range is an appropriate index of variability for measures having ordinal, interval, or ratio properties. As such, it can provide information about the amount of deviation from both the mean and median of a set of measures.

The main advantages of the range are that it is relatively easy to compute and interpret. To compute it you only have to identify the highest and lowest measures in a set. Its interpretation is more "intuitive" (i.e., understandable to persons who are not highly trained in statistical methodology) than any of the other indices of variability.

The main disadvantage of the range is that it can make a set of measures appear more variable than they are. A single measure that is relatively large or small compared to the others can increase the magnitude of the range a great deal. Suppose a group of 10 children earned the following scores on a language test:

75 80 80 85 85 85 90 95 95 135

The range of these scores would be 60 points (i.e., $135 - 75 = 60$). Except for one score (i.e., 135) these measures are not very variable. If it were deleted, the range would only be 20 points (i.e., $95 - 75 = 20$). Thus, one relatively extreme score resulted in a 300 percent increase in the magnitude of the range. This limitation of the range sometimes can be partially compensated for by reporting it both with and without the extreme values. In the above example this could be done as follows: "While the children's scores on the language test ranged from 75 to 135, their performances were not as heterogeneous as this would suggest. Excluding the child who earned a score of 135, the range was from 75 to 95."

Because of the susceptibility of the range to distortion by a few extreme measures, various restricted ranges (i.e., ranges in which a certain percentage of the measures are ignored) have been developed. The two such ranges most frequently used in speech and hearing research are the *interquartile range* and the *semi-interquartile range*. Both are based on the middle 50 percent of measures—i.e., the highest 25 percent and the lowest 25 percent are ignored. The relationship between them is that the semi-interquartile range is equal to the interquartile range divided by two. For the 10 language scores, the interquartile range would be 15 (i.e., 95 $-80 = 15$); the semi-interquartile range, 7.5.

The interquartile and semi-interquartile ranges can be used to answer questions such as the following:

    1. How well do speech-language pathologists agree when rating speech segments from persons who have cleft palates for degree of nasality?

    2. Do children's scores of Form A of a language test tend to be more variable than on Form B?

    3. Within what range of scores do the 25th and 75th percentiles fall for six-year-olds on a particular test of language performance?

Note that both ranges indicate the degree of separation between the 25th and 75th percentiles, i.e., they describe the variability of the middle 50 percent of measures.

The interquartile and semi-interquartile ranges are appropriate indices of variability for measures having ordinal, interval, or ratio properties. In this regard they are similar to the range. Since they are appropriate for measures with ordinal properties, they can provide an index of the dispersion of measures around the median.

The main advantage of these indices over the range is that they are not susceptible to distortion by a few extreme measures. They are therefore more *stable* indices of variability than the range. Their main disadvantage when compared to the range is that they are not as easily interpretable. While the interpretation of the range is relatively straightforward, even for someone with little or no statistical training, both interquartile and semi-interquartile ranges may be somewhat difficult to interpret even for someone who has had statistical training. This is particularly true for the interpretation of their absolute magnitudes (e.g., What do an interquartile range of 15 or a semi-interquartile range of 7.5 "mean"?). The interpretation of their relative magnitudes, however, may be straightforward (e.g., a set of scores with an interquartile range of 15 is less variable than one with an interquartile range of 30). For an illustration and application of this strategy for interpreting these indices, see Silverman, 1967b.

Another *possible* limitation of both the interquartile and semi-interquartile ranges is that they do not reflect the variability of all measures in a set, only the middle 50 percent. This is most likely to be a limitation in instances where it is necessary to describe the absolute (as opposed to the relative) variability of the measures in a set.

The final index of variability we will describe here, the *standard deviation*, does not have this limitation. It reflects the variability of all measures in a set. It also has an advantage over the range in that its magnitude is less likely to be distorted by a few extreme measures (assuming that the number of measures is relatively large). Partially for these reasons, the standard deviation has been the most frequently used measure of variability in speech, language, and hearing research.

The *magnitude* of a standard deviation indicates the degree of variability of the measures from which it was computed. The larger the standard deviation, the more variable the measures. The smallest possible standard deviation is 0, which, of course, indicates no variability. There is no upper limit on its size, or magnitude.

If the measures in a set are *normally distributed* (which is often the case for scores on standardized tests such as intelligence tests), the percentage, or proportion, of the population which deviates a given number of *standard deviation units* from the mean of that set can be estimated. The normal distribution is a symmetrical bell-shaped curve in which certain relationships hold regarding its height at specified distances from its center (see Figure 9.1). In a normal distribution, for example, approximately 68 percent of the measures are within one standard deviation of the mean. If the scores on a test that has a mean of 100 points and a standard deviation of 15 points are normally distributed, approximately 68 percent of persons from the population on which the test was standardized will have scores between 85 to 115.

The standard deviation can be used to answer such questions as the following:

1. How variable are the scores on a particular diagnostic test?
2. What range of scores would constitute "normal limits" on a particular diagnostic test (assuming that scores on this test are normally distributed)?
3. How far, on the average, did a person's thresholds for a 100 Hz tone deviate from this mean threshold for this tone? (The assumption is made here that this threshold was measured a number of times. Another way to ask the same question would be: "How representative was a person's mean threshold for 1000 Hz tone of those that were obtained on repeated testing?")

FIGURE 9.1   The normal curve, or distribution. The vertical line at the center designates the position of the mean, median, and mode, which are identical in this distribution. The other two vertical lines designate positions that are one standard deviation from the mean. Note that approximately 68 percent of the area under the curve falls between these two vertical lines.

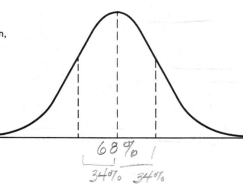

The first question illustrates the use of the standard deviation as a measure of variability. The second illustrates its use in estimating proportions of the population whose scores (or other measures) fall within certain limits. If you defined the lower boundary of "normal limits" on a particular test as that score that is equaled or exceeded by 90 percent of eight-year-olds, you could use the standard deviation to estimate that score. The third question illustrates its use in assessing the representativeness of the mean. The smaller the standard deviation (i.e., the less the average deviation of the scores from their mean), the more representative the mean.

The standard deviation is an appropriate index of variability for measures having interval or ratio properties. It is the most frequently used such index for the dispersion of measures around the mean.

The main *advantages* of the standard deviation over other indices of variability are: (1) it reflects the dispersion of all the measures in a set, and (2) it is the most stable index of variability and hence the most reliable such index. Also, if scores (or other measures) are normally distributed, the standard deviation provides more information about them than other indices of variability do.

The main *disadvantage* of the standard deviation as an index of variability is the same as that mentioned for the interquartile and semi-interquartile ranges. Unless measures are normally distributed, the *absolute* magnitude of their standard deviation may be difficult to interpret. To know that a set of measures that are not normally distributed has a standard deviation of 3.5 provides little information regarding their dispersion.

While the absolute magnitudes of standard deviations may be difficult to interpret, their *relative* magnitudes frequently provide useful information. If the means of the scores earned by two groups on a test of language functioning were approximately the same, but the standard deviations of their scores were quite different, this would indicate that the persons in one of the groups were more heterogeneous in their performance on this test than those in the other group.

The range, interquartile range, semi-interquartile range, and standard deviation are the only indices of variability used often enough in speech, language, and hearing research to be worth mentioning.

Measures of Association. These indices are used to describe the strength and direction of the relationships between sets of measures (these attributes of relationships are described in Chapter 6). They indicate how the attributes described by such sets of measures are related to each other, i.e., correlated. The numbers that are yielded by such indices are referred to as *correlation coefficients.* Computational formulas and worked examples for several types of correlation coefficients are in Appendix A.

Correlation coefficients typically provide several kinds of information about the relationships between the sets of numbers correlated. First, they provide information about the *strength* of the relationship between the attributes measured by such sets. The larger the correlation coefficient (i.e., the closer it is to 1.00), the stronger the relationship. The smaller the correlation coefficient (i.e., the closer it is to 0), the weaker the relationship. (If the correlation coefficient is 0, there is no relationship.)

Suppose you administered a test of auditory discrimination ability and a test of articulation proficiency to a kindergarten class and correlated the two sets of scores earned by the children on these tests. If the resulting correlation coefficient was 0.60, this would suggest that auditory discrimination ability and articulation proficiency were more closely associated, or related, for these children than would have been the case if the resulting correlation coefficient had been, for example, 0.15. The strength of this relationship, however, would *not* have been four times as great if the coefficient had been 0.60 rather than 0.15. Correlation coefficients have *ordinal* properties. Thus, a correlation coefficient of 0.50 indicates a greater degree of association than one of 0.30 and a lesser degree than one of 0.90.

Correlation coefficients may also provide a second kind of information about the relationships between sets of measures: the *direction* of the relationships between attributes measured by pairs of such sets. The direction of this kind of relationship can be either *positive* or *negative.* If it is positive, persons who tend to exhibit relative high (or low) levels of one of the attributes tend to exhibit corresponding levels of the other. Thus, height and weight are positively correlated (i.e., the taller a person is, the more he or she tends to weigh).

If the relationship between two attributes is negative, persons who tend to exhibit relatively high (or low) levels of one of the attributes tend to exhibit opposite levels of the other. Thus, chronological age and number of articulation errors is negatively correlated for elementary-school children (i.e., the older an elementary-school child, the fewer articulation errors he or she is likely to have). If a correlation coefficient is preceded by a minus sign, the relationship between the attributes correlated is negative.

Correlation coefficients usually range between -1.00 and $+1.00$. A correlation coefficient larger than 1.00 is impossible.

The correlation coefficients that are described in detail in this section and dealt with in Appendix A (i.e., the contingency coefficient, phi coefficient, Spearman rank-order coefficient, and Pearson product-moment correlation coefficient) are for assessing the association between pairs of attributes. While the most frequently used indices of association are of this type, they are not the only ones. Several other types—including multiple correlation and partial correlation—will be dealt with briefly at the end of this section.

The first measure of association we will describe is the *contingency coefficient.* It is an index of the degree of relationship, or association, between two attributes of events that had been assigned on the basis of these attributes to the cells of a contingency table. This is a table that contains two or more rows and two or more columns. The numbers of rows and columns do *not* have to be the same. Thus, a contingency table could have two rows and five columns, or five rows and two columns, or five rows and five columns, or two rows and two columns, and so on. (An example of a two-row and two-column contingency table is presented in Appendix A in the section on the contingency coefficient.)

The number of columns (or number of rows) in a contingency table is determined by the number of categories into which the scale for an attribute is divided, or segmented. For the attribute "biological sex," the scale would typically be divided into two categories: male and female. For the attribute "type of speech disorder," the scale could be divided into the following four categories: phonation, articulation, resonance, and fluency.

While the scales for attributes mentioned thus far have been nominal, those representing any level of measurement can be used in contingency tables. An example of an attribute with ordinal properties that could be used in such tables would be "grade level." The categories into which the scale for this attribute could be divided would include "first grade," "second grade," "third grade," and so on.

To illustrate the application of contingency tables and contingency coefficients, suppose you wished to determine whether the number of words repeated by elementary-school children tended to be related to their grade level. That is, you wished to determine whether older elementary-school children tended to repeat words less frequently than younger elementary-school children or vice versa. One approach you could use would be to determine the frequency of word repetitions per 100 words spoken by 10 first graders and 10 sixth graders and then compute the median word repetition frequency for the 20 first and sixth graders combined. Each of the 20 children would then be assigned to one of the four cells of a contingency table on the basis of: (1) whether he or she was a first or sixth grader, and (2) whether his or her word repetition frequency fell at or below the median or above the median. Three possible results from this assignment are depicted in Table 9.6. The configuration of A suggests a *strong positive* relationship between word repetition frequency and grade level; the 10 sixth graders all had higher word repetition frequencies than the 10 first graders. The configuration of B suggests *no* relationship between grade level and word repetition frequency; the sixth graders' word repetition frequencies exhibited no tendency to be systematically higher or lower than those of the first graders. The configuration of C, on the other hand, suggests a *strong negative* relationship between grade level and word repetition frequency; the 10 first graders all had higher word repetition frequencies than the 10 sixth graders. In most "real world" research, the relationships (or lack of them) would not be as clear-cut as those depicted in Table 9.6.

The procedure for computing the contingency coefficient is outlined in Appendix A. This procedure is applicable to a contingency table of any size.

TABLE 9.6   Three possible results from the assignment of 20 children to the cells of a contingency table on the basis of their word repetition frequencies and grade levels.

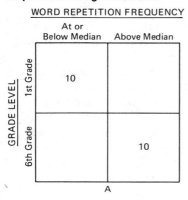

coefficient = .71

The contingency coefficient is zero when no relationship, or association, exists between the two variables. If the relationship between them is perfect (e.g., as depicted in parts A and C of Table 9.6), the value of the contingency coefficient will approach, but not equal, 1.00. How close it will come to 1.00 is a function of the size of the table; the larger the table, the closer it will come to 1.00. For a 2 × 2 table (which is the size of the tables in Table 9.6), the upper limit of the contingency coefficient is 0.71.

The nature of the relationship between the variables in a contingency table (i.e., positive or negative) has to be inferred from the configuration of the table, since it is impossible for a contingency coefficient to have a minus value. Thus, a contingency coefficient of 0.60 can indicate either a positive or a negative relationship between the attributes.

The contingency coefficient can be used to answer such questions as:

1. Is there a relationship between school grade and word repetition frequency for elementary-school children?

2. Is the acceptability of an electrolarynx associated with the socioeconomic level of the person who is laryngectomized?

A contingency table that could be used to answer the first question has
already been described (see Table 9.6). One that could be used to answer the
second question is presented in Table 9.7. Obviously, socioeconomic status
could have been categorized in other ways in this table.

The contingency coefficient can be computed from measures having
nominal, ordinal, interval, or ratio properties. It is the only measure of association that can be used with nominal data in contingency tables larger than
2 × 2.

While the contingency coefficient is a very useful index for assessing
degree of association in contingency tables larger than 2 × 2, it does have
several limitations. First, it is somewhat difficult to interpret because its upper limit is less than 1.00. Thus, a contingency coefficient of 0.70 could indicate either a perfect relationship or a fairly strong relationship between the
attributes, depending on the size of the contingency table.

A second possible limitation of this index is that contingency coefficients cannot be compared unless they are yielded by tables of the same size,
since the upper limits of contingency coefficients are a function of the sizes
of tables on which they are computed. Thus, a contingency coefficient of
0.70 for a 2 × 2 table would indicate a higher degree of association in between the attributes than one of 0.75 on a 3 × 3 table (the upper limit for a
contingency coefficient on such a table would be 0.82).

A third possible limitation of the contingency coefficient as an index of

**TABLE 9.7   A contingency table for
studying the association between
acceptability of an electrolarynx and
socioeconomic status.**

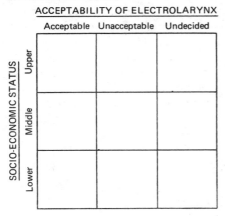

association, or correlation, is that its value is not directly comparable to those yielded by other such indices including the three dealt with in the computational appendix, i.e., the phi coefficient, the Spearman rank-order coefficient, and the Pearson product-moment correlation coefficient.

In summary, the contingency coefficient, in spite of its limitations, is a useful measure of association (or correlation) for contingency tables, particularly those larger than 2 × 2.

For contingency tables that are 2 × 2, an index of association that ordinarily would be preferable to the contingency coefficient is the *phi coefficient*. The phi coefficient has an upper limit of 1.00 (which would indicate a perfect relationship between the attributes), and the nature of the relationship between the attributes (positive or negative) is indicated by the sign of the coefficient. thus, in Table 9.6, the phi coefficient for A would be +1.00, for B would be 0.00, and for C would be −1.00. The phi coefficient is easier to interpret than the contingency coefficient, and its value is directly comparable to those yielded by the Spearman rank-order coefficient and the Pearson product-moment correlation coefficient. The coefficients yielded by these three indices on a given set of data, however, usually are not identical (a demonstration of this is provided in Appendix A, where all three were computed from the same set of data).

The procedure for computing the phi coefficient is outlined in Appendix A.

The phi coefficient can be used to answer the same types of questions as the contingency coefficient as long as the data can be cast into a 2 × 2 table.

The phi coefficient (like the contingency coefficient) can be computed from measures having nominal, ordinal, interval, or ratio properties. It is a particularly useful index of correlation between dichotomous attributes. (An example of a dichotomous attribute would be biological sex, which consists of the categories "male" and "female.")

The advantages of the phi coefficient over the contingency coefficient as an index of association for 2 × 2 contingency tables already have been mentioned.

In summary, the phi coefficient is a useful index of association, particularly for measures having nominal properties. The phi coefficient and the contingency coefficient are the only such indices described here that are appropriate for measures having nominal properties.

If the measures of the attributes you wish to determine the relationship between have at least ordinal properties, the *Spearman rank-order coefficient* can be used as an index of association. This coefficient is an index of the extent to which two sets of measures *rank order* a group of persons in the same manner. If both rank order the persons in the identical manner, this would indicate a *perfect positive* relationship between them, and the Spearman rank-order coefficient would be +1.00. On the other hand, if they rank order the persons in exactly the opposite manner, this would indicate a *perfect negative* relationship between them, and the Spearman rank-order coefficient would be -1.00. Spearman rank-order coefficients for less than perfect relationships fall between -1.00 and $+100$.

The procedure for computing the Spearman rank-order coefficient is outlined in Appendix A.

Suppose that in order to determine whether any relationship existed between the degree of recovery exhibited by receptive aphasics and their socioeconomic level, you rank ordered five receptive aphasics both on the basis of the amount of recovery they exhibited and their socioeconomic level. Three possible sets of orderings of the five aphasics on the basis of these attributes are presented in Table 9.8. The Spearman rank-order coefficient for the first set would be $+1.00$, for the second approximately 0.00, and for the third -1.00. Thus, the first set would suggest a *strong positive* relationship between improvement level and socioeconomic level, the second essentially *no* relationship between these variables, and the third a *strong negative* relationship between them.

The Spearman rank-order coefficient can be used to answer questions similar to these:

1. Is the amount of recovery exhibited by receptive aphasics related to their socioeconomic level?
2. Do the levels of children's performances of two particular tests of language functioning tend to be similar?
3. How well do two speech-language pathologists agree in their orderings of clients with regard to degree of improvement following a program of therapy?

Using the Spearman rank-order coefficient to answer the first question has already been described. Answering the second question would involve ordering the children on the basis of the two sets of language scores. And answer-

TABLE 9.8 Three possible sets of orderings for five receptive aphasics based on their socioeconomic levels and the amount of improvement they exhibited. The aphasics are designated by the letters A, B, C, D, and E.

Set I		Set II		Set III	
Socioeconomic Level	Improvement Level	Socioeconomic Level	Improvement Level	Socioeconomic Level	Improvement Level
A	A	A	E	A	E
C	C	C	A	C	D
B	B	B	D	B	B
D	D	D	C	D	C
E	E	E	B	E	A

ing the third would involve ordering the clients on the basis of each speech-language pathologist's ratings of degree of improvement.

The Spearman rank-order coefficient can be computed from measures having ordinal, interval, or ratio properties. It has been one of the most frequently used indices of association for measures having ordinal properties in speech-language pathology and audiology research.

The Spearman rank-order coefficient provides a satisfactory index of the degree of correspondence (or correlation) between two rank orderings of a group of persons. Thus, it is appropriate for measures having ordinal properties. While it is also appropriate for measures having interval or ratio properties, it has a limitation when used with such measures. This limitation is that the Spearman rank-order coefficient is insensitive to the sizes, or magnitudes, of the differences between measures. It is not possible with this procedure to detect the form of the relationship between a pair of attributes—i.e., whether the form is linear or nonlinear (see Figures 6.2, 6.5, and 6.6 and accompanying text for descriptions of linear and nonlinear relationships). To answer some questions, you must be able to determine whether the relationship between a pair of attributes is linear or nonlinear; to answer others, this information is not necessary. For answering questions of the second type, the Spearman rank-order coefficient would be satisfactory.

If the measures of the attributes you wish to determine the relationship between have interval or ratio properties and the relationship between them can be assumed to be linear (see Chapter 6), an index of association you can use for assessing this relationship is the *Pearson product-moment correlation coefficient*. This coefficient, which is also known as the *Pearson r*, is probably the most frequently used index of association (or correlation) in speech-language pathology and audiology research.

The Pearson *r* can be visualized, or interpreted, in several ways. First, it can be viewed as an index of how closely two sets of measures rank order a group of persons. Its magnitude is determined in large part by the extent to which the rank orderings are similar. As long as the relationship between a pair of attributes is not grossly nonlinear, the magnitude of the Pearson *r* will be quite similar to that of the Spearman rank-order coefficient.

The Person *r* also can be visualized as an index of the amount of deviation of the points in a scattergram (see Chapter 6) from the straight line from which they would deviate least. The more the points deviate from this line, the smaller will be the value of the Pearson *r*. If the points all lay on the line, the Pearson *r* would be $+1.00$ or -1.00. If the deviation of the points about such a line looked circular (i.e., if their deviation from this line was considerable), the Pearson *r* would be approximately 0.00. Scattergrams that depict these possibilities are presented in Figures 6.2 and 6.3.

The Pearson *r* is similar to the phi coefficient and Spearman rank-order coefficient in two ways: (1) its possible values fall between -1.00 and $+1.00$, and (2) the closer its value to $+1.00$ or -1.00, the stronger the association between the attributes.

The procedure for computing the Pearson r is outlined Appendix A. The Pearson r can be used to answer questions similar to these:

1. What is the nature of the relationship between preschoolers' auditory discrimination ability and their articulation proficiency?
2. To what extent are first graders' levels of performance on a particular test prior to participating in a therapy program *predictive* of their levels of performance on that test after completing the program?

Note that answering the first question involves assessing the relationship between performances of *different* tasks by a group of persons at the *same* point in time, and answering the second question involves assessing the relationship between performances of the *same* tasks by a group of persons at *different* points in time.

Strictly speaking, the Pearson r is only an appropriate index of association for measures having interval or ratio properties. Nevertheless, in speech-language pathology and audiology research, it has been used a great deal with measures that appear to have ordinal properties. Examples of such measures would be scores on tests of auditory discrimination ability and articulation proficiency. In most instances, probably no great harm is done if the Pearson r is used with measures that have ordinal properties. When it is used with such measures, the magnitude of a Pearson r can be interpreted as an *approximation* of what the coefficient describing the relationship would have been if the Spearman rank-order coefficient had been used.

To estimate the relative strength of the relationship indicated by a Pearson r, the *square* of its value (rather than its value) should be used. Squaring a Pearson r results in a reduction in its magnitude (except when its value is 1.00). The extent of this reduction can be surmised from Table 9.9, in which r^2 magnitudes are presented for selected r values. Note that a Pearson r of at least 0.70 is needed before even 50 percent of the variation observed in a scattergram can be accounted for on the basis of a linear relationship between the attributes. In fact, a Pearson r of 0.50 is needed before even 25

TABLE 9.9 r^2 **magnitudes for selected Pearson r values.**

r	r^2	r	r^2
0.05	0.00	0.55	0.30
0.10	0.01	0.60	0.36
0.15	0.02	0.65	0.42
0.20	0.04	0.70	0.49
0.25	0.06	0.75	0.56
0.30	0.09	0.80	0.64
0.35	0.12	0.85	0.72
0.40	0.16	0.90	0.81
0.45	0.20	0.95	0.90
0.50	0.25	1.00	1.00

percent of the variation observed in a scattergram can be accounted for on the basis of a linear relationship between the attributes.

How would you describe in words the strength of the relationship depicted by a particular Pearson *r*? While there is no universality of agreement among statisticians regarding strengths of relationships designated by particular Pearson *r* values, some rough guidelines exist, with which most statisticians probably would agree, that can be used for making such judgements including the following:

1. Pearson *r* coefficients of less than 0.30 usually indicate that for most *practical* purposes *no* linear relationship exists between the attributes.
2. Pearson *r* coefficients between 0.30 and 0.50 usually indicate a *weak* linear relationship between the attributes.
3. Pearson *r* coefficients between 0.51 and 0.85 usually indicate a *moderate* linear relationship between the attributes.
4. Pearson *r* coefficients between 0.86 and 0.95 usually indicate a *strong* linear relationship between the attributes.
5. Pearson *r* coefficients higher than 0.96 usually indicate an *extremely strong* linear relationship between the attributes.

In summary, the Pearson *r* is an extremely useful index of association between pairs of attributes when the measures of such attributes have interval or ratio properties and the relationship between them is fairly linear. It provides information concerning the strength, direction, and linearity of the relationship between pairs of attributes.

The indices of association described in this section are representative of a fairly large number of indices for assessing relationships between pairs of attributes that have been developed by mathematical statisticians. Descriptions of other such indices can be found in elementary and intermediate statistics texts intended for psychologists and sociologists.

Indices of association are not limited to describing the relationships between pairs of attributes when the relationship between the attributes is presumed to be linear. There are indices of association for other purposes or types of data, including the following:

1. *Indices of Association between Pairs of Attributes Where the Relationships between the Attributes are Presumed to be Nonlinear.* These indices can be used to answer the same kinds of questions that could be answered by means of a Pearson *r* if the relationship between the attributes were linear. To determine whether it would be most reasonable to assume that the relationship between two attributes were linear or nonlinear, you can plot the measures you made of them on a scattergram. If the line that best fits the configuration of the points does not appear to be a straight line, it might be safest to assume that the relationship between the attributes is nonlinear (a scattergram in which a nonlinear relationship exists between attributes is presented in Figure 6.5).

These indices assess the goodness of fit of the points plotted in a scattergram to various types of curved lines.

If you feel the relationship between a pair of attributes is nonlinear, show the scattergram to a statistician. He or she should be able to recommend an appropriate nonlinear correlation coefficient.

2. Indices of Association between Pairs of Attributes with the Effects of a Third Attribute Held Constant, or Eliminated.   Indices used for this purpose are referred to as coefficients of *partial correlation*. Suppose you wished to determine whether a relationship existed between auditory discrimination ability and articulation proficiency for the children in a kindergarten classroom. It is conceivable that there could appear to be a relationship between the two because both are related to mental age. The higher the mental age of a child, the better the child is likely to do on both tasks. You may therefore wish to answer the question: "Would there be any relationship between auditory discrimination ability and articulation proficiency if the effects of mental age were eliminated (i.e., held constant)?" Coefficients of partial correlation can be used to answer this type of question. See Shriberg and Kwiatkowski (1982) for an example of how coefficients of partial correlation can be used.

3. Indices of Association between an Attribute and the Composite of Two or More Other Attributes.   These indices are referred to as coefficients of *multiple correlation*. Suppose you wanted to identify the attributes of speaking behavior which influence judgments of stuttering severity. One approach would be to have speech samples from a number of stutterers rated for "degree of stuttering severity" by the method of direct magnitude-estimation (see Chapter 8). These samples would also be analyzed to determine the amounts of various attributes each possesses which might influence listeners' impressions of stuttering severity. Such attributes probably would include frequency of stuttering, average duration of moments of stuttering, and speaking rate. The composite of these three attributes would then be correlated with the ratings of stuttering severity by means of a coefficient of multiple correlation. If this coefficient were quite high (i.e., larger than 0.85), this would suggest that these attributes are likely to influence listeners' judgments of stuttering severity. For illustrations of the use of multiple correlation in speech and hearing research, see Young (1961), Katt and Sprague (1981), Shriberg and Kwiatkowski (1982), and Gelfand et al. (1983).

Programs for indices of multiple correlation are available at most computer centers. The statistical consultant should be able to advise you about which program is most appropriate for your purpose. The consultant should also be able to help you interpret the results of the computer analysis.

4. Indices of Association between More than Two Sets of Measures.
To answer a question, it is sometimes necessary to assess the degree of association,

or agreement, between a number of sets of measures. This need arises most often in speech and hearing research when an investigator wishes to determine how well a group of judges agree in their ratings of a set of stimuli. Suppose you wanted to determine how well the three agreed in their ratings of the children. Several indices of association could be used for this purpose. The Kendall coefficient of concordance (Siegel, 1956) would be appropriate if the ratings were assumed to be ordinal; the intraclass correlation coefficient (Ebel, 1951) would be appropriate if they were assumed to have interval or ratio properties.

Graphical Displays

Such displays are used frequently by speech-language pathologists and audiologists for organizing quantitative data. There are several types including line graphs, bar graphs, pie graphs, and column graphs. In *line graphs*, the scale for one attribute is presented on the horizontal (X) axis and the scale for the second on the vertical (Y) axis (see Figure 9.2). Each event is plotted at the point that would correspond to its value for the attributes. If its value for the first attribute was 3 and the second was 2, it would be plotted at the point indicated in Figure 9.2.

Several types of line graphs are often used by speech-language pathologists and audiologists. One of these, the *scattergram*, already has been described in considerable detail (see Chapter 6). Another used by both speech-

FIGURE 9.2 A line graph with one point plotted. After all the points were plotted, they would be connected.

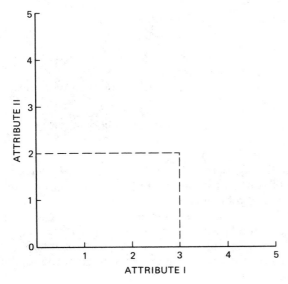

language pathologists and audiologists is the *pure-tone audiogram*. A third, which is frequently used by behaviorally oriented clinicians (particularly those who utilize operant conditioning), plots the frequency of occurrence of a specified behavior (or behaviors) over time. In Figure 9.2, *Attribute I* would be a time measure (e.g., seconds, minutes, hours, days, or weeks), and *Attribute II* would be frequency of occurrence (on a specified task or during a specified time period). Numerous examples of line graphs can be found in almost any volume of the *Journal of Speech and Hearing Research*.

Line graphs can be used to answer such questions as:

1. What is the nature of the relationship between number of articulation errors and chronological age?
2. What are a person's thresholds for pure tones of various frequencies?
3. What is the effect of response-contingent reinforcement on a particular behavior over a period of time?

The types of graphical displays that could be used for answering questions one through three respectively would be a scattergram, a pure-tone audiogram, and a behavior chart.

Line graphs can be used for organizing measures with ordinal, interval, ratio, or logarithmic properties.

A second type of graphical display that has been used by speech-language pathologists and audiologists for organizing and summarizing data is the *bar graph* (see Figure 9.3). These are similar to line graphs in that the scale for one attribute is presented on the horizontal axis and the scale for the second on the vertical axis (see Figure 9.3). Each event is depicted by a bar the length of which indicates its value on the horizontal scale. Thus, in Figure 9.3, the mean number of interjections per 100 words was approximately 2.0 for the nonstutterers and 3.0 for the stutterers.

Bar graphs can be used for answering questions such as:

1. Do stutterers differ from nonstutterers with regard to how likely they are to revise (i.e., correct their speaking errors)?
2. Do stutterers tend to repeat phrases as frequently as they repeat words?

Both questions can be answered using the data in Figure 9.3.

Bar graphs, like line graphs, can be used for organizing data with ordinal, interval, ratio, or logarithmic properties. They also can be used for organizing data with nominal properties.

A third type of graphical display that has been used by speech-language pathologists and audiologists to summarize data is the *pie graph* (see Figure 9.4). These depict the percentage of total events that fall into each of a series of categories (see Figure 9.4). Each category is represented by a "wedge" of pie: the higher the percentage of total events that fall into a particular category, the larger the "wedge." Thus, in Figure 9.4, the "wedge" for interjections is larger than that for revisions because a higher percentage of the total disfluencies were interjections.

FIGURE 9.3   A representative bar graph.

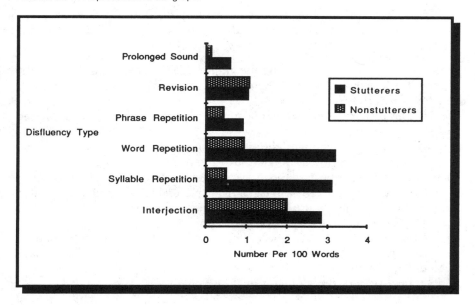

FIGURE 9.4   A representative pie graph.

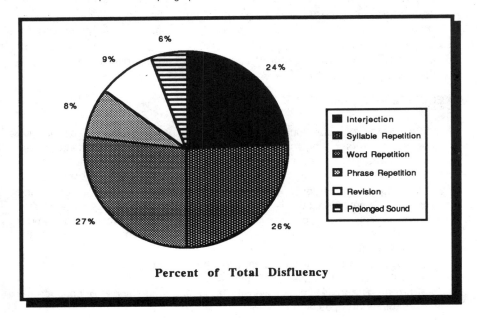

Pie graphs can be used for answering questions such as:

1. What types of disfluency tend to occur most often?
2. Do stutterers differ from nonstutterers with regard to the relative frequency of occurrence of various disfluency types?

The first could be answered using the graph in Figure 9.4. For answering the second it would be necessary to have two such graphs, one for stutterers and one for nonstutterers.

Pie graphs are used mainly for organizing data having nominal properties—e.g., frequency counts.

A fourth type of graphical display, the *column graph*, is identical to the bar graph except that everything is rotated 90 degrees—i.e., the bars are vertical rather than horizontal. It can be used for answering similar questions and for organizing data having the same properties. Bar graphs are preferable to column graphs when the categories on one axis are defined by words or phrases (see Figure 9.3). The reason is that it is unnecessary to rotate the graph to read them.

While these are not the only types of graphs that have been used by speech-language pathologists and audiologists, they are the ones that have been utilized by them most often. Others they have used include area charts and various types of three-dimensional displays.

Just as computers are useful tools for doing statistical analyses of numerical data, they are also useful tools for preparing graphs from such data. There are programs for most microcomputers that will draw any of the types of graphs mentioned in this section. These sometimes are referred to as presentation graphics or business graphics programs. Figures 9.3 and 9.4, for example, were drawn using the presentation graphics *Microsoft Chart* program (Lambert, 1984) on an Apple Macintosh computer.

For further information about the analysis and interpretation of graphical displays, see the chapter by Parsonson and Baer (1978).

EXERCISES AND DISCUSSION TOPICS

1. There are 23 computational exercises in Appendix A. The first 10 provide experience in computing most of the descriptive statistics mentioned in this chapter. Your instructor will tell you which to do and whether to do them with a calculator, a computer (with a statistical program package), or both.

2. The interpretation of descriptive statistics and graphical displays for answering questions is not "objective"—it is based on human judgment. Often a set of data can be interpreted to support several different answers to a question. Justify *both* a "yes" and a "no" answer to each of the following questions using the numerical or graphical data provided.

   a. Do stutterers exhibit the adaptation effect during a series of 15 consecutive readings of a passage? (The adaptation effect is the tendency for stutterers to become progressively more fluent during a series of consecutive readings of a passage.)

Observational Procedures. Ten adult stutterers each read a passage 15 times, one after the other. Their frequency of disfluency on each reading of the passage was determined.

Data. The mean frequency of disfluency on each of the 15 readings of the passage is presented graphically in Figure 9.5.

b. Do receptive aphasics tend to benefit from the *X* therapy program?

Observational Procedures. Ten receptive aphasics are administered the *Peabody Picture Vocabulary Test* (PPVT) both before and after participating in the *X* therapy program.

Data. The "before" and "after" PPVT scores for the 10 receptive aphasics are the following:

SUBJECT NUMBER	"BEFORE" PPVT SCORE	"AFTER" PPVT SCORE
1	40	39
2	79	79
3	25	20
4	50	51
5	15	12
6	15	90
7	75	73
8	65	65
9	38	36
10	48	49
MEAN	45	51

FIGURE 9.5 Frequency of disfluency on each of the 15 readings of the passage.

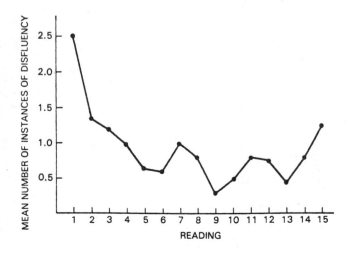

3. Why is knowledge of descriptive statistics important for evaluating therapy outcome research reports?

4. Which of the approaches mentioned in this chapter are usable for organizing qualitative and quantitative data in clinical evaluation reports?

10

Organizing Data for Answering Questions: Inferential Techniques

The statistical techniques discussed thus far are intended for summarizing, organizing, or describing aspects of a set of measures. They allow you to make statements and answer questions about a set of measures you have obtained.

Inferential statistical techniques allow you to answer several kinds of questions about a set of data that go beyond the analyses that were made of it. One such category of questions pertains to the *reliability* of differences or relationships observed in a set of data. Suppose you found that a group of children, on the average, made fewer articulation errors after participating in an experimental therapy program than before participating in it. This finding would allow you to answer the question: "Did the children in the experimental therapy program improve?" It would not by itself, however, permit you to answer the question: "If some other children similar to these children went through this experimental program, is it likely they also would improve?" The reason you could not answer this question is that the reliability of the difference between pre- and posttherapy measures would be uncertain. These measures would be unlikely to be identical even if the program had no effect. In fact, assuming the therapy had no effect, the children would stand a 50 percent chance of having the difference between their pre- and posttherapy measures suggest that it had an effect merely on the basis of "chance," or random fluctuation. The reason for the 50 percent chance is that there are only two outcomes possible here, both of which are equally likely—i.e., posttherapy measures "better" than pretherapy ones or vice versa. Before concluding, therefore, that an observed difference between pre- and posttherapy measures could have resulted from participating in a therapy program, it would be necessary to determine the likelihood that it could have resulted from random fluctuation. *Significance tests*, which are an aspect of statistical inference, can be used to estimate the probability that observed differences between means or medians (or other descriptive statistics) resulted from chance, or random fluctuation. These tests *do not* tell you whether an observed difference arose from this source, only the probability that it did so. Significance tests are described in the next section of this chapter, and computational formulas and worked examples for representative ones are in Appendix A.

Significance tests also can be used for assessing the reliability of observed *relationships*. Just as a difference between pretherapy and posttherapy measures would be unlikely to be zero if a therapy program had no effect, a correlation coefficient would be unlikely to be zero if there was no relationship between the attributes described by the measures correlated. By chance, a correlation coefficient can have a value between 0.01 and 1.00. Significance tests can be used for estimating the probability that nonzero correlation coefficients resulted from chance, or random fluctuation.

Another type of question that inferential statistical techniques allow you to answer concerns the *generality* of differences and relationships you observe in a set of data. Specifically, they allow you to answer the question: "How likely is it that the differences or relationships (or both) that I have observed in the sample of persons I've studied also are present in the *population* from which these persons were selected?" Suppose you developed a therapy program that seemed to be very effective for modifying some aspect of the communicative behavior of persons in your caseload, based on differences between the means (or medians) of measures made of this aspect of their communicative behavior both before and after they participated in the program. While the difference you observed would permit you to conclude that the program appeared to be effective for the average or typical person in your caseload on which it was used, it would not permit you to conclude it also would be effective for persons like them not in your caseload. Significance tests provide you with a way of estimating how safe you would be in concluding that differences or relationships you observed in a *sample* of persons also are present in the *population* to which these persons belong (assuming that your sample was *randomly selected* from this population). It should be noted, however, that such tests only indicate the likelihood that a difference or relationship observed in a sample is present in the population from which it comes. They do *not* provide an estimate of the *magnitude* of the difference or relationship in the population. You *cannot* assume that the magnitude of a difference or relationship present in a sample is a good estimate of that in the population from which the sample comes. This magnitude in the population may be considerably smaller or larger than that in the sample.

A third type of question that inferential statistical techniques allow you to answer pertains to estimating population values, or magnitudes, of descriptive statistics and of differences between descriptive statistics. Once you have established with a significance test that a difference or relationship in your sample is likely to be present in the population from which your sample was selected, you may wish to estimate the magnitude of the difference or the strength of the relationship in this population. Also, you may wish to estimate indices of central tendency and variability for it. Confidence intervals allow you to make such estimates. They will be described in some detail later in this chapter.

A fourth type of question that inferential statistical techniques help you to answer deals with inferences that are not related to population values of descriptive statistics. These include inferences about factors that influence a particular judgment (e.g., degree of nasality) or performance on a particular task (e.g., an aphasia test) or most reliably allow us to distinguish between groups (e.g., children who are normally disfluent and children who are beginning to stutter). Inferential statistical techniques for answering such questions are described at the end of the chapter.

SIGNIFICANCE TESTS

These statistics can be used for answering the following question: "How likely is it that a difference or relationship observed in a set of data is the result of chance, or random fluctuation?" The differences referred to could be between almost any types of measures including means, medians, modes, frequencies, percentages, proportions, standard deviations, and correlation coefficients. The relationships referred to involve correlation coefficients.

What does the chance, or random fluctuation, estimated by significance tests refer to? The most direct way to answer this question is through the use of probability theory. The basic point here is that measures that are not different or related can appear to be different or related. Suppose you had a stutterer perform a speaking task in two situations, and she stuttered on 10 percent of the words she spoke in Situation I and 13 percent of those she spoke in Situation II. Would it be safe to conclude that she tends to stutter more frequently in Situation II than in Situation I? The answer to this question would be no, because this outcome would occur by chance approximately 50 percent of the time. (We use the word *approximately* here because the two stuttering frequencies would be identical by chance a small percentage of the time.) For probability, the situation is analogous to tossing a coin. If you tossed a penny many times, approximately 50 percent of the time it would come up heads and approximately 50 percent of the time it would come up tails. A small percentage of time it may stand on edge, which would be analogous in our illustration to the two stuttering frequencies being identical.

Suppose you had the stutterer perform the speaking task a second time under the two conditions and the results were the same as the first time— i.e., she stuttered more frequently in Situation II than in Situation I. Would you then be able to conclude that she tends to stutter more frequently in Situation II than in Situation I? The approximate probability of this outcome being due to chance would be:

$$\frac{1}{2} \times \frac{1}{2} = \frac{1}{4}$$

While you would probably feel more confident concluding now than you would have after the first trial that she stutters more frequently in Situation II than in Situation I, the probability is still relatively high (i.e., one in four, or 25 percent) that the observed effect was due to chance, or random fluctuation. Most investigators would be unwilling to conclude that an observed effect (e.g., tending to stutter more frequently in one situation than another) was a "real" one unless the probability of its being due to chance was 5 percent or less. The probability that the observed difference between situations in our illustration was due to chance would be less than 5 percent if the stutterer stuttered more frequently in Situation II than in Situation I on five consecutive repetitions of the experimental task (i.e., speaking in two situations):

$$\frac{1}{2} \times \frac{1}{2} \times \frac{1}{2} \times \frac{1}{2} \times \frac{1}{2} = \frac{1}{32}$$

This outcome would only occur by chance approximately 3 percent of the time.

The above example illustrates the use of statistics for assessing the reliability of data when single subject designs are used. While using this procedure for estimating reliability with such designs is not controversial, using significance tests for this purpose is quite controversial, particularly in behavior-manipulation (e.g., operant conditioning) research (Levin, Marascuilo, and Hubert, 1978; Michael, 1974). Significance tests are not usually used for such research (McReynolds and Kearns, 1983; Tawney and Gast, 1984) and, consequently, journal editors do not ordinarily make their use a requirement for publication (as they do for research in which group designs are used). For further information about the use of significance tests with data from single subject designs see Edgington (1967, 1972, 1984), Gentile, Roden, and Klein (1972), Gottman (1981), Gottman and Glass (1978), Kratochwill (1978), Kratochwill and Brody (1978), Kratochwill and Levin (1980), Levin, Marascuilo, and Hubert (1978), Revusky (1967), and Rochon (1990).

Significance tests are the "tools" that are used most often in speech, language, and hearing research for determining whether the probability of an outcome being due to chance, or random fluctuation, is adequately small. They perform this function by estimating the likelihood of a *null hypothesis* being "true." Null hypotheses state that observed differences or relationships are due to chance, or random fluctuation. They state that if it were not for chance, or random fluctuation, the differences between the measures or the magnitudes of the correlation coefficients would have been 0.00. All significance tests have a single function—i.e., to determine the probability that null hypotheses are true. If the probability that a null hypothesis is true is small enough, it can be *rejected*. The investigator must decide before a significance test is "run" how small this probability has to be. The levels that are used most frequently for this purpose are 0.05 (5 percent probability of a null hypothesis being true) and 0.01 (1 percent probability of a null hypothesis being true). Obviously, the 0.01 level is more conservative than the 0.05 level since it is more difficult with it to reject a null hypothesis. The 0.05 level is sometimes selected for a study because by making it more likely that null hypotheses will be rejected it also makes it more likely that a report of the study will be accepted for publication—i.e., journals tend to view studies in which null hypotheses are rejected as being of greater value than those in which they are not (Greenwald, 1975).

In the statistical literature, the 1 percent level is referred to as the *0.01 level of confidence*, and the 5 percent level as the *0.05 level of confidence*. Thus, if a null hypothesis were rejected at the 0.01 level of confidence, it would be approximately 99 percent certain that the observed difference or relationship was not the result of chance, or random fluctuation.

Rejection of a null hypothesis only means that an observed difference or relationship is unlikely to have resulted from chance, or random fluctuation. It does not mean that it was due to the reason suggested by the experimenter in his or her *research hypothesis*. Often there is more than one possible explanation for an observed difference or relationship other than chance, or random fluctuation. Rejection of a null hypothesis provides no information about which such explanation is most viable. It only indicates that chance, or random fluctuation, is unlikely to be the explanation.

How do you decide on an explanation for an observed difference or relationship? Two approaches can be used: logical and logical-empirical. With a logical approach, you specify the possible explanations for a difference or relationship and, on the basis of the information that is available to you, decide which explanation (or combination of explanations) is most plausible. One obvious limitation of this approach is that the "real" explanation (or explanations) may not have occurred to you and hence would not have been among those you considered. Under this circumstance, the most plausible explanation would not be the most plausible explanation.

The logical-empirical approach goes one step beyond the logical approach. After the explanation for a difference or relationship that appears to be the most plausible is identified by a reasoning process, an experiment or a series of experiments is conducted to assess its viability. If the findings of the experiment or experiments are consistent with the explanation, you could have more confidence in its viability than if it were arrived at by a reasoning process alone.

Failure to reject a null hypothesis does *not* necessarily mean that the difference or relationship observed was the result of chance, or random fluctuation. There are at least two other possible explanations:

1. The difference or relationship was a real one, but because its magnitude was relatively small, the significance test was not *powerful* enough to detect it. The smaller a difference or weaker a relationship, the larger the number of subjects or observations needed to detect it, i.e., cause the null hypothesis to be rejected. While a significance test on the difference between the means of two groups, each consisting of 10 persons, may not lead to rejection of the null hypothesis, the same significance test on the difference between the same means could lead to this outcome if the groups consisted of 25 persons. For further discussion of this issue, see Lieber (1990).

2. The "real" difference or relationship (i.e., the one in the population) is larger in magnitude than the observed difference or relationship. By chance, subjects representing the extremes of the population distribution (or distributions) were not adequately represented in the sample. If the sample had been more representative, the difference between the means would have been larger, or the relationship stronger, and the null hypothesis would have been rejected.

Failure to reject a null hypothesis when it should be rejected is known as a *Type II error*. This is one of the two types of error that can occur in a decision on a null hypothesis. The other, a *Type I error*, occurs when a null hypothesis is rejected when it should not have been rejected—i.e., when the observed difference or relationship really was the result of chance, or random fluctuation.

A Type I error can occur for several reasons. First, on the basis of random fluctuation you will occasionally obtain a difference large enough, or a relationship strong enough, for a null hypothesis to be rejected. Thus, if a significance test were run at a 5 percent *alpha level* (i.e., a 0.05 level of confidence), the probability of the null hypothesis being rejected on the basis of chance alone would be 5 percent. You would expect 5 percent of the null hypotheses you test to be rejected when they should not be rejected—i.e., when they are true.

A Type I error may also occur because the measures on which a significance test is performed are biased. One of the most common sources of such bias is the investigator's expectations regarding the results of the research. Such expectations can consciously or unconsciously influence measurements. This is particularly apt to happen in therapy outcome research. Clinicians may feel such a strong need for their therapy to appear effective that they may unconsciously manipulate pre- and posttherapy measures so that the magnitude of the difference between them is increased. This could cause a true null hypothesis to be rejected.

Suppose that in order to assess the impact of a therapy program on a group of stutterers, you measured 25 aspects of their behavior both before and after participating in the program and tested the reliability of the difference between the means of each of these 25 pairs of measures at the 5 percent (i.e., 0.05) level of confidence. Suppose, further, that the difference between only one of these 25 sets of pre- and posttherapy means was *statistically significant*—i.e., was large enough for the null hypothesis to be rejected. Could you conclude that the behavior this measure measured had changed? The answer to this question is no, because you would expect approximately one out of every 20 true null hypotheses tested at the 0.05 level of confidence to be rejected. The probability of a Type I error having occurred when this null hypothesis was rejected is *not* 5 percent (the probability if only one null hypothesis had been tested) but *close to 100 percent*. It is necessary to consider the *experiment-wise error rate*, then, when interpreting the results of studies in which more than one null hypothesis is tested. The level of confidence at which a given null hypothesis is tested applies only if a single null hypothesis is tested. Otherwise, it is higher.

Many types of significance tests have been developed for testing null hypotheses. A representative sample of such tests is presented in Table 10.1. Computational formulas for them are in Appendix A. There is a test in this table that would be appropriate for most occasions when a speech-language pathologist or audiologist wished to assess the statistical significance of differences between sample means or medians. Some representative studies from

TABLE 10.1 Significance tests categorized on the basis of: (1) their level of measurement, (2) whether they are intended for independent or related samples, and (3) whether they are intended for the two-sample case or the more than two-sample case.

Level of Measurement	Two-Sample Case		More than Two-Sample Case	
	Related Samples	*Independent Samples*	*Related Samples*	*Independent Samples*
Nominal		Chi square		Chi square
Ordinal	Sign test	Mann-Whitney U test	Friedman two-way analysis of variance	Kruskal-Wallis one-way analysis of variance
Interval and Ratio	*t*-Test for related measures	*t*-Test for independent measures	One-way analysis of variance for dependent measures	One-way analysis of variance for independent measures

the communicative disorders literature in which the tests presented in Table 10.1 were used are listed in Table 10.2.

How do you identify an appropriate significance test? To do this, you need several pieces of information about the data on which the significance test is to be performed:

1. the level of measurement of the measures
2. whether the measures are independent or related
3. the number of means, medians, or other measures you wish to test the differences between

With this information, you can probably locate an appropriate significance test in Table 10.1.

The level of measurement of the measures refers to whether they possess nominal, ordinal, interval, or ratio properties (see Chapter 7). There are different significance tests for nominal, ordinal, and interval-ratio measures (see Table 10.1). The same significance tests are used for both interval and ratio measures. While is is permissible to use a significance test appropriate for a lower level of measurement than that present in the data, this is usually not done, because such a test would probably be less *powerful* than one appropriate for the level of measurement present in the data. (Nominal would be a lower level of measurement than ordinal, ordinal would be a lower level of measurement than interval, and so on.) One consequence of using a less powerful test is that more subjects (i.e., larger groups) are needed to detect differences of a given size—i.e., cause a false null hypothesis to be rejected at a given level of confidence. The less powerful the test you use, the more likely you are to commit a Type II error (i.e., retain a false null hypothesis).

Another piece of information you need about the data to select an appropriate significance test is whether the sets of measures which you wish to assess the difference (or differences) between are independent or related. If the sets of measures were made on the same persons, they are *related*. Thus, if you wished to assess the difference between measures made on a group of persons before and after participating in a therapy program, you would have to use a significance test appropriate for related measures.

If the sets of measures were made on different persons, they *usually* would be regarded as *independent*. Thus, if you wished to compare a group of persons who had spastic dysarthria to a group of persons who did not have spastic dysarthria on some measure, ordinarily you would have to use a significance test appropriate for independent measures. We use the qualifier *ordinarily* here because there is one circumstance when this would not be true. If the persons on whom the sets of measures were made were *very closely matched* for all relevant variables, the sets of measures could be treated as related. About the only time you can be reasonably confident that this level of matching has been achieved is when the persons in the group are

TABLE 10.2   Representative studies in the communicative disorders literature in which certain inferential statistics were used.

Statistic	References
Binomial test	Tomes and Shelton (1989)
Chi square	Townsend and Olson (1982); Daniloff et al. (1982); Holland (1982); Holland et al. (1989)
Confidence intervals	Bennett and Weatherby (1982); Hirshoren et al. (1979); Steele et al. (1978)
Discriminant function analysis	Elliott et al. (1989); Katt and Sprague (1981); Rizzo and Stephens (1981)
Factor analysis	Fimian et al. (1991); Iler et al. (1982); Linville et al. (1989); Lewis (1991); Luick et al. (1982); Metz et al. (1990); Pauloski et al. (1989); Pezzei and Oratio (1991); Smith and Anderson (1982); Wilson et al. (1991)
Fisher exact test	Kelly and Dale (1989)
Friedman two-way analysis of variance	Ladouceur et al. (1982); Clark and Stemple (1982); Mower et al. (1978)
Kruskal-Wallis one-way analysis of variance	Ladouceur et al. (1982); Portnoy and Aronson (1982); Kubaska and Keating (1981); Kelly and Dale (1989)
Mann-Whitney U test	Lasky and Klopp (1982); Mallard et al. (1982); Kelly and Dale (1989)
Meta-analysis	Fitz-Gibbon (1986); Wachter and Straf (1990)
Multidimensional scaling	Doyle et al. (1990); Kempster et al. (1991); Tyler et al. (1989)
Multiple regression	Holland et al. (1989); Nelson and Pavlov (1989); Sommers (1991)
One-way analysis of variance for dependent measures	Helm-Estabrooks et al. (1982); Clark and Stemple (1982); Klitch and May (1982)
One-way analysis of variance for independent measures	Daniloff et al. (1982); Zinkus and Gottlieb (1983); Murray (1978)
t-test for independent measures	Seymour and Seymour (1981); Weismer and Elbert (1982); Zinkus and Gottlieb (1983)
t-test for related measures	Daniloff et al. (1982); Iwan and Siegel (1982); Clark and Stemple (1982)
Wilcoxon signed-ranks matched-pairs test	Weston et al. (1989); Ohlsson et al. (1989)

identical twins (where one twin from each set would be in each group). If there is any doubt whether groups are closely matched, it probably would be safest to treat them as independent.

The third piece of information you need to select an appropriate significance test is the *number* of sets of means, medians, or other measures you wish to assess differences between. If this number is *two*, one set of significance tests is appropriate; if it is *more than two*, a second set is appropriate.

For "before and after" therapy measures a significance test for two sets would be appropriate, and for "before and after" therapy plus follow-up measures (three sets) a significance test for more than two sets would be appropriate.

With these three pieces of information, you may enter Table 10.1 to identify an appropriate significance test. To illustrate how to use this table, let us suppose you administered a picture vocabulary test to a group of children twice, once preceding and once following their participation in a therapy program. Most likely you would wish to determine whether a difference you observed between medians of the two sets of scores were large enough for chance, or random fluctuation, to be unlikely as an explanation. It would probably be safest to assume that the scores on such a vocabulary test have *ordinal* properties. The sets of measures would be *related* because they were made on the same persons, and the number of sets would be *two*. The significance test in Table 10.1 appropriate for two sets of measures having ordinal properties is the *sign test*.

Table 10.1 does not present any tests for sets of related measures having nominal properties. There appear to be no commonly used tests for such measures in speech and hearing research. Significance tests have, however, been developed for such measures—e.g., the McNemar test for the significance of change (Siegel, 1956)—and a statistician should be consulted to help identify the most appropriate for a given instance.

Table 10.1 also does not include tests appropriate for relatively complex comparisons between means or medians. Such tests would be required to answer questions similar to this one: "Was the effect of a speech-improvement program that was administered to a group of kindergarten children different for boys than for girls?" If a difference did exist, it would probably be inadvisable to combine outcome data from boys and girls. A complex analysis-of-variance design could be used to assess the likelihood that the program affects boys and girls differently (i.e., to test the null hypothesis that the differences between boys and girls arose from chance, or random fluctuation). You should consult with someone knowledgeable about analysis-of-variance and related multivariate techniques (e.g., a statistician) if the comparisons you want to make are relatively complex.

You also should consult with someone knowledgeable about these techniques if you want to follow-up an analysis-of-variance in which you reject the null hypothesis. Rejecting the null hypothesis in this case indicates that at least one of the possible differences between means is unlikely to be due to chance. It does not indicate that all of them are likely to be "real" ones! To determine which one (or ones) is, you would test the differences between the various pairs of means that were included in the analysis-of-variance. *T*-tests are *not* appropriate for this purpose. Appropriate ones include the Newman-Keuls post hoc tests, the Sheffe post hoc tests, and the Tukey post hoc tests. (Examples that illustrate the use of these tests can be found on the following pages in the 1989 volume of the *Journal of Speech and Hearing Research*: 36,

333, 447, 506, 629, 710, 718, 768, 819, 833, 838, and 841.) Programs for computing one or more of these are included in most analysis-of-variance computer software packages.

All of the significance tests dealt with thus far have been for *differences* between means, medians, and other descriptive statistics. As indicated earlier, there are also significance tests for assessing the likelihood that observed *relationships* (as designated by nonzero correlation coefficients) arose from chance, or random fluctuation. A test of this type appropriate for Pearson product-moment correlation coefficients is included in Appendix A. For tests of this type appropriate for other correlation coefficients, consult a statistician or someone knowledgeable about inferential statistics.

After the statistic for a significance test has been computed, it is necessary to determine whether the probability of its occurrence is smaller than the level of confidence selected. If the value of this statistic (e.g., x^2, x, z, t, or F) is such that the probability of its occurrence as a result of chance is less than (i.e., smaller than) this level, the null hypothesis is rejected. Otherwise, it is retained. For example, if the level of confidence selected was 0.05 and the probability for the statistic computed resulting from chance was 0.03, the null hypothesis would be rejected. On the other hand, if the level of confidence selected was 0.01 and the probability for the statistic computed resulting from chance was 0.03, the null hypothesis would be retained.

How do you determine whether the value computed for a significance test statistic has a small enough probability of occurrence under the null hypothesis to reject it? To do this, you use a *table* in which you can locate either: (1) the probability associated with the value for the test statistic that the difference or relationship was due to chance, or (2) the value the test statistic would have to *exceed* before you could conclude that the probability of the difference or relationship being due to chance was equal to or less than the level of confidence selected. The tables in Appendix A for the binomial distribution (Table A.3) and the normal distribution (Table A.4) provide probability values, and those for the chi square distribution (Table A.2), the *t*-distribution (Table A.5), and the *F*-distribution (Table A.6) provide values that have to be exceeded.

You are likely to need several pieces of information before you can enter a table to determine if the outcome of a statistical test permits the null hypothesis to be rejected. Those required most often include:

1. the appropriate distribution to use
2. the alpha level, or level of confidence, at which the null hypothesis is being tested
3. the degrees of freedom (*df*)
4. whether the test is to be one-tailed or two-tailed
5. the value computed for the test statistic

The first thing you need to know before you can determine if the outcome of a statistical test permits the null hypothesis to be rejected is what distribution to use. The appropriate distribution, or table, for a particular test statistic is usually indicated in the description of that statistic. Tables containing the most frequently used distributions are presented at the end of Appendix A.

A second piece of information you will almost always need is the alpha level, or level of confidence, at which the null hypothesis is being tested. Though any level 0.05 or smaller is considered acceptable by the editors of scientific and professional journals, most investigators limit themselves to the 0.05 and 0.01 levels. The tabled distributions at the end of Appendix A can all be entered at these two alpha levels.

A third piece of information you may need to enter a table is the number of degrees of freedom (df) in your data. Tables that require this information to enter them (e.g., $x2$, t, and F) contain a *number* of distributions, one for each df value designated in them. The df value for a set of data designates the distribution in a table that contains the *critical value* of the statistic that the one computed on the data must *exceed* before the null hypothesis can be rejected. With the exception of contingency tables, degrees of freedom for the significance tests in Appendix A are based on (but not equal to) the number of subjects. For contingency tables, df values are based on the numbers of rows and columns in a table rather than on the numbers of subjects contained in them.

The procedure for determining the df value for a particular test is indicated in the description of the computational procedure for that test. (Such procedures are indicated in Appendix A for all significance tests that require df values.) Note that the table for the F-distribution (Table A.6) requires two df values rather than one to locate critical values of the statistic.

A fourth piece of information sometimes necessary to determine if the outcome of a statistical test permits the null hypothesis to be rejected is whether the test is *one-tailed* or *two-tailed*. If, to answer a question, you must only be able to detect a difference in one direction, a one-tailed test can be used. The following are representative questions that can be answered with a one-tailed test:

1. Are stutterers more anxious than nonstutterers in a particular situation?
2. Do children evince fewer articulation errors after participating in a particular therapy program?

To answer the first question, it would not be necessary to determine whether nonstutterers are more anxious than stutterers. To answer the second question, it would not be necessary to determine whether children exhibit more articulation errors after participating in the therapy program.

If you must be able to detect a difference in either direction to answer a question, you must use a two-tailed test. The following are representative questions that can be answered with a two-tailed test:

1. Do stutterers and nonstutterers *differ* with regard to intelligence (IQ)?
2. Do aphasics' word-finding abilities tend to be *different* two years after they terminate a particular therapy program than when they terminated it?

To answer these questions, it would be necessary to be able to detect differences in both directions. Stutterers would differ from nonstutterers if their IQ were either higher or lower. Also, the aphasics' word-finding abilities two years following termination of treatment would be different, regardless of whether they were better or poorer than at termination.

It is advantageous to use a one-tailed test *if it is appropriate to do so* because the probability of committing a Type II error is less than for a two-tailed test. For detecting differences in a single direction using a *one-tailed* test, the 0.05 level of confidence really would be the 0.05 level of confidence. However, for detecting differences in a single direction using a *two-tailed* test, the 0.05 level of confidence would become the 0.025 level of confidence. Hence, the probability of committing a Type II error for a particular sample size would be greater.

If you wish to use a one-tailed test (or tests), you are required by the assumptions underlying statistical inference to decide on the direction in which you want to be able to detect a difference *before beginning to collect data.* It is not legitimate to change your mind or decide on the direction after you have seen your data. If you do either, the probability of a Type I error will be higher than the level of confidence would indicate.

There is a direct way of entering some tabled distributions for two-tailed tests. For other such tables, there is no direct way. In these instances, critical values for two-tailed tests can be obtained by adjusting the level of confidence. For a two-tailed test at the 0.05 level, you would enter the table at the 0.025 level. For a two-tailed test at the 0.01 level, you would enter the table at the 0.005 level. Note that the larger values of a test statistic are necessary to reject a null hypothesis if a two-tailed test rather than a one-tailed test is used.

A final piece of information that may be essential for determining whether the null hypothesis can be rejected is the value computed for the test statistic. This information is required for significance tests that use the normal distribution (Table A.4) or the binomial distribution (Table A.3).

Once you have the necessary information to enter the appropriate table for a test statistic, you can determine whether the null hypothesis should be rejected. The procedure for entering each table in Appendix A is as follows:

1. *Chi Square Distribution (Table A.2).* Enter this table with the appropriate *df* value for your data and the level of confidence at which the null

hypothesis is to be tested. The *df* values are indicated in the first column and levels of confidence in the top row. To identify the critical value of chi square for testing the null hypotheses, you first locate the row containing the appropriate *df* value and then the column for the level of confidence you wish to use. The value of chi square that appears at the intersection of this row and column is the critical value for testing the null hypothesis. If the value you computed is larger, the null hypothesis can be rejected. The levels of confidence are for one-tailed tests. Two-tailed tests are rarely, if ever, used for contingency tables. Rejection of the null hypothesis permits you to conclude that the configuration of frequencies in a contingency table is unlikely to have resulted from chance, or random fluctuation.

2. *Binomial Test (Table A.3)*. Enter this table with the value of *x* for your data (see sign test in Appendix A) and the number of subjects (N) whose data are being tested for statistical significance. Numbers of subjects are indicated in the first column and *x* values are indicated in the top row. To determine the *probability* that a value of *x* resulted from chance, or random fluctuation, you locate the row for the appropriate number of subjects and the column for the obtained *x* value. The probability value that appears at the intersection of this row and column is the probability that the obtained value of *x* resulted from chance, or random fluctuation. If this probability is smaller than the level of confidence you selected, the null hypothesis should be rejected. These probability values can be used for either one-tailed or two-tailed tests.

3. *Normal Distribution (Table A.4)*. Enter this table with the value you compute for *z*. Note that *z* values to one decimal place are indicated in the first column and those to two decimal places in the top row. The numbers in the table are probabilities that given *z* values resulted from chance, or random fluctuation. For a one-tailed test at the 0.05 level, if the probability associated with a given *z* is less than 0.05, the null hypothesis is rejected. For a two-tailed test at the 0.05 level, if the probability associated with a given *z* is less than 0.025, the null hypothesis is rejected.

4. *t-Distribution (Table A.5)*. Enter this table with the appropriate *df* value for your data and the level of confidence at which the null hypothesis is to be tested. The *df* values appear in the first column. The levels of significance, or confidence, for one-tailed tests appear in the top row and those for two-tailed tests in the second row. To identify the critical value of *t* for testing the null hypothesis, you locate the row containing the appropriate *df* value and the column for the level of confidence you wish to use. (Note that different columns are used for one-tailed and two-tailed tests.). The value of *t* that appears at the intersection of the row and column is the critical value for testing the null hypothesis. If the value you computed is larger, the null hypothesis should be rejected.

5. *F-Distribution (Table A.6)*. Enter this table with two *df* values: df_1 is the degrees of freedom for columns (or between group or treatment variation) and df_2 is the degrees of freedom for rows (or within group or treatment

variation). The set of numbers which appears at the intersection of the df_1 column and df_2 row are critical values of F for selected levels of confidence, including 1 percent and 5 percent levels. If the value you compute is larger than that in the table for the level of confidence you are using, the null hypothesis should be rejected.

CONFIDENCE INTERVALS

Thus far, we have dealt with the use of statistical inference for determining whether a difference or relationship exists. This section will describe the use of statistical inference for estimating its *magnitude* after it has been shown (by rejecting the null hypothesis) to exist. Rejecting the null hypothesis merely indicates it is likely that a difference or relationship exists—it provides no information about its magnitude. *You cannot assume that the observed magnitude is the real one!* The *confidence interval* is the inferential statistic used for estimating magnitudes. Several studies from the communicative disorders literature in which it was utilized are listed in Table 10.2.

Why might you want to use a confidence interval? There are several reasons. First, you may need to estimate the population value of a descriptive statistic. The following are representative of questions requiring such an estimate to answer:

1. By what age do 50 percent of children perform a particular task correctly?
2. What percentage of persons with a particular communicative disorder derive benefit from a particular therapy program?
3. How predictive is a person's score on a test before he or she participates in a therapy program of what it will be after he or she participates in the program?

To answer the first question, you have to estimate a *population median*; to answer the second, a *population percentage*; and to answer the third, a *population correlation coefficient* (between the scores of a group of persons before and after participating in the program).

A second reason to use a confidence interval is to estimate the population value of a difference between descriptive statistics. Once a null hypothesis has been rejected, indicating that an observed difference is likely to be a real one, it *may* be important to estimate the magnitude of the difference. Such an estimate may be helpful for judging its importance—i.e., for deciding whether it is likely to be a large enough difference to make a difference in the "real world" (Gardner and Altman, 1990; Murray, 1989). Aphasics may make gains if they participate in a particular intensive therapy program (judging by the results of a significance test on the difference between pre- and posttherapy scores), but the magnitudes of these gains may not be sufficient to effect any real improvement in their ability to communicate. To determine if this were likely to be the case, the magnitude of the difference between pre- and posttherapy scores could be estimated by means of a confidence interval (assuming that the results of a test of the difference between pre- and posttherapy measures resulted in rejection of the null hypothesis). Unless the null hypothesis were rejected, indicating that the observed difference is likely to be a real one, it would make no sense to estimate its magnitude!

The following are representative of questions about differences between descriptive statistics that could be answered by means of a confidence interval:

1. How much of a reduction in the severity of a particular communicative disorder could be expected to result from participation in a particular therapy program?
2. How much of a difference is there apt to be between persons who have a particular communicative disorder and those who do not have it in the performance of a particular task?

Both questions can be answered by a confidence interval for the difference between the mean (or median) performances of the groups.

What are confidence intervals? These are intervals designated by two values (a lower limit and an upper limit) between which we can be a given percent certain (usually 95 percent or 99 percent) that the magnitude of a descriptive statistic or a difference between them falls. Thus, based on confidence intervals, we might conclude it is 95 percent certain that the mean IQ for a population falls between 90 and 105, or it is 99 percent certain that the mean amount sixth-grade children who stutter are behind their peers in academic achievement is between five and 12 months. In the second example, the difference between two means is being estimated—i.e., the difference between the mean of the scores of sixth-grade stutterers on a test of academic achievement and that of their peers.

The most most frequently used levels for confidence intervals are 95 percent and 99 percent. With the first, you can be 95 percent certain that the population value falls between the specified limits, and with the second, you can be 99 percent certain that it falls between these limits. These interpretations, of course, would only be valid if the subjects in the sample from whose data the confidence interval was computed were representative of those in the population to which the interpretations referred—i.e., if they at least approximated a random sample from this population.

A 95 percent confidence interval always would be *narrower* than a 99 percent confidence interval. The *higher* the degree of confidence that the population value of the descriptive statistic (or difference between descriptive statistics) computed lies within the confidence interval (i.e., between its upper and lower limits), the *wider* it will be.

Another factor that influences the widths of confidence intervals is *sample size*. The larger the number of subjects in the sample, the narrower the confidence level.

The narrower a confidence interval, the more useful the information it provides. Knowing that the mean IQ for children in a population (e.g., those who have cleft palates) is probably somewhere between 90 and 95 is likely to provide more useful information than knowing it is somewhere between 80 and 105.

What can you do to ensure that the width of a confidence interval will be minimized? One way would be to use a 95 rather than a 99 percent confidence level and another would be to use as many subjects (i.e., as large an N) as possible.

Confidence intervals can be computed from measures having ordinal, interval, or ratio properties. The confidence interval for the median (see Appendix A) is one that can be computed from measures having ordinal properties. Those for the mean and differences between means (see Appendix A) can be computed from measures having interval or ratio properties.

It is possible to compute a confidence interval for almost any descriptive statistic and for the differences between almost any descriptive statistics. A statistician should be able to provide the necessary formulas.

OTHER INFERENTIAL STATISTICAL TECHNIQUES

This section will briefly describe several inferential statistical techniques which can be useful for answering questions pertaining to communicative disorders. These are factor analysis, discriminant function analysis, multidimensional scaling, and meta-analysis. The computations for all four can be done on a computer. The necessary software is available for microcomputers, as well as minicomputers and mainframes (Silverman, 1987).

Factor Analysis

Factor analysis is a technique for identifying general factors, or abilities, that influence performance on a series of tasks (e.g., psychological or language tests). Suppose, for example, you *told* an aphasic to do the following tasks: (1) point to the objects named, (2) name the objects shown, and (3) protrude his or her tongue. A general factor, or ability, that underlies the performance of all three can be labeled "language comprehension." To be successful in performing them it is necessary to understand the instructions you are given.

Factor analysis can be used for answering questions about: (1) general abilities, or factors, that underlie the performance of a series of tasks, and (2) tasks that can be used to evaluate (test) for each such factor.

Suppose you wanted to develop a comprehensive test for evaluating aphasics. This test would consist of a series of tasks, and there would be a great many tasks that could be included. To help you decide which to include, you would want to know: (1) the aspects, or dimensions, of speech and language that are apt to be impaired as a result of the condition, and (2) the task, or tasks, best suited to evaluate for each. This information could be obtained with factor analysis as follows:

1. A large number of possible tasks for such a test would be administered to a fairly large group of aphasics. All of the various types of tasks that have been used to evaluate aphasics would be represented.
2. The scores earned by the aphasics on all possible pairs of tasks would be correlated and displayed in a *correlation matrix*. A correlation matrix for five such tasks is depicted in Table 10.3. A correlation coefficient would appear in each square marked with an X. The type of correlation coefficient most often used for this purpose is the Pearson *r* (see Chapter 9 and Appendix A).
3. The correlation matrix would be factor analyzed using a computer with appropriate software.

The printout from the computer will contain information about: (1) the number of general factors, or abilities, identified by the program which presumably influenced the aphasics' performances of the tasks, and (2) the spe-

TABLE 10.3   A correlation matrix for five tasks. Each square marked with an X would contain a correlation coefficient.

	Task I	Task II	Task III	Task IV	Task V
Task I		X	X	X	X
Task II			X	X	X
Task III				X	X
Task IV					X
Task V					

cific tasks that had relatively "high loadings" and "low loadings" for each. A task with a "high loading" for a particular factor, or ability, would be good for assessing that factor, or ability. Conversely, a task with a "low loading" for a particular factor, or ability, would not be very good for assessing that factor, or ability. You would probably want to include at least one task in your aphasia test that had a relatively high loading for each factor.

How can you identify the ability that each factor represents? The computer does not label the factors. It does provide information, however, that can be used for inferring the ability each represents. Suppose two tasks had relatively high loadings and three had relatively low loadings for a particular factor. To determine what it represented, you would attempt to identify the ability that successful completion of the two tasks with high loadings required that was not required of the three with low loadings. Obviously, labels assigned to factors by such a reasoning process have to be regarded as tentative because tasks with relatively high loadings may require *more than one* ability that is not required of those with relatively low loadings.

In summary, factor analysis can be a useful exploratory procedure for identifying general abilities that underlie the performance of a series of tasks. For further information on this technique, you may find books by Cureton and D'Agostino (1983), Gorsuch (1983), and McDonald (1985) helpful.

For illustrations of the use of factor analysis in speech, language, and hearing research, see Table 10.2.

Discriminant Function Analysis

Discriminant function analysis is a statistical procedure used to assign people to categories, usually dichotomous categories. The following are examples of pairs of categories to which discriminant function analysis might be used for assigning persons:

1. "beginning stuttering" versus "normally disfluent speech"
2. "adequate velopharyngeal closure" versus "inadequate velopharyngeal closure" for speech

Programs for performing a discriminant function analysis should be available at most college or university computer centers.

The types of questions that discriminant function analysis may be useful for answering include:

1. Is a given four-year-old exhibiting "beginning stuttering" or "normally disfluent speech"?
2. What variables best differentiate "beginning stuttering" from "normally disfluent speech" for four-year-olds?
3. Is the velopharyngeal closure of a given child who has a cleft palate

"adequate" or "inadequate" to support speech that has normal nasal resonance?

4. What measures best differentiate "adequate" from "inadequate" velopharyngeal closure?

While these questions all involve discriminating between two categories, discriminant function analysis is not limited to the two-category situation. Computer programs are available for discriminating among three or more categories.

The general strategy underlying discriminant function analysis for the two-category case can be summarized as follows:

1. A series of tasks (e.g., tests), which there is some reason to believe might discriminate between persons who fall into the two categories, are administered to two groups. Each consists of persons who fall into one of the categories. For the first question, one group would consist of four-year-olds who are known to be beginning to stutter and the other would consist of four-year-olds who have no history of a stuttering problem.

2. A discriminant function analysis is performed on the measures (e.g., test scores). The results of this analysis indicate which task, or combination of tasks, best discriminates between the groups (assuming that both groups did not perform essentially the same on the tasks).

3. The task, or combination of tasks, identified by the analysis can be used for determining the category, or group, to assign a person when the group to which he or she should be assigned is unknown. The analysis provides an equation for this purpose. In this equation, the person's score on each task (S) is multiplied by a weight (W) that is determined by the program and the products of these multiplications are summed algebraically. The form of a typical such equation would be similar to:

$$X - S_1W_1 + S_2W_2$$

In words, you would multiply the person's score on task one by the weight assigned to that task and add this to his or her score on task two multiplied by the weight assigned to task two.

The value of X would indicate the category to which the person should be assigned. If it exceeds one given in the computer printout, the person would be assigned to one category; if it is smaller than this value, the person would be assigned to the other category. The computer printout also provides information on the likelihood of category assignments being incorrect.

The procedure for a discriminant function analysis involving more than two categories is essentially the same as that outlined here.

In summary, discriminant function analysis can be a useful procedure for: (1) identifying the way, or ways, in which the members of a group differ, and (2) identifying the categories, or groups, to which people belong.

For illustrations of the use of discriminant function analysis in speech, language, and hearing research, see Table 10.2.

Multidimensional Scaling

Multidimensional scaling is a procedure for identifying the attributes of stimuli (or events) to which people attend, i.e., the attributes which they abstract. Suppose you wanted to identify the attributes of moments of stuttering to which people attend. To do this, you could collect "moments of stuttering" from a number of stutterers on videotape. You would then have these taped moments of stuttering rated for *degree of similarity* by a fairly large number of observers. The similarity ratings could be made in several ways. One that appears to be used most often is called the "method of triads." With this method, all possible combinations of the moments of stuttering taken *three* at a time would be formed. Observers would be asked to indicate the two moments of stuttering in each group of three that are most similar. The resulting similarity ratings would be subjected to several computer analyses, including a factor analysis. The attributes of the stimuli to which the observers consciously or unconsciously attended while making their similarity ratings can be inferred from the factors identified by the factor analysis.

Multidimensional scaling has been used by speech-language pathologists and audiologists for answering certain questions (see Table 10.2). Information about it can be obtained from a number of sources, including books by Davison (1983), Green (1989), and Schiffman, Reynolds, and Young (1981).

Meta-Analysis

Meta-analysis (Fitz-Gibbon, 1984, 1986; Glass, McGaw, and Smith, 1981; Hedges and Olkin, 1985; Hennekens, Buring, and Hebert, 1987; Hunter, 1982; Hunter and Schmidt, 1990; Laird and Mosteller, 1990; Matt, 1989; Wachter and Straf, 1990; Wolf, 1986) is a statistical approach, of relatively recent origin, for combining data from separate studies for the purpose of obtaining information that cannot be derived from the individual studies. It is used to integrate information from different studies of a given problem. Hence, it differs from the other statistical methods described in this chapter in that it is not used for analyzing the data from a single study. It has been used extensively in psychology and medicine for integrating and interpreting the results of outcome studies on specific intervention strategies (Hsu, 1989; Matt, 1989; Simes, 1990; Wachter and Straf, 1990).

Why is a methodology like meta-analysis needed? The reason is that questions, particularly those pertaining to therapy outcome, can rarely be answered unequivocally with a single set of data (i.e., by a single study). There are several reasons. First, the subjects used in a particular study may not constitute a truly random sample from the population to which the question refers, and the sample size may be relatively small. Second, if a group design was used, rejection of the null hypothesis may have resulted from a Type I error or its retention from a Type II one (Hennekens, Buring, and Hebert, 1987). Third, if a single subject design was used, the generality of the findings would be uncertain. Finally, an effect (or a lack of one) could have resulted from experimenter or subject bias (see Chapter 13) or from extraneous variables that were not adequately controlled for and biased the data.

The approach used with meta-analysis for summarizing research findings can be summarized as follows:

> To investigate the effects of an experimental treatment ... *all* studies concerned with that treatment—published and unpublished studies, statistically significant or not, well-designed or not—are collected for analysis. Each study is regarded as providing a sample estimate for the population parameter of interest, the Effect Size. . . . The Effect Size is an index of how much difference the treatment made. . . . In addition to obtaining Effect Sizes from studies, each study is coded for all variables that might affect the reported outcome of the treatment, such as the site, year of publication, the adequacy of the design, reliability of instruments, treatment characteristics, personnel involved etc. The obtained Effect Sizes are then related to the characteristics of the experiments from which they arose. The aim is not to say that a treatment has an effect with a certain probability that a Type I error has been avoided, but to provide estimates of the size of effects in various circumstances, with various subjects. (Fitz-Gibbon, 1986, p. 118)

Statistical procedures for computing Effect Sizes and combining them—i.e., for performing a meta-analysis—are described in publications by Glass, McGaw, and Smith (1981), Hedges and Olkin (1985), and Laird and Mosteller (1990).

Meta-analysis can be used for the same purpose as a confidence interval—i.e., to estimate the magnitude of a difference (an Effect Size). Hence, it can be used for answering the same types of questions. In some cases, confidence intervals are used in conjunction with Effect Size estimates.

While meta-analysis appears to be the most frequently used methodology for combining the results of independent studies, it is not the only one. For descriptions of several others, see Rosenthal (1978).

Meta-analysis did not appear to have been utilized a great deal in speech-language pathology and audiology research when this chapter was written. The only references I was able to find to it pertained to its use in aphasia therapy outcome research (Fitz-Gibbon, 1986; Wachter and Straf, 1990). One reason undoubtedly is that the technique is so new. Nevertheless, judging by the literature pertaining to its utilization in psychotherapy and medical intervention research, it should be a useful tool for investigators in our field who are attempting to answer questions concerning treatment efficacy.

EXERCISES AND DISCUSSION TOPICS

1. There are 13 computational exercises in Appendix A that provide experience in computing significance tests and confidence intervals. Your instructor will tell you which to do and whether to do them with a calculator, a computer (using a statistical program package),or both.

2. The interpretation of inferential statistics for answering questions is not "objective"—it is based on human judgment. Often a set of data can be interpreted to support several different answers to a question. Justify *both* a "yes" and a "no" answer to the following question using the data provided.

   Do persons who have a sensorineural hearing loss understand speech better if they use an X-type hearing aid?

   Observational Procedures. Three persons who had sensorineural hearing losses were administered a different 50-item PB word list while wearing an X-type hearing aid and without it.

   Data. Of the 50 PB words on a list, the numbers accurately repeated by each subject under each condition were the following:

SUBJECT NUMBER	NUMBER CORRECT WITHOUT AID	NUMBER CORRECT WITH AID
1	15	38
2	25	43
3	20	35
Mean	20	39

   A *t*-test for two related samples (see Appendix A) was performed in these data. The value of *t* computed was not large enough to reject the null hypothesis at the 0.01 level of confidence (alpha level).

3. Why is knowledge of inferential statistics important for evaluating therapy outcome research reports?

11

Evaluating Research

Consumers of research have to be able to evaluate the adequacy of findings (i.e., answers to questions) reported in journal literature as well as the cogency of interpretations and generalizations made from them. It is not safe to assume that the findings reported in a journal article allow the questions asked to be answered in the ways they were answered, or the answers to be interpreted in the ways they were interpreted, merely because the study was published. Even though most journals subject submitted manuscripts to a careful review process, and many are rejected as a consequence of this process (Culatta, 1984), papers are nevertheless published in which the answers to the questions asked or the interpretations made of these answers are either not appropriate or are not the only possible answers or interpretations.

Sometimes when readers detect an error in the authors' answers or interpretations, they write a letter to the editor in which they indicate alternative ones. Letters to the editor about research papers are published in the *American Journal of Audiology: A Journal of Clinical Practice*, the *American Journal of Speech-Language Pathology: A Journal of Clinical Practice, Asha,* the *Journal of Speech and Hearing Disorders,* the *Journal of Speech and Hearing Research,* and *Language, Speech, and Hearing Services in Schools.* However, this is not always done. One reason is that most journals permit an author to reply to a letter critical of his or her paper, and this rebuttal is printed along with it. In his or her rebuttal, the author can answer the points raised in a manner that makes it appear the criticisms are not valid when in fact they are. Unfortunately, the writer of the letter to the editor usually is not given an opportunity to respond to the author's rebuttal. This situation obviously would discourage some persons who come upon "errors" and inappropriate interpretations from writing letters to the editor.

You should approach published research with an attitude of *healthy skepticism*. Doing so is particularly important for that which could affect your clinical functioning.

Criteria for interpreting, or evaluating, answers to questions are also relevant for *producers* of research. Once an investigator has answered a question, he or she usually attempts to relate the answer to the existing body of knowledge. The investigator may use it to fill a gap or gaps and/or to question the accuracy of certain information contained in it.

DIMENSIONS TO CONSIDER
WHEN EVALUATING RESEARCH

What dimensions should you consider when evaluating answers to determine the interpretations and generalizations that can legitimately be made from them? The three most important are *validity*, *reliability*, and *generality*.

Validity

The validity of observations refers to their *appropriateness* for answering the questions they are used to answer. If they are not appropriate, the answers they yield *may* be inaccurate.

Because the observations used to answer a question are inappropriate does not necessarily mean that the answer will be inaccurate. An investigator will occasionally arrive at the right answer for the wrong reason—i.e., through the use of invalid observations. A classic example previously mentioned (see Chapter 3) is Gall's conclusion, on the basis of a friend's eyes being widely separated, that the anterior portion of the brain is important for motor speech (Head, 1963).

If the observations used to answer a question appear to be invalid, it probably would make most sense to regard the question as *not having been answered* (at least as far as the observations reported are concerned). It would *not* be appropriate to regard the question as having been incorrectly answered, since a certain percentage of the time an investigator will arrive at a correct answer from invalid observations. As a matter of fact, if a question could only be answered in two ways (e.g., yes or no), you could arrive at a correct answer *without even knowing the question* approximately 50 percent of the time.

The probability of a correct answer by chance would be the reciprocal of the number of ways a question could be answered. If a question could be answered in three ways, the probability of a correct answer by chance would be $\frac{1}{3}$ or 0.33.

In summary, if the observations used for answering a question are appropriate, the odds will be *greater than chance* that the answer reported is correct. On the other hand, if the observations used for answering a question are inappropriate, the odds will be approximately *equal to chance* that the answer reported is correct.

Reliability

The reliability of the observations used for answering questions refers to their *repeatability*. The more repeatable (or replicable) a set of observations, the greater will be their reliability.

The extent to which observations can be repeated, or replicated, is a function of how similarly a *given observer* would describe them on *different* occasions, or how similarly a *group of observers* would describe them on the *same occasion* (or occasions). Descriptions can consist of words, numbers, or a combination of the two. The more similar the descriptions, the more reliable the observations.

The level of reliability of the observations used for answering a question influences the odds that the answer will be correct. How reliable the observations have to be for these odds to be acceptable depends on the question. For questions concerning *differences* (e.g., "Were the language formulation abilities of a group of children better on the average after participating in a particular therapy program than prior to participating in it?"), more reliable observations are required if a difference is relatively small than if it is relatively large. Similarly, for questions concerning *relationships* (e.g., "Is there a relationship between the scores earned by a group of persons who have a particular type of communicative disorder on two tests of auditory functioning?"), more reliable observations are required if a relationship is relatively weak than if it is relatively strong.

Because the observations used for answering a question are not adequately reliable does not necessarily mean that the answer will be incorrect. The answer can be correct by chance alone. As I indicated in the discussion of validity, the probability of an answer being correct by chance is the reciprocal of the number of ways the question can be answered. Also, the observations may be more reliable than they appear to be. Some types of observations typically tend to be viewed as less reliable than they actually are. An example would be ratings obtained through the application of psychological scaling methods (see Chapter 8).

One consequence of observations not being adequately reliable is a relatively high probability of a Type II error (see Chapter 10). Briefly, this means concluding that there is no real difference or relationship when there is. Usually, when an investigator fails to reject a null hypothesis, he or she does not indicate the probability that this failure was due to the measures used not being sufficiently reliable to detect the difference or relationship present. It is quite likely there are some instances in the speech-language pathology and audiology literature when the null hypothesis was not rejected that the reason was a Type II error arising from the use of measures which were not adequately reliable.

Regardless of the reason for a null hypothesis not being rejected, it is inappropriate to interpret failure to do so as *proving* there is no difference (see the discussion of the null hypothesis in Chapter 10). Studies by speech-language pathologists and audiologists have been criticized on this basis (Finn and Glow, 1990; Meyers, 1990). Of course, if there is no difference between the means or medians (or only a minute one), it is more likely that there really is none than that there is a Type II error. But failure to reject the null hypothesis does not prove it!

In summary, the impact of the reliability of the observations used for answering a question on the accuracy of the answer obtained may not be clear-cut. Observations that do not appear to be adequately reliable can yield both correct and incorrect answers. Judgments concerning the accuracy of answers to questions, therefore, should be regarded as tentative until the data used to answer them have been replicated (preferably by other investigators at other institutions).

Generality

A third factor to be considered when evaluating answers to questions and interpretations made from them is the *generality* of the observations used to answer the questions. This refers to the extent to which the persons or events observed are representative of those in the population designated by the question. The more representative of this population they are, the more viable will be the generalizations made from them.

The persons or events observed to answer a question are most likely to be representative of those in the designated population if they constitute a *random sample* from that population. The only way you can be reasonably certain they constitute such a sample is if they were selected from the population by a table of random numbers (see Appendix B) or by a series of random digits generated by a computer. If they were not selected in this manner, their generality would be uncertain *to some degree*. Of course, even if they were selected by a random process, it still is possible they would not be representative because of a sampling error.

The persons and events observed in speech-language pathology and audiology research often do not constitute a random sample from the population to which the investigator(s) want to generalize. While this population consists of *all persons* who have a particular communicative disorder, the population sampled may consist of *all persons available to the investigator* who have that communicative disorder.

If an investigator wishes to limit generalizations to the *subpopulation* of persons who have a particular communicative disorder from which he or she sampled (e.g., a caseload), then so long as the persons were randomly selected from this subpopulation, the generalizations made should be viable. There are instances, of course, when it would be meaningful to generalize to such a subpopulation. One such instance would be when you wished to assess the impact of participation in a treatment program on a group of persons at your own institution. Rather than assessing the impact of the program on all participants, it may be more economical and efficient to limit the assessment to a random sample. Inferences could be made about the impact of the program on all participants from observations made on this sample. With the probable continuing interest of administrators of clinical speech, language, and hearing programs in "accountability," such inferences could be quite useful.

If investigators do not want to limit their generalizations to the subpopulations from which their samples were drawn, or if their samples were not randomly selected from the populations to which they wish to generalize, the cogency of their generalizations will be uncertain. To have a reasonable degree of confidence in the viability of such generalizations, it is necessary to assume that the persons observed constitute a *representative*, or random, sample from the population to which they are being made. In some instances, this assumption will seem reasonable; in others, it will not seem reasonable; in still others, insufficient information will be presented in the report about the persons observed for any judgment to be made regarding its reasonableness. Knowing, for example, that they were all receiving therapy at a particular rehabilitation center without knowing the characteristics (i.e., physical, intellectual, emotional, socioeconomic, etc.) of those who do so is likely to leave you uncertain about the reasonableness of this assumption.

Can generalizations legitimately be made from observations of persons who were not randomly selected from the population to which it was desired to generalize? The answer to this question would be yes if: (1) a single subject design were used, and (2) you were willing to assume it is highly unlikely that the only persons in the population who would perform as these subjects did under the experimental condition (or conditions) are these subjects. If you are willing to make this assumption, it would seem reasonable to conclude that the performance of the subjects is representative of that of a *segment* of the population from which they were selected. It wouldn't be possible, however, to specify the size of this segment on the basis of a single sample that was selected in this manner.

Because the interpretations and generalizations made by an author from his or her data seem inappropriate does not necessarily mean they are incorrect. An author can arrive at a correct conclusion for the wrong reasons. In fact, an accurate interpretation or generalization can be arrived at by chance alone.

CRITERIA FOR EVALUATING VALIDITY, RELIABILITY, AND GENERALITY

Now that we have commented upon the relevance of validity, reliability, and generality for assessing accuracy, we will consider some questions that should be asked when judging them. The answers to these questions provide a basis for making judgments about the accuracy of answers to research questions as well as the cogency of interpretations and generalizations made from them.

Validity

A necessary question to answer when you want to assess the validity of the observations used for answering a question is: "Were the observations made appropriate for answering the question asked?" That is, did the investigator observe and describe the attribute (or attributes) of the events that he or she wanted to observe and describe? If the investigator did, the observations will be valid to some degree. If the investigator did not, they will be invalid.

An investigator may not have observed the attribute or attributes needed to answer a question because the filter used to isolate it did not do so (see Chapter 1). This could have resulted from using an inappropriate or inaccurately calibrated instrument or from failing to take on an appropriate set. An inappropriate instrument in this context would be one that would not permit the investigator to isolate the attribute he or she wanted to observe and describe. Such an instrument could be a part of an electronic instrumentation measurement scheme, or it could be a psychological or educational performance test or task (see Chapter 8). An example of using inappropriate electronic instrumentation to isolate a target attribute would be using an electromyographic (EMG) recorder with *surface electrodes* to study the differential activity of the internal and external intercostal muscles during breathing for speech. (*Needle electrodes* would be needed at least at some sites to study the differential activity of these muscles.) An example of an inappropriate application of educational or psychological tests for isolating and describing a target attribute would be using articulation test performance to infer intelligence level. (While both are related in a general way to overall development, articulation test performance does not appear to be a particularly valid index of intelligence level.)

An *inaccurately calibrated* instrument in this context would be one which when properly adjusted, or calibrated, would permit the investigator to isolate the attribute he or she wanted to observe and describe. If the target attribute was "thresholds for pure tones" and the audiometer used was not properly calibrated, the investigator would be unable to describe this attribute validly on the basis of the thresholds obtained. The investigator would, of course, be able to describe the attribute with this type of instrumentation if it were properly calibrated.

An *inappropriate set* in this context would be one an observer assumes that does not "target" the attribute he or she wants to observe and describe. On psychological scaling tasks (see Chapter 8), for example, where observers are asked to rate a series of speech segments for two attributes *separately* (e.g., degree of "articulation defectiveness" and degree of "nasality"), they may be unable to assume the appropriate sets. That is, they may be unable to ignore one of them (e.g., nasality) while rating the speech segments for the other (e.g., articulation defectiveness).

Reliability

A necessary question to answer when assessing the reliability of observations is: "Were the observations made sufficiently free from random and systematic measurement error (including experimenter bias) to answer reliably the question asked?" The sources from which both types of error arise have already been discussed (see Chapter 8). If the answer to this question is yes, the observations are likely to be sufficiently free of error to answer reliably the question asked. If, on the other hand, it appears to be no, the answer should be regarded as suspect.

Impact of Random Measurement Error on Reliability. Random measurement error can influence the accuracy of answers to questions on differences and relationships (and hence the interpretations made of them) by increasing the probability of a Type II error—i.e., the probability of not rejecting the null hypothesis when it should be rejected (see Chapter 10). Obviously, if the null hypothesis is rejected, this source of error could not have influenced the accuracy of the answer. If the null hypothesis is retained, however, random measurement error could have been responsible. That is, rather than retaining the null hypothesis, which indicates that an observed difference or relationship probably resulted from chance, or random fluctuation, it merely may indicate that the level of random error was too high to detect a difference or relationship of the magnitude present with the number of subjects used. If more subjects had been used, the null hypothesis might have been rejected. (The larger the sample size, the less likely you are to retain a false null hypothesis because of random error). For this reason, whenever you are interpreting an answer to a question that was based on failure to reject the null hypothesis, one possibility you must always consider is a Type II error. (A statistician should be able to provide you with the appropriate formula for estimating this probability for a given significance test.) Unfortunately, most journals don't require authors to specify the probability of a Type II error when they fail to reject the null hypothesis.

A Type II error is particularly likely to explain retaining the null hypothesis if at least two of the following three statements apply:

1. The sample size was relatively small.
2. The observed difference or correlation was relatively small.
3. The alpha level (i.e., level of confidence) used was relatively small (e.g., 0.01).

In summary, unless it was possible to demonstrate the probability of a Type II error was acceptably small (i.e., 0.05 or smaller), it would be inappropriate to interpret failure to reject the null hypothesis as indicating that an observed difference or relationship is not a "real" one.

Impact of Systematic Measurement Error on Reliability. Systematic measurement error can influence the accuracy of answers to questions (and hence the interpretations made of them) by biasing the observations used to answer them. It can make it appear that a difference or relationship exists where there is none, or that no difference or relationship exists where there is one.

Therapy outcome research is particularly vulnerable to systematic measurement error (e.g., Beasley and Manning, 1973; Meitus, Ringel, House, and Hotchkiss, 1973). It is especially likely to occur if the person or persons doing the research have an ego investment in the outcome (e.g., Rosenthal, 1963, 1966, 1969). An investigator may strongly desire that a therapy be shown to be effective, or vice versa. This is especially true in studies where an investigator is comparing several therapies, one of which he or she has emotionally identified with and hopes (or expects) to be the most effective. The bias may be subtle, and the investigator may not be conscious of it.

How might an investigator bias his or her therapy outcome research? One way is by choosing criterion measures and designs that are most likely to make the approach in which he or she has an ego investment appear superior to those to which it is being compared. Suppose, for example, an investigator was comparing the impact of a stuttering therapy program he or she helped to develop to the impact of another one. The investigator might use as a criterion measure stuttering frequency before and after participating in a program. The results may indicate that the stutterers who participated in the investigator's program had a greater reduction in stuttering frequency than those who participated in the other program. Therefore, based on a stuttering frequency criterion measure, it would seem reasonable to conclude that the investigator's program was more effective than the other one. However, if a different criterion measure had been used, the conclusion might have been different. Another criterion measure that could have been used is "avoidance of speaking when stuttering is anticipated." Perhaps the other therapy would have been more effective in treating this aspect of the stuttering problem. Also, if the stuttering frequency criterion measure had been used with a different design—e.g., one that included a two-year follow-up—the outcome could have been different. That is, the amount of relapse for the program which seemed to be the most effective at the point therapy was terminated could have been considerably greater than for the other.

An investigator can bias the results of therapy outcome research in other ways as well. If he or she attempted to evaluate retrospectively the effectiveness of a therapy program, several types of distortion could bias the evaluation. The investigator may be more successful, for example, in remembering factors that suggest the therapy was effective than factors that suggest

FIGURE 11.1   Evaluation checklist for validity, reliability, and generality.

Indicate beside each statement whether or not it appears to be true. If insufficient information is presented to judge whether a statement is true, place a checkmark in the ? column.

YES	NO	?		STATEMENT
___	___	___	1.	The question, or questions, that the investigator(s) attempted to answer are "answerable" (see Chapter 5).
___	___	___	2.	The investigator(s) selected the appropriate type of design–single subject and/or group–for answering the question, or questions (see Chapter 6)
___	___	___	3	The investigator(s) selected attributes of events to observe that are appropriate for answering the question, or questions (see Chapter 7).
___	___	___	4.	The specific observations that the investigator(s) made were of the attributes referred to in Statement 3, rather than some other attributes (see Chapter 7).
___	___	___	5.	The persons on whom the observations were made—i.e., the research subjects—were appropriate ones for answering the question, or questions (see Chapter 7).
___	___	___	6.	The subjects were selected by a method that should have made them *representative* of persons in the population referred to in the question, or questions—e.g.. by means of a random sampling procedure (see Chapter 6).
___	___	___	7.	It appears unlikely that the theoretical and clinical biases of the investigator(s) consciously or unconsciously influenced the methodology used (i.e., the selection of subjects, the choice of observations to be made, and/or the manner in which the observations were made) in a manner that would have been likely to bias the data (see Chapter 11).
___	___	___	8.	Evidence is presented which indicates that electronic instrumentation used for measuring attributes of events was properly calibrated (see Chapter 8).
___	___	___	9.	Evidence is presented which indicates that the observations made possess an acceptable level of reliability (see Chapter 11).
___	___	___	10.	It appears unlikely that the observations were biased by order or sequence effects (see Chapter 6).

FIGURE 11.1 Continued

YES	NO	?		STATEMENT
___	___	___	11.	It appears unlikely that the observations were biased by how the subjects thought the investigator(s) wanted them to respond or by what they thought was the purpose of the study (see Chapter 8).
___	___	___	12.	The descriptive statistics, tables, or graphical displays used were appropriate for organizing the data to answer the question, or questions (see Chapter 9).
___	___	___	13.	The manner in which the descriptive statistics, tables, graphical displays, and other data were *interpreted* was appropriate for answering the question, or questions (see Chapter 9).
___	___	___	14.	The conclusions that were drawn from the descriptive statistics, tables, graphical displays, and other data appear to be the most plausible ones (see Chapter 9).
___	___	___	15.	The inferential statistical procedures used were appropriate ones (see Chapter 10).
___	___	___	16.	Failure to reject the null hypothesis does not appear to have been due to a Type II error (see Chapter 10).
___	___	___	17.	Failure to reject the null hypothesis is not interpreted as indicating that there is no difference (see Chapter 10).
___	___	___	18.	The magnitude of the difference between the descriptive statistics (e.g., between the means or between the medians) is not interpreted as being the magnitude of the difference in the population unless a confidence interval has been computed which indicates that it is (see Chapter 10).
___	___	___	19.	The population to which the findings are generalized is an appropriate one (see Chapter 11).
___	___	___	20.	Observed differences and relationships are not interpreted as being clinically or theoretically meaningful just because they are "statistically significant" (see Chapter 10).
___	___	___	21.	The theoretical and clinical biases of the investigator(s) do not appear to have influenced the manner in which the findings were interpreted (see Chapter 11).

it was ineffective, or vice versa. Or the investigator could conclude that a reduction in the severity of a person's communicative disorder has occurred because the investigator has "adapted" to it (e.g., Trotter and Kools, 1955). A person with a severe phonological disorder could seem more intelligible to his or her clinician following a period of therapy because the clinician has learned the lawful ways in which the person's language usage differs from the standard. And a stutterer's stuttering could seem less severe to his clinician because the clinician has grown accustomed to it (Trotter and Kools, 1955).

Another way an investigator can bias the results of such research is by not reporting the effects of the therapy on all persons on whom it was tried. While it is sometimes justifiable (and indeed necessary) to exclude clients from reports of therapy outcome because the therapy was not administered to them in the prescribed manner, such exclusion should be done only when absolutely necessary—i.e., when not excluding them would *almost certainly* lead to a biased evaluation. Unfortunately, it is usually relatively easy to rationalize the elimination of any client from a study of therapy outcome who does not respond to the therapy as the investigator desires—i.e., who would have to be classified as a "failure."

Therapy outcome research also can be biased when the findings are interpreted. Data pertaining to the effectiveness of a program can often be interpreted in more than one way. In fact, a given finding can often be interpreted *both* to support the conclusion that a therapy was effective and to support the conclusion that it was ineffective. It depends on whether one wishes to view the proverbial cup as half full or half empty. Suppose a particular stuttering therapy was found to reduce stuttering frequency by 10 percent. This could be used both to support the conclusion that the therapy was effective (i.e., it reduced stuttering frequency) and to support the conclusion that it was ineffective (i.e., it didn't produce enough of a reduction in stuttering frequency to make a meaningful difference in how clients are likely to be perceived and reacted to). Both interpretations are defensible. When you are reading and evaluating outcome research, therefore, it is important that you seek out the data on which conclusions and interpretations are based.

Generality

The question you must answer to assess generality is: "Did the subjects observed at least approximate a random sample from the population to which the question refers—i.e., the one to which generalizations are being made?" If the subjects observed were chosen by a random process (e.g., by a table of random numbers—see Appendix B) from the population to which a question refers, it is highly likely that they constitute a random sample from that population.

If subjects were not randomly selected from the population to which a question refers, it would be *uncertain* whether they constitute a random sample from that population. Any inferences, conclusions, and generalizations made from observations of such subjects would have to be regarded as *quite tentative.*

CHECKLIST FOR EVALUATING THE VALIDITY, RELIABILITY, AND GENERALITY OF RESEARCH FINDINGS

A number of considerations are mentioned in this chapter and elsewhere in the book for evaluating the validity, reliability, and generality of research findings. A checklist (Figure 11.1) is presented on page 230 that can be helpful when evaluating for these. The checklist consists of a series of statements which if true suggest that the findings being evaluated possess adequate levels of validity, reliability, and generality.

EXERCISES AND DISCUSSION TOPICS

1. Use the Evaluation Checklist (Figure 11.1) to assess the validity, reliability, and generality of the findings presented in *three* research reports published in the *Journal of Speech and Hearing Research.* At least one of these reports should deal with clinical research.

2. Which of the statements on the Evaluation Checklist could be used for assessing the validity, reliability, and generality of the findings reported in clinical evaluation reports if the word *clinician* were substituted for the word *investigator?* Give your reasons for your decisions.

3. John's mother was asked the age at which he said his first word. She looked in his "baby book" and found that the age she had recorded for his first word was 18 months. Based on this evidence, the clinician stated in his report that John said his first word at 18 months. Assess both the validity and reliability of this conclusion, using the criteria presented in this chapter.

4. A clinician wishes to determine whether Mrs. Smith, a stroke patient, is having any difficulty understanding speech. He asks her to point to a series of objects that he names. She does so without error. He concludes that she is having no difficulty understanding speech. Assess both the validity and generality of this conclusion using the criteria presented in this chapter.

12
Communicating Research

Once a question has been formulated and answered and the answer has been interpreted, the next step is to communicate the question, answer, and interpretation to potential consumers of the information. This is the final step in the research process. If you do clinical (e.g., therapy outcome) research and your findings are not disseminated formally, their potential to be of help to people who are communicatively impaired is likely to be restricted to your caseload and those of your colleagues to whom you informally communicate them.

MODES FOR DISSEMINATING RESEARCH FINDINGS

There are two main modes for disseminating research findings: written reports and convention presentations. Written reports usually consist of papers published in journals and books. Convention presentations usually consist of talks and exhibits (including poster sessions) at local, state, national, and international meetings. Other modes for disseminating research findings include motion picture films, videotapes, audiotapes, self-published reports, and computer conferencing.

Written Reports

Written reports are the most frequently used mode for disseminating research findings in speech-language pathology and audiology. They are published in a variety of journals, including those of state speech, language, and hearing associations; the American Speech-Language-Hearing Association; international speech, language, and hearing associations (e.g., the International Society for Logopedics and Phoniatrics); specialty speech, language, and hearing associations (e.g., Computer Users in Speech and Hearing and the International Society for Augmentative and Alternative Communication); as well as ones published by educational, psychological, sociological, medical, physics, speech communication, and linguistics associations. To identify journals that have published, and presumably will continue to publish, papers dealing with certain aspects of communicative disorders, search for them in a relevant computer database (e.g., Medline) or look them up in the indexes of several recent volumes of a relevant abstract's journal, such as *Linguistics and Language Behavior Abstracts,* and note the journals in which papers concerned with them have been published. A 1991 ASHA publication, *Journals in Communication Sciences and Disorders,* can also be helpful here.

Written reports can range in length from less than a page to more than 100 pages. Most are between four and 12 journal pages in length. They may be classified as articles, reports, clinical exchange reports, case reports, points of view, or letters to the editor.

Journals that classify papers as articles and reports usually distinguish between these two categories on the basis of length—longer papers are classified as articles. The magnitude of the research reported also may be a consideration. Papers that report a single study may tend to be classified as reports and those that report a series of related studies as articles. Organization is the same for both types of papers.

Clinical exchange contributions tend to be relatively short reports that are clinically relevant—i.e., deal with diagnostic or therapy procedures. They are published by several journals, including the *American Journal of Audiology: A Journal of Clinical Practice,* the *American Journal of Speech-Language Pathology: A Journal of Clinical Practice,* and *Language, Speech, and Hearing Services in the Schools.*

Case reports (i.e., case studies) are descriptions of individuals who are noteworthy for some reason. The symptomatology or etiology of their communicative disorder may be unusual in some respect; they may have responded in an unexpected manner to a diagnostic or therapeutic procedure; or an unusual diagnostic or therapeutic procedure may have been administered to them. Such papers may contain a single case study or several related case studies.

Point-of-view papers are not intended primarily for the dissemination of research findings. They are sometimes included, however, as support for the contentions, or points of view, presented.

Letters to the editor are occasionally used to disseminate research findings. They are particularly likely to be used for this purpose when an investigator has data to report that are relevant to a question answered in a published paper. The investigator may write a letter to the editor of the journal that published the paper reporting data that either replicate those used to answer the question or suggest a different answer to the question. Letters to the editor are sometimes also used to disseminate research findings unrelated to any that have been reported when such findings can be presented in a few paragraphs.

Convention Presentations

Convention presentations are the second most frequently used mode for disseminating research findings in speech-language pathology and audiology. They can be made in a variety of settings, including state speech and hearing association and American Speech-Language-Hearing Association conventions. The three most common types are talks, poster presentations, and scientific exhibits.

The typical convention presentation consists of a ten- or fifteen-minute talk and a question-and-answer period (usually five minutes or less). The organization of this kind of talk is similar to that of a written report; however, the language is usually less formal and more conversational, and the presentation is usually less detailed and more redundant, than that of a written report.

The poster presentation is a relatively recent addition to convention programs. Each presenter is usually assigned to a poster board for at least an hour. The presenter mounts research findings on this board in graphical, tabular, photographic, or narrative form and then stands beside this "poster" for the period assigned and answers questions about it (see Figure 12.1).

Scientific exhibits, such as those at American Speech-Language-Hearing Association conventions, can be used to disseminate research findings. They are generally similar to poster presentations. However, scientific exhibits can be larger and more elaborate and last a longer period of time than poster presentations.

Other Approaches to Disseminating Research Findings

While written reports and convention presentations are the modes that have been used most frequently by speech-language pathologists and audiologists or disseminating research findings, they are not the only ones. Others include motion picture films, videotapes, audiotapes, self-published reports, and computer conferencing.

Motion picture films have been used by speech-language pathologists and audiologists to disseminate research findings for a relatively long period of time. They also have used videotapes for this purpose. The latter are now being used for it more frequently than the former because the technology is less expensive and more accessible.

Audiotapes have been used for disseminating research findings. For example, presentations at state and national speech, language, and hearing con-

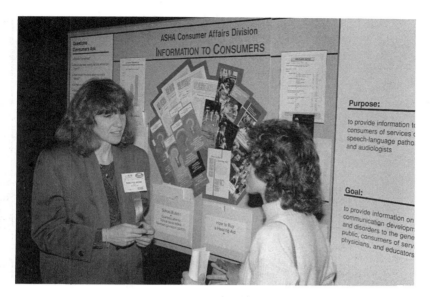

FIGURE 12.1 A poster session at an American Speech-Language-Hearing Association Convention.

ventions (including ASHA conventions) have been audiotaped and copies made available to interested persons at relatively low cost.

Some individuals and institutions disseminate research findings by publishing their own reports. A university speech and hearing program, for example, may periodically publish reports of research by its students and faculty. Or investigators who have written final reports for agencies that have funded their research may make them available, in whole or part, to interested persons. Because of easy access in most institutions to microcomputers with software for desktop publishing and laser printers, publications of this type that look very professional (e.g., see Miles, 1987) can be produced relatively inexpensively. Research disseminated in this manner may, at a later time, be communicated through journal articles and/or convention presentations.

Findings reported in convention presentations often are disseminated in self-published reports. This is particularly likely to be the case if they are viewed as "preliminary" and, therefore, not appropriate for reporting in a journal article. Copies of convention papers, incidentally, often are obtainable from their authors. A form that can be used for requesting copies of such papers, as well as reprints of published ones, is reproduced in Figure 12.2.

Computer conferencing is a relatively new approach for disseminating research findings. Persons interested in a particular disorder (e.g., stuttering) or a particular intervention approach (e.g., augmentative communication) communicate with each other by linking their personal microcomputers, via

---

MARQUETTE UNIVERSITY
Department of Speech Pathology and Audiology
Milwaukee, Wisconsin 53233

Dear

    I would appreciate receiving . . . .

. . . .

. . . .

. . . .

and any related papers if available.

                           Cordially,

FIGURE 12.2   A form for requesting copies of convention papers and reprints of journal articles.

modem, to minicomputers (e.g., Vax computers) or mainframe ones that provide access to networks such as BITNET (CREN) and INTERNET. These networks link computers around the world. An example of such a discussion group is STUTT-L which is for researchers and clinicians working on the problem of stuttering (*STUTT-L for researchers, clinicians,* 1990). The advantage of disseminating findings in this manner is that it can be done more quickly than by other means. Findings and their interpretations can be communicated within days after being acquired and formulated, rather than months or years. The disadvantage of doing so is that they are communicated to only a relatively small number of persons—i.e., those who have access to the network. Of course, findings and interpretations disseminated in this manner can later be communicated by more traditional ones—through journal articles and convention presentations.

OBJECTIVES OF SCIENTIFIC COMMUNICATION

Certain types of information should be communicated when disseminating research findings regardless of the mode used. These are discussed here with reference to objectives of scientific communication.

Overall Purpose of Scientific Communication

Before discussing the specific objectives of scientific communication, let's briefly consider its overall purpose, i.e., *communication.* Information should be provided about questions, answers, and interpretations as unambiguously as possible. Anything that facilitates communication is desirable; anything that impedes it is undesirable.

What factors can affect the adequacy of scientific communication? The answer to this question would be partially dependent on the mode used. Factors likely to impede communication in oral presentations differ somewhat from those likely to do so in written reports or videotapes.

While some factors that affect the adequacy of scientific communication are specific to the medium used, there are two that tend to do so in all of them. The first is *organization.* If the information to be disseminated is not organized in a manner that can be easily comprehended, the adequacy of the communication will be reduced. For this reason, the organization (or structure) of both written and oral research reports has been standardized to a degree. (This organization is described elsewhere in the chapter.)

The second factor that tends to affect the adequacy of scientific communication in all media is *language usage.* Accurate, detailed verbal "maps" facilitate communication, and inaccurate or vague ones impede it (see Chapter 7 for a discussion of map-territory relationships).

Specific Objectives of Scientific Communication

To be effective, scientific communication requires the following:

1. Each question to be answered must be stated as unambiguously as possible.
2. The importance of answering each question must be demonstrated, thereby establishing scientific justification.
3. The manner in which the observations were made to answer each question must be described as clearly as possible.
4. The observations made that are relevant for answering each question must be reported (i.e., each question be answered).
5. Some implications (clinical, theoretical, or both) of the answer to each question must be indicated.

We will now consider the contribution made by each of these to the effective communication of research findings.

One of the more important requirements for effective scientific communication is that each question the investigator(s) attempted to answer be stated as clearly as possible at the beginning of the report, regardless of the medium used. If potential consumers of information being reported do not know the specific questions it is intended to answer (i.e., the purpose of the study), they are unlikely to fully understand the answers (or findings) and the conclusions and generalizations made from them.

A second requirement is that the importance of answering each question be made explicit at the beginning of the report. This involves providing cogent answers for the "so what" or "who cares" questions—i.e., establishing *scientific justification* for the research. If potential consumers of the research feel, rightly or wrongly, that an answer to a particular question does not affect them (i.e., is not relevant), they will probably pay little, if any, attention to the answer. It is risky to assume that they will see the importance of answering it without this being pointed out to them. The more explicitly scientific justification is established, the more likely the information presented will be attended to and utilized, regardless of the communication mode used.

A third requirement is a description of how the observations were made to answer each question which is sufficiently detailed to enable someone else to replicate the process. Basic to the scientific method is *intersubjective testability* (see Chapter 3), the requirement that the observations used to answer questions be verifiable by other investigators. For this to be possible, there must be adequate descriptions of both the subjects observed and the procedures used to observe them.

A detailed description of methodology also is necessary to allow potential consumers of the observations reported to estimate their levels of validity, reliability, and generality (see Chapter 11).

A fourth requirement is reporting the observations made to answer each question as clearly (unambiguously) as possible. The observations relevant to answering a particular question should be organized for reporting in such a manner that the reason or reasons for the answer given are obvious (see Chapters 9 and 10).

Finally, a fifth requirement is an indication of possible implications of the answer to each question for the existing body of knowledge. Where possible, both theoretical and clinical implications should be suggested. It is usually not safe to assume that consumers of the research reported will see the implications of the findings without their being pointed out. And, of course, if your audience is unaware of the implications of the findings, they are unlikely to influence either theory or clinical practice.

ORGANIZATION OF WRITTEN REPORTS

We will now describe the organization of one of the two most commonly used modes of scientific communication: written reports. (The other is oral convention reports.) The information presented in such reports usually is organized in the manner described here because it facilitates communication. There are several reasons why this sort of organization tends to do so. First, the sequence in which the topics are presented is a logical one. It begins with the questions and the reasons for wanting to answer them. The sequence then moves to a description of how the observations were made to answer each question. Next is the presentation of the observations that answer each question. Last, possible theoretical and clinical implications of the answers are suggested.

There is another reason why this organization facilitates communication. With it, a reader will know where within a report to locate desired information. Information about the subjects observed, for example, is almost always presented in the *Methods* section.

The traditional research report has most, if not all, of the following parts:

1. title
2. abstract (or summary)
3. introduction
4. methodology
5. results
6. discussion
7. acknowledgments
8. references
9. appendixes

The purpose and content of each is described below.

Title

A title is very important. If the information presented in a research report is not indicated by its title, the report may not reach potential consumers, for several reasons. First, the title is one of the main sources of information used for indexing articles in abstracts journals and computer databases (see Chapter 4). Papers dealing with communicative disorders are indexed in a number of such journals and databases, including ones in linguistics, biology, physics, engineering, education, psychology, and medicine. If the title does not clearly indicate the content of an article, it is likely to be indexed improperly.

A title is also important because people scan titles (in bibliographies, tables of contents, and so forth) to identify papers they wish to read. If the content of a paper is not evident from its title, the paper may not be read by potential consumers of the information presented in it.

What should you keep in mind when writing a title for a paper? First, the wording should indicate as explicitly as possible the content of the paper—i.e., the questions dealt with. It should indicate both the specific population or populations studied (e.g., adults over the age of 50 who have cerebellar ataxia) and what was studied (e.g., the outcome of a particular therapy.) Both types of information can be combined to form a title such as:

Therapy X: Impact on Adults over the Age of Fifty with Cerebellar Ataxia

Second, be as concise as possible. All unnecessary words should be eliminated. Consider this title:

A Study of the Impact of Therapy X on Adults over the Age of Fifty with Cerebellar Ataxia

The first four words ("A Study of the . . .") can probably be deleted without altering what the title is intended to communicate.

Third, order the words appropriately. The first word (or words) in a title should at least partially define the topic. Consider the two titles suggested in this section for a study of the impact of a therapy on persons over the age of 50 who have cerebellar ataxia. Even if the first four words of the second were eliminated, the first would still be better than the second because it begins with a word that is more important for communicating the content of the paper—i.e., the name of the therapy.

Abstract

The abstract (or summary) provides the reader (usually in less than 150 words) with concise information about the question or questions asked, the procedures used to answer them, the answers obtained, and how the answers were interpreted. In most journals, it appears below the title. One of its most important functions is to indicate—in conjunction with the title—the content of the article to users of abstracts journals and computer literature-search databases (see Chapter 4). The titles and abstracts of almost all recent papers dealing with communicative disorders (as well as some not-so-recent ones) are in at least one of these journals and databases. An investigator doing a search of the communicative disorders literature usually uses more than one because there are none that are likely to include all literature relevant to a topic. If the title and abstract of a paper do not accurately and unambiguously indicate its content, the information in it is likely to be lost to at least some potential users.

There are two basic types of abstracts. The first (and most commonly used) *summarizes* the content of the paper—i.e., the question or questions asked, the observational procedures, the observations made, the answers to the questions, and the interpretations made. Here is a representative abstract of this type:

> The effect of adaptation on the masking of tinnitus was investigated. Six patients with tinnitus performed two 5-min tracking tasks, each replicated six times. The first task investigated the masking of tinnitus by tracking the intensity of a pure tone required to mask the tinnitus. The second task examined adaptation of a suprathreshold tone by tracking the intensity of a pure tone required for constant loudness. For 3 patients, the change required for constant loudness did not differ from the change required for constant maskability. For 3 patients, however, these two changes were different. Possible implications of these results for determining the locus of tinnitus and for the use of tinnitus maskers are discussed. (Penner and Bilger, 1989, p. 339)

The second type of abstract, which is used less often than the first, *describes* the content of the paper. It indicates the topics that were dealt with.

This type of abstract frequently is used for relatively long papers where the content cannot be summarized in the number of words allowed. It also sometimes is used for one- or two-page papers because a long abstract could look ridiculous when printed in one this short. Here is a representative abstract of this type:

> This paper describes a dimension of the stuttering problem of elementary-school children—less frequent revision of reading errors than their nonstuttering peers. (Silverman and Williams, 1973, p. 584)

What should you keep in mind when writing an abstract (or summary)? The main thing is that it must indicate the content of the paper as accurately and completely as possible within the length (i.e., word) limit imposed by the journal. Also, the writing should be as concise as possible. The most appropriate (e.g., descriptive, concrete) words for conveying what you wish to convey should be used. All unnecessary words should be eliminated. You may find it helpful to read a number of abstracts (e.g., all those in several issues of the *Journal of Speech and Hearing Research*) one after the other. This intensive reading should help you develop an intuitive feeling for how they are written.

Introduction

In the introduction to a paper, you indicate *what* you were trying to do and *why* you were trying to do it. That is, you indicate the questions you attempted to answer and why you felt it important to attempt to answer each. Stating the importance of answering each question establishes the *scientific justification* for the study.

It is very important to demonstrate as explicitly as possible the relevance of the research you are reporting—i.e., the questions you are answering. You should indicate as many *cogent* theoretical and clinical implications of possible answers to your questions as you can. Lead your readers to the point where they would agree that the questions you sought to answer were worth answering. As mentioned previously, it is not safe to assume that readers will understand the implications of answers to questions without having these implications pointed out to them.

In the introduction you also review the literature that is *relevant to the questions you were attempting to answer.* Specifically, you indicate any data you are aware of that directly or indirectly suggest an answer to these questions. These data, of course, may suggest different answers to specific questions (which would make any answer to them equivocal). An investigator usually attempts to indicate in the literature review why the available data only permit the questions asked to be partially answered and/or why it is important to gather additional data so that they can be answered unequivocally. If, based on a careful review of relevant literature, it appears that no data have been reported that suggest an answer to the questions asked, this should be indicated.

Before you attempt to write an introduction, you might find it helpful to read a number of them, one after the other, in articles published in an issue of the *American Journal of Audiology: A Journal of Clinical Practice,* the *American Journal of Speech-Language Pathology: A Journal of Clinical Practice,* or the *Journal of Speech and Hearing Research.* Doing so should help you to develop an intuitive understanding of how they are structured.

Methodology

In the methods section of a research report, you indicate *who* you observed and *how* you observed them. That is, you describe the subjects who were observed and the procedures followed in observing them. Both should be described in enough detail that another investigator could replicate your observations, but not in so much detail that this section would become unnecessarily long and confusing.

How do you decide what information should be included in a methods section? The sole criterion for any bit of information is whether it is necessary to someone who wished to replicate your observations. If you feel a given piece of information is likely to be necessary for this purpose, it should be included. If you do not feel it is necessary for this purpose, you can probably safely exclude it. If you are uncertain whether it is necessary, however, it should be included. Problems caused by not providing adequate information about subjects in aphasia research have been described in Brookshire (1983).

Before you attempt to write a methods section, you may find it helpful to scan a number of them in an issue of the *Journal of Speech and Hearing Research,* one after the other, paying particular attention to how they are organized.

Results

In the results section of a research report, you describe *what* was observed—i.e., the observations that were made to answer each question. You organize these observations in a manner that should make the answer to each question fairly obvious to most readers. In this section you answer each question and report the data upon which your answers are based.

Interpretations of the data are usually made not in this section but in the discussion one. There are instances, however, when it is desirable to interpret the data while they are being presented. A combined results and discussion section can be used in these cases.

Discussion

In the discussion section of a research report, you indicate *possible implications*—both theoretical and clinical—of the answers you obtained. You indicate both the ways in which your answers appear to be consistent with existing theory and clinical practice and the ways in which they raise questions concerning the validity of aspects of existing theory and clinical practice.

It is particularly important, in the discussion section, to deal with the possible implications of the research mentioned in the introduction to establish scientific justification. You should summarize the answers to the questions and indicate their implications for these aspects of theory and clinical practice.

Questions for future research are sometimes suggested in the discussion section. A study may raise more questions than it answers. By mentioning such questions and indicating why each would be important to answer, you can help an investigator who wishes to attempt to answer them establish scientific justification. That is, he or she can cite your paper when attempting to do so.

Acknowledgments

The primary purpose of an acknowledgments section is to credit and recognize the financial and other support of individuals and organizations you received while doing the research and preparing the research report. Any financial assistance should be acknowledged, as should any persons who significantly contributed to the research by performing such functions as locating subjects, administering the experimental treatments, or assisting in the process of data analysis. Other persons you may wish to acknowledge are consultants, investigators who provided you with unpublished data, administrators who in some manner facilitated the research process, and persons who read the manuscript critically and offered suggestions for improvement.

Another type of information that may be presented in an acknowledgment section is the author's current institutional affiliation if it differs from that given at the beginning of the article. Some journals also include in this section the name and address of the person to whom requests for reprints should be directed.

References

All papers and books mentioned in the paper should be listed here. Since there is no standard reference style, you should acquaint yourself with the style used by the journal to which you plan to submit the paper before preparing this section. ASHA journals use that of the American Psychological Association (*Publication Manual of the American Psychological Association*, 1983).

Appendixes

Appendixes usually contain unpublished documents pertaining to the methodology used for gathering data. An example would be an unpublished test or other assessment instrument.

ORGANIZATION OF ORAL PRESENTATIONS

The organization described for written reports is generally suitable for oral presentations. The two main ways in which oral reports differ from written ones are *length* and *style*. Because an investigator is usually permitted only a short period of time at most conventions and other professional meetings to report the research, he or she must summarize methodology and results briefly rather than describing them in detail.

A second difference is that the style of oral reports is usually less formal and more redundant than the style of written reports. The language of an oral report should be as conversational as possible, because the goal is to communicate with the audience. If the language of a paper read aloud is similar to that of a formal, written research report, at least some members of the audience will not pay as much attention as they would otherwise.

To communicate effectively, an oral report must be more repetitious than a written one. If you do not understand something in a written report, you can reread it. This is not possible with an oral presentation, unless it is on audiotape or videotape. One strategy that is helpful for providing the necessary redundancy in oral reports is to begin by summarizing what you are going to say, then saying it, and ending by summarizing what you have said.

PREPARATION OF WRITTEN AND ORAL REPORTS

Besides reading a number of already published reports for organization and wording, you can learn to prepare reports by consulting references on scientific writing. There are several relevant books and articles you may find helpful for this purpose. The *Publication Manual for the American Psychological Association* (1983) is a highly useful source of such information. So are *A Manual Guide for Writers in Communicative Disorders* (Shipley, 1982), "Guidelines for Nonsexist Language in Journals of ASHA" (1979), and *The Publication Process: A Guide for Authors* (1991). Other publications you might wish to consult are those of Forscher and Wertz (1970), Jerger (1962), Moore (1969), and Weiss-Lambrou (1989).

Before preparing a written report that you intend to submit for publication, you should read the information to contributors provided by the journal you plan to submit it to. Some journals publish this information in every issue; others publish it at regular intervals (e.g., one issue a year); still others do not publish it but send copies on request. The information usually provided in the section on information to contributors includes the following:

1. types of papers the journal prints (e.g., research review papers) and their topics (e.g., hearing problems, cleft lip and palate)

2. instructions for preparing tables and figures and for typing the manuscript
3. maximum length for the abstract
4. reference style
5. number of copies that should be submitted
6. name of the editor to whom the copies of the manuscript should be
submitted

LOCATING OUTLETS FOR SPEECH-LANGUAGE PATHOLOGY AND AUDIOLOGY RESEARCH

Your final task in the research process is disseminating your questions, answers, and interpretations where they are likely to reach potential consumers
of the information. This process usually involves either locating a journal to
which to submit a written report or locating a professional meeting (e.g., a
convention of an organization) at which to present a report (or both, since
many papers presented at professional meetings are later published).

The outlets probably most often used by speech-language pathologists
and audiologists for disseminating research findings are the publications and
convention programs of the American Speech-Language-Hearing Association
(ASHA). The ASHA journals include:

- *American Journal of Audiology: A Journal of Clinical Practice*
- *American Journal of Speech-Language Pathology: A Journal of Clinical
Practice*
- *Journal of Speech and Hearing Disorders* (Combined with the *Journal of
Speech and Hearing Research* in 1991)
- *Journal of Speech and Hearing Research*
- *Language, Speech, and Hearing Services in Schools*
- *Asha*
- *ASHA Monographs*
- *ASHA Reports*

Each issue of these journals contains a statement of the types of research
reports it will consider. One advantage of publishing in ASHA journals is that
you are quite likely to reach most speech-language pathologists and audiologists who would be potential consumers of your research.

More than 500 research reports dealing with all aspects of speech-
language pathology and audiology are usually included in the program of the
annual convention of the American Speech-Language-Hearing Association.
For a research report to be considered for inclusion in the convention program, a summary and abstract of the research have to be submitted to the
program committee. Additional information can be found in the annual "Call
for Papers," which is usually published in the February issue of *Asha*.

State speech and hearing association publications and convention programs are also outlets for disseminating research findings. Their main limitation is that the audience you can reach through them is geographically limited.

A number of other associations publish research relevant to speech-
language pathology or audiology in their journals and include such reports in
their convention programs. The following is a representative, not an inclusive, list of such organizations:

- Academy of Aphasia
- Academy of Cerebral Palsy
- Acoustical Society of America
- Alexander Graham Bell Association
- American Cleft Palate Association
- American Psychological Association
- Canadian Speech and Hearing Association
- College of Speech Therapists (London)
- Computer Users in Speech and Hearing
- Council of Exceptional Children
- International Association of Logopedics and Phoniatrics
- International Fluency Association
- International Society for Augmentative and Alternative
  Communication
- Societa Italiana di Foniatria e Logopedia

Finally, several journals not published by scientific and professional associations can serve as outlets for speech-language pathology and audiology
research. Two examples would be the *Journal of Communication Disorders*
and *Perceptual and Motor Skills*.

Perhaps the best strategy for identifying possible journals to submit a
particular research report to is to scan abstracts dealing with the same general
topic in the Medline computer database or in *Index Medicus, Linguistics and
Language Behavior Abstracts,* or *Psychological Abstracts* and note the journals
in which the papers have been published.

Some journals are regarded as better than others. A survey of faculty
members of 116 colleges and universities (Goodwin, 1982) revealed that the
following journals were regarded as the 20 best for speech-language pathologists; that is, these are the journals in which they felt it was most desirable
to publish and/or in which they would expect most material important to
them as a speech-language pathologist to appear. The order indicates their
ranking within the group.

- *Journal of Speech and Hearing Disorders*
- *Journal of Speech and Hearing Research*

- *Asha*
- *Journal of Child Language*
- *Language, Speech, and Hearing Services in Schools*
- *Journal of Communication Disorders*
- *Brain and Language*
- *Cleft Palate Journal*
- *Journal of the Acoustical Society of America*
- *Folia Phoniatrica*
- *Journal of Verbal Learning and Verbal Behavior*
- *Cortex*
- *Journal of Fluency Disorders*
- *Journal of Psycholinguistic Research*
- *Journal of Learning Disabilities*
- *Language and Speech*
- *Brain*
- *Archives of Otolaryngology*
- *Laryngoscope*
- *Acta Oto-Laryngologia*

Those regarded as the 20 best for audiologists were ranked as follows:

- *Journal of Speech and Hearing Research*
- *Journal of Speech and Hearing Disorders*
- *Journal of the Acoustical Society of America*
- *Archives of Otolaryngology*
- *Ear and Hearing*
- *Audiology (International)*
- *Acta Oto-Laryngologia*
- *Journal of Auditory Research*
- *Annals of Otology, Rhinology, and Laryngology*
- *Asha*
- *Laryngoscope*
- *Hearing Instruments*
- *Volta Review*
- *American Annals of the Deaf*
- *Audiology and Hearing Education*
- *Scandinavian Audiology*
- *Language, Speech, and Hearing Services in Schools*
- *Archives of Oto-Rhino-Laryngology*
- *Hearing Aid Journal*
- *Brain and Language*

One limitation of both lists, of course, is that journals were not considered that begin after the survey was completed such as the *American Journal of*

Audiology: A Journal of Clinical Practice, the *American Journal of Speech-Language Pathology: A Journal of Clinical Practice, Augmentative and Alternative Communication*, and the *Journal for Computer Users in Speech and Hearing.*

EDITORIAL PROCESSING OF MANUSCRIPTS

How is a manuscript processed after it has been submitted to a journal to be considered for publication? After receiving the copies of the manuscript, the editor usually sends a form letter to the author indicating that the manuscript has been received and that the decision concerning it will be relayed as soon as the manuscript has been reviewed. The editor usually sends copies of the manuscript to at least two editorial consultants, or reviewers, who the editor feels are competent to assess the suitability of the manuscript for publication. The editor asks them for a recommendation on the disposition of the manuscript (accept as is, accept if revised according to instructions, reject, etc.), the reason or reasons for their recommendation, and suggestions for revising the manuscript. After receiving the reviewers' recommendations and reading the manuscript, the editor decides on the disposition of the manuscript and informs the author of the decision and the reason or reasons for it. If the editor feels that parts of the manuscript need to be rewritten before it is suitable for publication, he or she will indicate to the author the parts that have to be rewritten and may offer some suggestions for rewriting them. (Almost all manuscripts, incidentally, require some rewriting.) The review process can take anywhere from a few weeks to more than a year; in most cases it takes between two and six months.

What should you do if a manuscript you write is rejected by a journal? Few people enjoy being rejected; and if a manuscript you write is rejected, it can hurt your ego. Since some journals have rejection rates of more than 75 percent, most (if not all) investigators are going to have papers rejected sooner or later. What you should do with such a manuscript depends on the reason or reasons for its rejection (as well as this can be determined from the editor's and reviewers' comments). A manuscript could be rejected for the following reasons:

1. The author(s) failed to establish scientific justification for the study (i.e., the reviewers regarded it as trivial).
2. The observational procedures used would probably not permit the question or questions to be answered with an adequate level of validity, reliability, and generality.
3. The data analyses procedures were inappropriate.
4. The writing did not meet minimum standards for publication.
5. The content of the manuscript was inappropriate for the journal.

6. The reviewers did not like the question or questions the author(s) asked and/or how the findings were interpreted.

If your manuscript is rejected because you failed to establish adequate scientific justification for the study in it, you should attempt to rewrite the introduction to demonstrate the relevance of the study. Assuming this was the *only* reason why the manuscript appeared to have been rejected, and you feel that you have established adequate scientific justification for the study in your rewrite of the introduction, you may wish to resubmit the manuscript to the journal with a note indicating how it has been revised. Or you may wish to submit it to another journal.

If your manuscript is rejected because something was wrong with the methodology used to make the observations, and you agree that the reviewers' criticisms are valid, you may want to rerun the study using observational procedures that were modified as recommended. However, if you feel that the reviewers' criticisms are not valid, you may wish to send a rebuttal to the editor indicating why you felt your methodology was adequate and requesting that the editor reconsider the manuscript. Or you may wish to submit the manuscript to another journal.

If your manuscript is rejected because something was wrong with how the data were analyzed, you should reanalyze the data and either resubmit the corrected manuscript to the journal or submit it to some other journal. If you feel, however, that the data have been appropriately analyzed, you may wish to write the editor indicating why you feel your analyses were appropriate, including, if possible, supporting statements from one or more statisticians.

If your manuscript is rejected because it was badly written, it should be rewritten (with particular consideration given to relevant comments by reviewers) and either resubmitted to the journal or submitted to some other journal. Hopefully, some person at your institution experienced in writing research reports could assist you with the rewriting.

If your manuscript is rejected because the content was inappropriate for the journal to which it was submitted, it should be submitted to a journal for which the content would be appropriate. You may be able to identify one by scanning several volumes of an abstracts journal for papers with similar content.

Occasionally, a manuscript is rejected by a journal because the reviewers did not like the questions the author asked or the interpretation of the findings. This is particularly likely to occur when an author's findings challenge accepted theory or clinical practice. An author who feels a manuscript has been rejected on this basis should submit it to another journal.

For further information about why articles are rejected, see the paper by Culatta (1984). In it he analyzed why articles were turned down by *Asha*.

FIGURE 12.3 Evaluation checklist for quality of communication.

Indicate beside each statement whether or not it appears to be true.

Yes	No		Statement
＿＿	＿＿	1.	The need (i.e., scientific justification) for the research is clearly explained at the beginning of the report.
＿＿	＿＿	2.	The questions that the research seeks to answer are clearly stated.
＿＿	＿＿	3.	The relationship of the research to previous research is clearly explained.
＿＿	＿＿	4.	The observational procedures that were used for answering the questions are clearly described. A reader or listener should not "lose the forest for the trees" because too much detail is being presented. This is particularly likely to happen during oral presentations such as convention papers.
＿＿	＿＿	5.	The population from which the subjects were sampled is clearly described.
＿＿	＿＿	6.	The data which were generated by the observational procedures are clearly presented. A listener or reader should not "lose the forest for the trees" because (a) data are presented that are not relevant for answering the questions being asked or (b) data are not organized in a manner that can be readily understood by readers or listeners. The latter is particularly likely to happen during oral presentations, particularly if complex figures or tables are used.
＿＿	＿＿	7.	The answers to the questions are clearly stated and it is clear how the answers were derived from the data.
＿＿	＿＿	8.	Theoretical and clinical implications of the answers are clearly stated, even the ones which seem obvious. An implication that seems obvious to the investigator may not be so to a listener or reader. Implications may seem obvious to investigators because they have thought about them a great deal.
＿＿	＿＿	9.	The language used is appropriate for the situation. It is intended to communicate rather than impress. Technical terms with which some readers or listeners are likely to be unfamiliar are either avoided or defined. This is particularly important for oral presentations, since listeners obviously cannot look words up immediately. Also, a writing style should be used that will make the paper interesting to most listeners or readers. An "oral" writing style will do this. To determine whether a paper is written in an oral style read it *aloud*. If it doesn't sound the way you or another human being would talk (i.e., if the sentences seem awkward), it probably is not written in an oral style.

EVALUATION CHECKLIST FOR QUALITY OF COMMUNICATION

The quality of the communication in a journal article or convention paper can profoundly influence the impact that the research reported in it will have on consumers. Several undesirable consequences can occur if the quality of the communication is low. The findings of the research may not be fully understood or their theoretical and clinical implications may be unclear. Either can significantly reduce the probability that particular research findings will be helpful to persons who are communicatively impaired.

There are a number of things which investigators can do to maximize the quality of the communication in their written reports and oral presentations. Some of them are mentioned in the evaluation checklist (see Figure 12.3). Investigators can use it as a guide when *preparing* written reports (including journal articles) and oral presentations (including convention papers). It also can be used as a guide for *evaluating* journal articles and convention papers if used in conjunction with the checklist in Chapter 11.

EXERCISES AND DISCUSSION TOPICS

1. Use the Evaluation Checklist (Figure 12.3) to assess the quality of the communication in three papers from a recent issue of the *Journal of Speech and Hearing Research.*

2. Listen to tape recordings of two convention papers and assess the quality of the communication in them, using the Evaluation Checklist.

3. What statements in the Evaluation Checklist can be used for assessing the quality of the communication in clinical evaluation reports?

13

Assessing the Effects of Intervention Strategies

To continue to grow as clinicians, we must continually evaluate the impacts of our intervention strategies—both positive and negative—on our clients. Without the information such an evaluation gives, we are apt to use either a small number over and over again or continuously seek out the "newest" ones. Our reason for adopting or rejecting a particular intervention strategy is likely to be its acceptance or rejection by an "authority," such as the author of a textbook we are familiar with, rather than its impact on clients' behavior, particularly their communicative behavior.

We can make one of two presumptions about the impact of an intervention strategy on behaviors contributing to a client's communicative disorder: (1) we can consider it effective until it is proven ineffective, or (2) we can consider it ineffective until it has been proven effective. The choice between them is somewhat analogous to that in law between considering a person innocent until proven guilty and considering him or her guilty until proven innocent.

What are the consequences of choosing each presumption? There are two types of consequence. The first is *clinical*. Each presumption has associated with it a type of treatment error. That is, considering an intervention strategy effective until there is reasonable evidence that it is ineffective exposes a client to an intervention strategy that could have no effect, or an undesirable effect, on him or her. On the other hand, considering an intervention strategy ineffective until there is reasonable evidence that it is effective could result in a client who could be helped by it not being so.

The presumption that would be most likely to lead to undesirable consequences for a client would not be the same in all instances. To illustrate this point, let's consider two instances in which we might be tempted to try an intervention strategy that seems sound theoretically but has not yet been proven effective. In instance A, there is at least one other intervention strategy that has been proven effective; in instance B, there are no intervention strategies that have been proven effective. The consequences of *using* the new approach in instance A and finding it ineffective are likely to be more undesirable than not using it when it would have been effective. On the other hand, the consequences of *not using* this approach in instance B are likely to be less desirable than using it and finding it ineffective.

The second type of consequence can be referred to as *logical*. A logical consequence is one related to the choice of research design, particularly statistical inference. If our presumption is that an intervention strategy is ineffective until it is proven effective, we can use traditional statistical hypothesis testing procedures to determine the likelihood that it has been effective (see Chapter 10). Recall that the null hypothesis—the hypothesis tested by all traditional statistical significance tests—states that a treatment has produced no difference, i.e., has had no effect. For determining whether an intervention strategy has influenced behavior, the null hypothesis would state that any impacts the intervention strategy appears to have had are not real but the result of random fluctuation or sampling error. In other words, differences in behavior following intervention are not sufficiently *reliable* to be attributed to it.

Rejecting the null hypothesis provides some support for the alternative, or research hypothesis, that intervention has been effective—i.e., has resulted in behavioral change. However, it is necessary to keep constantly in mind that rejecting a null hypothesis or null hypotheses only indicates that any behavioral changes observed following intervention are unlikely to have been the result of random fluctuation or sampling error (see Chapter 10). It does not establish that such changes resulted from intervention. Other events occurring while a client was in therapy could be responsible for the observed behavioral change. Examples of such events would be: (1) maturation (particularly of concern when evaluating intervention strategies for children who have a language disorder), (2) improved self-concept (particularly of concern when evaluating intervention strategies for stuttering), (3) spontaneous recovery (particularly of concern when evaluating intervention strategies for aphasia, agnosia, apraxia, and dysarthria), and (4) events, other than those that were a part of the program, that occurred while it was being administered.

We will now consider the logical consequences of the alternative presumption—i.e., considering an intervention strategy effective until it is proven ineffective. This is comparable to interpreting failure to reject a null hypothesis as support for a strategy's effectiveness. As you may recall from our previous discussion of the null hypothesis, it is inappropriate to interpret failure to reject a null hypothesis as support for a research hypothesis (in this case, an intervention strategy being effective).

In most instances considering an intervention strategy ineffective until there is considerable evidence that it is effective would probably be more defensible than the alternative presumption, i.e., considering it effective until there is considerable evidence to the contrary.

QUESTIONS TO CONSIDER WHEN EVALUATING AN INTERVENTION STRATEGY

A basic premise of this book is that research can be viewed as a process of answering "answerable" questions. Systematic research to assess the effects of an intervention strategy upon persons who have a communicative disorder should provide answers to a series of such questions, including the following:

1. What Are the Impacts of the Intervention Strategy on Specific Behaviors That Contribute to a Client's Communicative Disorder at Given Points in Space-Time? Here "specific behaviors" include what are traditionally called "attitudes" and "feelings." We become aware of attitudes and feelings by observing behavior—that is, attitudes and feelings are *explanations* for behavior. "Points in space-time" refers to how the impacts of an intervention strategy on specific behaviors vary, over a period of time and according to situation. *Space-time* is hyphenated to indicate (as Einstein and others have pointed out) that time cannot be separated from space but provides the fourth dimension necessary to specify the location, or coordinates, of an event.

2. What Are the Impacts of the Intervention Strategy on Other Attributes of a Client's Communicative Behavior at Given Points in Space-Time? An intervention strategy that has a desirable impact on behaviors that contribute to a client's communicative disorder can affect other attributes of his or her communicative behavior in undesirable and desirable ways—i.e., it can have good and/or bad *side effects*. Other attributes affected might include: (1) speaking rate, (2) auditory acuity, (3) speech rhythm, (4) speech articulation, (5) voice intensity, (6) voice quality, (7) language formulation, (8) verbal output, (9) spontaneity, and (10) credibility as a communicator. If, for example, a stutterer is taught to monitor his speech for moments of stuttering and voluntarily reduce their severity, this may not only result in a reduction in his stuttering severity but in his speaking rate, spontaneity, and inflection as well. If a client's communicative behavior after intervention with a particular strategy called more adverse attention to itself than before receiving it, this would be an undesirable side effect. On the other hand, if a mentally retarded child who had little or no speech was taught to communicate manually (e.g., with American Sign Language) and as a consequence significantly increased his or her verbal output—which happens in approximately one-third of cases (Silverman, 1989)—this side effect would be highly desirable.

3. What Are the Impacts of the Intervention Strategy on a Client Other Than Those Directly Related to Communicative Behavior at Given Points in Space-Time?

The intent of this question is similar to the second, since it is concerned with identifying undesirable and desirable side effects of the strategy. The side effects we are concerned with here would include impacts on: (1) self- concept, (2) peer acceptance, and (3) anxiety. A client given an instrumental aid (such as an electrolarynx or miniature metronome with which to pace his speech) might be able to communicate better with the device but might also feel there is something wrong with him for having to rely on it rather than being able to overcome the problem by "force of will." On the other hand, a severely motor handicapped client who cannot speak but learns to do so using a laptop microcomputer with a speech synthesizer is likely to be more accepted by peers than previously and, as a consequence, develop a better self-concept (Silverman, 1989).

4. What Are the Client's Attitudes Toward the Intervention Strategy and Its Impacts on His or Her Communicative and Other Behaviors at Given Points in Space-Time?

A client's attitude toward an intervention strategy and its impacts on his or her behavior can influence (reduce or enhance) the effectiveness of the strategy. If, for example, a person with a hearing loss refused to wear a hearing aid, the use of this strategy could not be effective in reducing the severity of the communicative disorder (unless, of course, the person's attitude could be changed). On the other hand, a client with a strong belief that an intervention strategy could benefit him or her would invest more time and energy in the program which, in turn, would tend to enhance its effectiveness.

5. What Are the Attitudes of a Client's Clinician, Family, Friends, and Others Toward the Intervention Strategy and Toward Its Impacts on the Client's Communicative Behavior and Other Attributes of Behavior at Given Points in a Space-Time?

The attitudes of persons with whom a client interacts toward an intervention strategy the client is receiving and toward its effects on his or her behavior can influence the probable success of that strategy. A clinician who does not believe that an intervention strategy will be effective is likely to communicate this attitude to the client and thereby reduce the likelihood that the client will benefit from it. If, for example, a clinician were directly or indirectly to communicate to a client who is severely communicatively impaired and could benefit from using a conversation board that he or she considered the use of such a device a last resort, this might reduce the likelihood that the client would use the device and thereby benefit from it. On the other hand, if such a client's family and friends were to spend more time with him or her after he or she has begun using a conversation board, this would increase the likelihood that the client would continue using the device and thereby benefit from it.

6. What Investment is Required of Client and Clinician at Given Points in Space-Time?   Several types of investment can be required, including: (1) financial, (2) time and energy, and (3) willingness to be uncomfortable, i.e., to do things one does not want to do (things that tend to make a person uncomfortable or increase his or her anxiety level). An intervention strategy may be effective but may be too demanding in cost or time to be practical for many clients. An example of such a strategy would be traditional psychoanalysis, in which the client may be required to be seen by the psychoanalyst daily for a period of several years. Also, a strategy may be effective but may cause clients to be so uncomfortable that few would be willing to make the necessary investment. One such strategy would be voluntary stuttering— "fake stuttering"—outside the clinic situation. Many stutterers find this activity extremely noxious and refuse to do so when asked by their clinician.

7. What is the Probability of Relapse Following Termination of Therapy?   Persons with communicative disorders, particularly stutterers, may relapse to some degree when they stop seeing their clinicians on a regular basis. While a person exposed to almost any intervention approach can relapse, the probability of relapse tends to be higher for some approaches than for others. If the positive impacts of an intervention approach were quite likely to wear off after termination of therapy, it would be of questionable value. It is important, then, when evaluating an intervention strategy to take the probability of relapse into consideration.

RESEARCH DESIGN CONSIDERATIONS FOR ASSESSING
THE IMPACTS OF INTERVENTION STRATEGIES

This section suggests some issues to consider when designing research to answer the questions raised in the preceding one. Most of the topics that have already been discussed—particularly descriptive statistics, inferential statistics, and measurement—are relevant for answering such questions. The comments here pertain mostly to ones that have not previously been discussed.

While there has not been much methodological research dealing specifically with considerations when assessing the impacts of intervention strategies on persons who have communicative disorders, considerable relevant methodological research has been published in education, clinical psychology, and psychiatry journals. Since the problems involved in assessing the impacts of teaching methods and psychotherapies are much the same as those involved in assessing the impacts of intervention on communicative disorders, some of this methodological research will be referred to in this discussion.

What Are the Impacts of the Intervention Strategy on Specific Behaviors That Contribute to a Client's Communicative Disorder at Given Points in Space-Time?

There are a number of things we must do when we wish to assess systematically the impacts of an intervention strategy on behaviors contributing to a client's communicative disorder, including the following:

1. choosing a criterion measure or measures
2. establishing a baseline
3. establishing a measurement interval
4. selecting criteria for deciding whether an intervention strategy has been effective
5. identifying viable alternatives to the hypothesis that an intervention strategy was responsible for an effect, if an effect is observed
6. reducing the effects of the experimenter's expectations and theoretical biases on the data
7. identifying relevant organismic variables
8. identifying relevant therapist variables
9. controlling positive and negative placebo effect contamination

We will now consider some issues that are applicable to each of them.

Choosing a Criterion Measure or Measures. The choice of a criterion measure or measures is one of the most important considerations when designing research to assess the impacts of intervention strategies on persons who have communicative disorders. If a criterion measure selected is not sufficiently reliable and valid, it can make an effective strategy appear ineffective.

One way to maximize the probability that an effective strategy will be judged effective is to use more than one criterion measure. If, for example, we wish to determine whether an intervention strategy for ameliorating an articulation error is effective, we might use as criterion measures the percent correct production of the "error" phoneme on several types of speaking tasks.

Establishing a Baseline. To determine whether an intervention strategy has been effective, an attribute of a client's behavior after being exposed to the strategy is compared to what it was either before being exposed to it or at an earlier point—or points—in therapy (e.g., the beginning of the semester). The measure or measures of that attribute to which those following intervention are compared constitute the baseline. The simplest baseline would consist of a single criterion measure made once before beginning intervention. More complex baselines would consist of: (1) a single criterion measure made more than once, (2) multiple criterion measures made once, or (3) multiple criterion measures made more than once. For further information about these, see Chapter 6.

Establishing a Measurement Interval.   One consideration in designing therapy outcome research is how frequently to make the criterion measure. The measurement interval probably used most frequently in such research is twice—once preceding a period of intervention and once following it. This is the traditional *pretest-posttest* design. This design is not a particularly good one for several reasons. First, it is more likely than most designs to result in a Type II error, since relatively high levels of random measurement error are possible when comparisons are made between single measures. Second, it is more difficult to interpret than most others. If a client's communicative disorder is less severe in the posttest than in the pretest, there may be plausible explanations for this difference other than its resulting from the intervention. Among the classes of extraneous variables that could account for such a difference, according to Campbell, are the following:

1. *History:* the other specific events occurring between the first and the second measurement in addition to the experimental variable [i.e., the intervention strategy].
2. *Maturation:* processes within the respondents [clients] operating as a function of the passage of time *per se* (not specific to the particular events), including growing older, growing hungrier, growing more tired, and the like.
3. *Testing:* the effects of taking a test upon the scores of a second testing.
4. *Instrumentation:* changes in the calibration of a measuring instrument or changes in the observers or scorers which may produce changes in the obtained measurements.
5. *Statistical regression:* regression operating when groups have been selected on the basis of their extreme scores.
6. *The reactive* or *interactive effect of testing,* in which a pretest might increase or decrease the respondent's sensitivity or responsiveness to the experimental variable and thus make the results obtained for a pretested population unrepresentative of the effects of the experimental variable for the unpretested universe from which the experimental respondents were selected. (Campbell, 1963, p. 215)

The effects of three of these causes—maturation, testing, and statistical regression—can be at least partially controlled by substituting a *time series* design such as the one illustrated for a pretest-posttest design (the notation used here is the same as that used in Chapter 6):

$A_1\ A_2\ A_3\ A_4\ A_5\ A_6\ A_7\ A_8$

With this design, a baseline measurement is made a predetermined number of times (in the above example, eight) at a set time interval. The duration of the interval between measures would be approximately equal to the duration of the intervention approach being evaluated. The clients receive the intervention (B) during the interval between two measures (in the example, they would receive it between measures of four and five). The criterion measures are then plotted, and the pattern of the resulting trendline is interpreted to indicate whether the intervention has had an impact (see Figure 13.1). This

FIGURE 13.1   Some possible outcome patterns from the introduction of an experimental variable at point B into a time series of measurements, A_1–A_8. Except for 4, the A_4–A_5 gain is the same for all time series, while the legitimacy of inferring an effect varies widely, being strongest in 1 and 2 and totally unjustified in 5, 6, and 7. (Adapted from Campbell, 1963, and reproduced with permission of the publisher.)

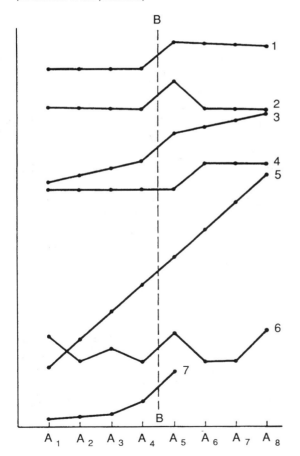

design is most practical for intervention approaches of relatively short duration.

A treatment does not have to occur at the midpoint of a time series. It could occur toward the beginning:

$$A_1 \ A_2 \ B \ A_3 \ A_4 \ A_5 \ A_6 \ A_7 \ A_8$$

Such a design could be useful for assessing the long-term impacts of an intervention strategy.

A variation of the time series design, the *multiple time series* (Campbell, 1963, p. 232), is even more effective in controlling for the effects of extraneous variables. Such a design is illustrated graphically by the following:

$$\text{GROUP 1 } A_1 \ A_2 \ A_3 \ A_4 \ B \ A_5 \ A_6 \ A_7 \ A_8$$

$$\text{GROUP 2 } A_1 \ A_2 \ A_3 \ A_4 \quad A_5 \ A_6 \ A_7 \ A_8$$

This design controls at least partially for five of the six classes of extraneous variables to which the pretest-posttest design is sensitive—history, maturation, testing, instrumentation, and statistical regression.

With a multiple time series design, the measures made on the members of a group with whom a particular intervention strategy is used (in the example, Group 1) are compared to those made on the members of a comparable group who do not receive that type of intervention (in the example, Group 2). The measures are made on both groups at the same time intervals. The measures made on the control group provide a secondary baseline against which to assess those made on the experimental group. The primary baseline is the same as for the pretest- posttest and single time series designs, i.e., the measures made prior to intervention.

The control, or secondary, baseline can be helpful in interpreting several of the outcome patterns in Figure 13.1. If, for example, the eight measures made on the members of a control group were approximately equal (i.e., the control baseline was relatively flat), Pattern 4 would indicate that the intervention strategy had been effective.

One limitation of the multiple time series design is the need for a control group. We could probably have reservations about withholding therapy from a group of clients who need it. There are circumstances, however, when this ethical consideration would not occur. One would be when enough people are on a waiting list who: (1) have the same type of communicative disorder as the members of the experimental group, and (2) do not differ systematically from them in relevant organismic variables such as age and intellectual level. A second circumstance would be when intervention is of relatively short duration. Delaying its start in this instance would probably do no harm.

For further information about these and other time series designs, see Chapter 6.

Selecting Criteria for Deciding Whether the Intervention Strategy Has Been Effective.   Before concluding that an intervention strategy has been effective, it is necessary to demonstrate a difference between pre- and post-intervention measures that: (1) is unlikely to have resulted from random, or chance, fluctuation, and (2) is more likely to have resulted from intervention than from extraneous variables. Demonstrating the first requires the use of statistical inference, specifically tests of the null hypothesis that no difference exists between client's pre- and post-intervention measures that is unlikely to have been the result of random, or chance, fluctuation. Considerations in selecting and interpreting such tests are discussed in Chapter 10. One point that must be stressed again is the importance of specifying and keeping relatively low the probability of a Type II error. In therapy outcome research, the size of the experimental group (and of the control group, if one is used) is apt to be relatively small, and hence the probability of a Type II error is apt to be relatively high.

If a null hypothesis is rejected, the next step is to demonstrate that the observed difference between pre- and post-intervention measures is more likely to have resulted from intervention than from extraneous variables. The ease with which it is possible to accomplish this objective is partially a function of the measurement interval used. It would be much simpler to accomplish, for example, with a time series than with a pretest-posttest design. With a pretest-posttest design, it is doubtful that you could be reasonably certain that an observed difference was the result of intervention rather than of extraneous variables.

Identifying Viable Alternatives to the Hypothesis That Intervention Was Responsible for an Impact, If One Was Observed.   The identification of viable alternative hypotheses is not, strictly speaking, a problem of research design or statistics. To identify factors that could explain an observed difference other than the intervention strategy being evaluated, an investigator must do a careful search of relevant literature.

Reducing the Effects of the Experimenter's Expectations and Theoretical Biases on the Data.   A number of investigations have demonstrated that an experimenter's expectations and biases can influence the results (Rosenthal and Rosnow, 1969; Whitaker, Dill, and Whitaker Jr., 1990). The nature of this influence is such that the investigator may not be consciously aware of it. While it is probably not possible in most instances to eliminate these effects completely from therapy outcome research, there are ways to reduce their influence, including the following:

1. Have someone *other than the experimenter* conduct the therapy session(s) and make and interpret the criterion measures. Ideally, the ex-

pectation of the person who performs these tasks should be relatively neutral with regard to the effectiveness of the therapy being evaluated.

2. Whenever possible, the person who makes and interprets criterion measures should not know when the material being measured and interpreted was collected. This can be done when the criterion measures are ratings of audiotapes or videotapes. The observers rating the tapes should not know whether any given tape was recorded prior to, during, or following intervention. This approach also can be used when the criterion measures are from physiological data readouts and psychological test protocols.

3. If the design used has both experimental and control group subjects— i.e., both subjects who receive and do not receive the therapy—the person who makes and interprets the measures should not know in any given instance which group a subject belongs to.

4. In studies of the relative effectiveness of several intervention strategies, it would be best if the same clinician did not administer all of them. A clinician may expect one to be more effective than the others, which could influence the data on their relative effectiveness.

Identifying Relevant Organismic Variables.   Organismic variables are properties or attributes of the individual (Edwards and Cronbach, 1966). Examples are sex, chronological age, socioeconomic status, intellectual level, and educational level. The degree of effectiveness of a therapy may be influenced by such variables. A particular approach to teaching the American Sign Language, for example, may be more effective with adults than with children.

There are at least two reasons for identifying relevant organismic variables in therapy outcome research. First, organismic variables may help define the subpopulation for which a given intervention strategy is effective. If there are no relevant organismic variables, one that is effective with some persons who have a particular communicative disorder should be effective with most, if not all, of those who have it (assuming the disorder has only one cause). On the other hand, if the effectiveness of a strategy is influenced by one or more organismic variables, the strategy *may* only be usable with a subset of the population. The word *may* was italicized because even though a strategy may not be as effective with some persons who have a particular disorder as it is with others, it still may be the most effective one to use with them.

A second reason for identifying relevant organismic variables is concerned with the meaningfulness of combining subjects into groups. The effects of an intervention strategy can be cancelled by combining data from subjects who differ with respect to relevant organismic variables. If an intervention strategy were effective with children and not with adults, for example, combining data from children and adults could make it appear to have been ineffective (particularly if there were more adults than children in the sample).

Identifying Relevant Therapist Variables. An intervention strategy administered by one therapist may not have the same effect as the same one administered by a second therapist. Certain attitudes and attributes of therapists can enhance or reduce the effectiveness of intervention strategies. One such attribute is amount of clinical experience. An intervention strategy administered by a clinician with considerable experience may be more effective than the same one administered by a beginning clinician. Also, a clinician who expects an intervention strategy to be effective may get a different result than one who expects it to be ineffective. Other therapist variables that could influence the effectiveness of an intervention strategy are sex, chronological age, socioeconomic status, degree of confidence in self, ability to communicate, and professional title (Dr. versus Mr., Ms., Miss, or Mrs.).

If the effectiveness of an intervention strategy is at least partially a function of therapist variables, this has several implications. First, it limits the generality of research findings on the effectiveness of that strategy. Perhaps an intervention strategy would only be recommended for clinicians with considerable experience or for those with considerable confidence in its effectiveness. Second, it may not be possible to combine, or "lump," data from different clinicians. If such data are combined, an intervention strategy that is effective for certain clinicians may appear to be ineffective, particularly if it is ineffective for the majority of clinicians.

Controlling Positive and Negative Placebo Effect Contamination. A placebo is

> ... any therapeutic procedure (or that component of any therapeutic procedure) which is given deliberately to have an effect, or unknowingly has an effect on a patient, symptom, syndrome, or disease, but which is objectively without *specific* activity for the condition being treated. The therapeutic procedure may be given with or without conscious knowledge that the procedure is a placebo, may be an active (non-inert) or nonactive (inert) procedure, and include, therefore, all medical procedures no matter how specific—oral and parenteral medication, topical preparations, inhalants, and mechanical, surgical, and psychotherapeutic procedures. The placebo must be differentiated from the placebo effect which may or may not occur and which may be favorable or unfavorable. The placebo effect is defined as the changes produced by placebos. (Shapiro, 1964, p. 75)

Thus, the placebo effect can either enhance or reduce the effectiveness of an intervention strategy. That is, the placebo effect can make it appear more effective or less effective than it really is. In therapy outcome research, therefore, one should recognize the possibility of, and control for, the placebo effect whenever possible (Rosenthal and Frank, 1956).

What factors may be responsible for the placebo effect? According to Shapiro (1964), any of the following can result in a placebo effect:

1. The client's faith in the ability of the clinician, the therapy, or both, to help him. This can result in either a positive or a negative placebo effect.

2. The clinician's attitude toward the intervention strategy—his or her faith or confidence in its effectiveness. This also can result in either a positive or a negative placebo effect.
3. The clinician's relationship to the client. The interested clinician "who imparts confidence, who performs a thorough examination, and who is not anxious, conflicted, or guilty about the patient or his treatment is more likely to elicit positive placebo reactions. Negative placebo reactions are more likely when the doctor [or clinician] is angry, rejecting, and contemptuous toward patients or seriously preoccupied with his own problems" (Shapiro, 1964, p. 77).

How can a placebo effect be distinguished from an effect resulting from intervention? One approach would be to replicate the therapy with a client and clinician who are relatively neutral in their expectations concerning its effectiveness. If the therapy was ineffective when replicated, this would suggest (not prove) that the previous positive results were a function of something other than it. On the other hand, if the same results were obtained, this would provide additional support for the hypothesis that the intervention strategy is effective.

What are the Impacts of the Intervention Strategy on Other Attributes of a Client's Communicative Behavior at Given Points in Space-Time?

What are the Impacts of the Intervention Strategy on a Client Other Than Those Directly Related to Communicative Behavior at Given Points in Space- Time?

The considerations in designing research to assess systematically the impacts of an intervention strategy on attributes of a client's communicative disorder other than those being studied are the same as for assessing the impacts of one on behaviors that contribute directly to a client's communicative disorder. The same would be true for designing research to assess systematically the impacts of an intervention strategy on a client other than those related directly to communicative behavior.

What Are the Client's Attitudes toward the Intervention Strategy and Its Impacts on His Communicative and Other Behaviors at Given Points in Space- Time?

Many of the considerations discussed previously are relevant in designing research to answer this question. One that has not yet been dealt with in this chapter is the selection of a methodology for "measuring" attitudes. Several methodologies that have been developed and used for this purpose—including the *semantic differential* technique (Osgood, Suci, and Tannenbaum, 1957)—are described in Chapter 8.

What Are the Attitudes of a Client's Clinician, Family, Friends, and Others toward the Intervention Strategy and toward Its Impacts on the Client's Communicative Behavior at Given Points in Space-Time?

The considerations in designing research to answer this question are the same as for the previous question. The semantic differential in Figure 8.10 was developed to partially answer this question for a stuttering intervention strategy (Silverman and Trotter, 1973b).

What Investment Is Required of Client and Clinician at Given Points in Space-Time?

To answer this question, both the client and the clinician will have to keep careful records of their time and financial investment in the intervention approach being evaluated. The client's emotional investment in an intervention approach can be partially inferred from comments he or she makes to the clinician during the course of therapy and from interviews conducted by the clinician (or someone else) following its termination.

What Is the Probability of Relapse Following Termination of Therapy?

An investigator should assess the long-term effects of an intervention strategy in addition to its immediate effects. Clinicians would be naive to assume that their client's status following termination of therapy will necessarily remain unchanged over a relatively long period of time.

Investigators who wish to incorporate some type of follow-up into their design—i.e., who wish to continue to make criterion measures following termination of therapy—will have to make three decisions: (1) which measures to make, (2) the intervals at which to make these measures, and (3) the length of time to continue to make these measures.

You should decide whether your design will include follow-up before you select criterion measures. Some measures that would be sufficiently reliable and valid for your purposes would be difficult or impossible to make following termination of therapy, particularly for those clients who live some distance from where they received therapy. It may be necessary, therefore, to select criterion measures that can be made by telephone or by using a "paper and pencil" task.

How frequently should criterion measures be made following termination of therapy? This is a decision for which it is difficult to provide guidelines. However, if the design included periodic sampling during the course of therapy (e.g., a time series design), it may be both desirable and possible to make measures following termination of therapy at the same interval as during therapy—particularly for the first year.

The final decision—the length of time to follow-up—is also a difficult one for which to provide guidelines. There is insufficient data on the long-term effects of intervention approaches for communicative disorders to pro-

FIGURE 13.2   Evaluation checklist for adequacy of therapy outcome research.

Indicate beside each finding whether its validity, reliability, and generality appear adequate for answering the question. If the validity, reliability, or generality of a finding is uncertain, place a question mark in the appropriate space. Room is provided on the form for evaluating two findings that are relevant to each question.

     1. WHAT ARE THE EFFECTS OF THE INTERVENTION PROGRAM UPON SPECIFIC BEHAVIORS THAT CONTRIBUTE TO A CLIENT'S COMMUNICATIVE DISORDER AT GIVEN POINTS IN SPACE-TIME?

     FINDING #1:

     VALIDITY_____   RELIABILITY_____   GENERALITY_____

     FINDING #2:

     VALIDITY_____   RELIABILITY_____   GENERALITY_____

     2. WHAT ARE THE EFFECTS OF THE INTERVENTION PROGRAM UPON OTHER ATTRIBUTES OF A CLIENT'S COMMUNICATIVE BEHAVIOR AT GIVEN POINTS IN SPACE-TIME?

     FINDING #1:

     VALIDITY_____   RELIABILITY_____   GENERALITY_____

     FINDING #2:

     VALIDITY_____   RELIABILITY_____   GENERALITY_____

(Continued)

FIGURE 13.2   Continued

3. WHAT ARE THE EFFECTS OF THE INTERVENTION PRO-
GRAM ON A CLIENT OTHER THAN THOSE DIRECTLY RELATED TO
HIS COMMUNICATIVE BEHAVIOR AT GIVEN POINTS IN SPACE-TIME?
   FINDING #1:

   VALIDITY_____   RELIABILITY_____   GENERALITY_____

   FINDING #2:

   VALIDITY_____   RELIABILITY_____   GENERALITY_____

4. WHAT ARE THE CLIENT'S ATTITUDES TOWARD THE INTER-
VENTION PROGRAM AND ITS EFFECTS UPON HIS OR HER COMMUNI-
CATIVE AND OTHER BEHAVIORS AT GIVEN POINTS IN SPACE-TIME?
   FINDING #1:

   VALIDITY_____   RELIABILITY_____   GENERALITY_____

   FINDING #2:

   VALIDITY_____   RELIABILITY_____   GENERALITY_____

5. WHAT ARE THE ATTITUDES OF A CLIENT'S CLINICIAN,
FAMILY, FRIENDS, AND OTHERS WITH WHOM HE OR SHE COM-
MUNICATES TOWARD THE INTERVENTION PROGRAM AND ITS EF-
FECTS UPON HIS OR HER COMMUNICATIVE BEHAVIOR AND OTHER
BEHAVIOR AT GIVEN POINTS IN SPACE-TIME?
   FINDING #1:

FIGURE 13.2   Continued

VALIDITY_____   RELIABILITY_____   GENERALITY_____

FINDING #2:

VALIDITY_____   RELIABILITY_____   GENERALITY_____

6.   WHAT INVESTMENT IS REQUIRED BY A CLIENT AND HIS OR HER CLINICIAN AT GIVEN POINTS IN SPACE-TIME?

FINDING #1:

VALIDITY_____   RELIABILITY_____   GENERALITY_____

FINDING #2:

VALIDITY_____   RELIABILITY_____   GENERALITY_____

7.   WHAT IS THE PROBABILITY OF "RELAPSE" FOLLOWING TERMINATION OF THE INTERVENTION PROGRAM?

FINDING #1:

VALIDITY_____   RELIABILITY_____   GENERALITY_____

FINDING #2:

VALIDITY_____   RELIABILITY_____   GENERALITY_____

vide a sound basis for making this decision. Perhaps until adequate data are available, it would be advisable to be conservative and adopt a five-year follow-up period, as have many investigators in the fields of medicine and psychotherapy as well as in speech-language pathology (e.g., Van Riper, 1958).

EVALUATION CHECKLIST FOR ASSESSING THE ADEQUACY OF THERAPY OUTCOME RESEARCH

Seven questions are mentioned in this chapter that should be answered when assessing the adequacy of almost any clinical intervention program. This checklist (see Figure 13.2) can be used for evaluating the adequacy of available research findings that are relevant for answering each of these questions. The word *adequacy* here refers to the validity, reliability, and generality (see Chapter 11) of such findings. For further information about this checklist, see Silverman (1977b).

EXERCISES AND DISCUSSION TOPICS

1. Use the checklist in this chapter for evaluating some of the outcome research on an intervention program (therapy method) of your choice.
2. What items on the checklist included in this chapter are usable *clinically* for evaluating therapy outcome?
3. Use the semantic differential reproduced in Chapter 8 for evaluating the attitudes of three persons toward one of your clients. Have them listen to an audiotape or videotape (preferably the latter) of your client speaking.

14

Legal and Ethical Considerations In Clinical Research

Almost all of the research conducted by speech-language pathologists and audiologists involves the use of human subjects. Persons who have participated in such research have been harmed by the failure of investigators to foresee possible undesirable effects of their experimental procedures on them (e.g., Silverman, 1988). There has been considerable interest since the Nuremberg trials (which were conducted after World War II) in the mental and physical welfare of persons who serve as subjects in research studies. This interest has resulted in the creation of regulations on both national and international levels (see Appendix D) that are intended to protect the rights of such persons. It also has stimulated considerable discussion about ethical aspects of how human subjects are used in clinical research (see, e.g., Freund, 1970).

A number of legal and ethical considerations in clinical research are discussed in this chapter. Much of this discussion is also applicable to other kinds of research in which human subjects are used.

NEED FOR PROTECTING RESEARCH SUBJECTS

Persons who volunteer to serve as subjects are likely to assume that they will be *protected by the experimenter* from being harmed in any way. They would be particularly likely to make this assumption if they are volunteering to participate in an experiment from which they could not expect to benefit personally. (Subjects can benefit personally by participating in an experiment in several ways, such as gaining knowledge, improving physical and/or mental health, or being paid.) They also would be particularly likely to make it if the research was being conducted under the auspices of a respected institution (such as a university or hospital).

While subjects may assume that there is no possibility of their being harmed by participating in an experiment, such an assumption would not be valid. It is impossible to design an experiment that is entirely risk-free. One of the most difficult components of the ethical review of research proposals by institutional review boards (IRBs) is assessing potential risks of harm to research participants (Meslin, 1990; Thompson, 1990).

Although it would be unrealistic for subjects to assume that their participation in an experiment is entirely risk free, it would not be unreasonable for them to assume that their risk of being harmed is almost nonexistent if they are not informed to the contrary. Hence, an experimenter who exposed subjects to more than extremely minimal risks of harm *without first informing them* about these risks would probably be viewed as behaving irresponsibly. The subjects, if they were harmed, could sue both the experimenter and the institution under whose auspices the research was conducted for negligence and/or some other tort (possibly battery) with a reasonable expectation of winning (Silverman, 1983). This is one of the reasons why institutions have committees to evaluate research proposals.

It is important that the actual risk of harm to a subject be consistent with the subject's assumption regarding the nature of this risk. How can one ensure that this will be the case? Several approaches can be used to ensure that a subject's *consent* to participate in an experiment is *informed.* One would be to rely on the *experimenter* both to minimize risks to subjects and to inform them voluntarily about the risks remaining. While this would be the simplest (and probably is the most common) approach, it has several limitations. Perhaps its main limitation is that the goals of collecting desired data and of protecting the persons from whom these data are being collected may not be compatible. Ordinarily an experimenter's primary objective is to gather the data needed to answer specific questions or to test specific hypotheses. While few experimenters would knowingly expose their subjects to highly dangerous experimental conditions without informing them about the risks, they might be tempted to be less forthright when there are potential risks associated with them that have not been demonstrated unequivocally to exist. Experimenters may hesitate to inform potential subjects about such risks because it could discourage enough of them from volunteering to make it impossible for the study to be undertaken or completed.

A second approach that can be used for ensuring that a subject's consent to participate is informed and that potential risks have been minimized and are within acceptable limits is to require the designs of all research studies that wish to use institutional clients as subjects to be scrutinized by an

institutional review board (IRB). The mission of this board would be to identify potential risks and to determine both whether they are within acceptable
limits and whether subjects will be fully informed about them (Metz and
Folkins, 1985). This approach has been adopted by many institutions, including school systems, universities, and hospitals. Requiring such a board to ap-
prove the design for a study can protect subjects in several ways. First, it
would probably motivate the experimenter to design the study so as to minimize the risks to subjects and thus maximize the odds of the proposal's being
approved by the committee. Also, the experimenter would hesitate to pro-
pose a study that would expose subjects to unacceptably high risks of harm
because doing so could damage his or her professional reputation. Second,
such a board provides a mechanism for monitoring the degree to which subjects are informed about potential hazards and hence the degree to which
their consent constitutes *informed consent*. Institutional review boards may
require experimenters to submit to them copies of the consent forms that
subjects will be asked to sign. The committee would then decide whether
the presentation of possible hazards on them is sufficiently complete and
accurate for a subject's consent to constitute fully informed consent. If a
subject is not fully informed about potential hazards before signing a consent
form, his or her consent probably would not be recognized by a court (Fried,
1974). The concept of informed consent is dealt with in-depth elsewhere in
this chapter.

    While the second approach (using institutional review boards) tends to
be superior to the first (relying solely on the experimenter) for protecting the
rights of subjects, it is not perfect. One of its limitations is that board members may not be familiar with the methodology an investigator proposes to
use, and, hence, they may fail to recognize potential hazards to subjects. It
is even conceivable that no board members will be familiar with the methodology outlined in a proposal.

INFORMED CONSENT AS A VEHICLE FOR PROTECTING
INVESTIGATORS AND INSTITUTIONS

Clinical research in the previous section was viewed from the perspective of
the need for protecting the rights of research subjects. In this section it will
be viewed from a different perspective—that of the need for protecting the
rights of investigators and the institutions under whose auspices they are
doing their research. If our legal system did not protect these rights, little (if
any) clinical research would be undertaken, which would have an obvious
detrimental impact on the health of persons in our society.

    Securing subjects' *informed consent* to participate in a study can pro-
vide both the investigator(s) and the institution under whose auspices the
research is being conducted with some protection against litigation arising
from allegations that they were physically or mentally harmed by doing so. If

they were aware of a particular risk before consenting to participate in the study and if they were harmed in a manner predictable from this risk, they would be unlikely to be successful if they sued either the investigator or the institution.

One of the main types of litigation against which a subject's informed consent to participate in a study can provide some protection is *battery*. According to Fried:

> The central concept of battery is the offense to personal dignity that occurs when another impinges on one's bodily integrity without full and valid consent. A punch in the stomach or being doused with a pail of water are classic examples. It is not necessary to show that one has been physically injured, much less that one has suffered financial loss. The injury is to dignity. That being the case, law suits have been brought and won against doctors who performed needed and successful operations, but without consent of their patients. (Fried, p. 15)

Hence, experimenting on people without their "full and valid consent" can result in litigation for battery even if they were not physically injured and even if they did not suffer financial loss. Such litigation also can result from subjecting clients to *therapy programs* without their "full and valid consent." For further information about battery and other torts for which an investigator can be sued, see Chapter 6 in Silverman (1992).

The requirement that must be satisfied to justify intentionally invading another's bodily integrity is securing his or her *free and informed* consent to do so. According to Fried:

> To be effective the consent must be to the particular contact with the person in question, and if procured by "fraud or mistake as to the essential character" of the conduct it is invalid. . . . And it is not just active fraud or concealment which destroys consent. The doctor [or experimenter] who obtains consent has the duty to give the facts the patient [or subject] needs to make an informed choice. . . . He must tell the patient [or subject] about the benefits and risks of the treatment [or experimental condition(s)], and how likely they are. And some courts have said that the patient must also be told about the hazards and advantages of alternative forms of treatment. (Fried, 1974, pp. 19–20)

Hence, for consent to participate in an experiment to be regarded by a court as having been *free and informed*, the experimenter would have to be able to prove that subjects were not coerced into giving their consent and that they had been fully informed about the risks involved before they gave it.

Under some circumstances a subject's free and informed consent to participate in a study *may* not be essential. One such circumstance would be when the subject is a *child*, particularly a very young child who would be unable to understand the study and hence would be incapable of giving informed consent. Consent in such a circumstance would have to be obtained from the child's legal guardian, who in most instances would be a parent. However, a guardian's ability to consent to a child's serving as a research subject is limited: "The tendency of the law has been to limit what may be done to children and incompetents just because they are unable to give effective consent. And those who act for them are strictly charged to act only in the manifest interests of these persons. They may not, for instance, volunteer them for experimentation which will *not directly* [italics mine] benefit them" (Fried, 1974, p. 23). The message here appears to be that securing a guardian's consent for his or her child to serve as a subject may not be adequate to protect against litigation against either the experimenter or the institution under whose auspices the research is being conducted.

A subject's free and informed consent also may not be essential if he or she is an adult whom the court would classify as *incompetent*. Adults are likely to be classified as incompetent if they are thought to be unable to make rational decisions regarding their own welfare. Persons diagnosed as psychotic or severely mentally retarded are likely to be classified as incompetent. Persons who are *severely communicatively handicapped* (e.g., global aphasics) also may be classified as incompetent. A court-appointed guardian could consent to such a person's serving as a subject. The restrictions on the guardian's ability to do so are the same as were given for guardians of children.

A subject can *withdraw* consent to participate in a study at any time, even if the subject promised when giving consent not to withdraw it (Fried, 1974). The National Institute of Health policy statement on the protection of human subjects, in fact, not only mandates that subjects be allowed to withdraw consent at any time but requires that subjects *be informed* that they have this right.

LEGAL-ETHICAL IMPLICATIONS
OF THE THERAPEUTIC-NONTHERAPEUTIC
CONTINUUM IN CLINICAL RESEARCH

The legal doctrines that apply to a particular clinical study are determined in part by whether the experimental conditions administered to subjects are intended to be therapeutic to them. Some studies are *entirely therapeutic* in their intent. An example would be a study of the impacts of a particular intervention program that the clinician would have used even if the research was not being done.

At the other end of the continuum would be studies in which the investigator had *no therapeutic intent*. The subjects in such studies would be unlikely to benefit personally from participating in them. They may, however, be providing data that could contribute to improving therapy programs for others with similar communicative disorders at some future date. An example would be an investigation by an audiologist of the responses of persons having a particular type of lesion in the auditory system to a particular type of auditory test. The audiologist's intent is to use their responses to the test stimuli to refine the test rather than to benefit them directly.

There are clinical studies that fall on the continuum between these extremes. In these studies some of the experimental conditions have a therapeutic intent and others do not. Or the experimental conditions are intended to be therapeutic for some subjects but not for others. An example of the first would be a study in which clients are given one or more diagnostic tests in addition to those they would ordinarily be given for clinical purposes. Those that ordinarily would be administered for clinical purposes constitute experimental conditions having a therapeutic intent; the others constitute experimental conditions that are not intended to be therapeutic.

An example of a clinical study in which the experimental conditions are intended to be therapeutic for some subjects but not for others would be a study in which subjects are *randomly assigned* to one of two treatment groups. The subjects assigned to the first group (the experimental group) would be administered a treatment (experimental condition) that was intended to be therapeutic and hence could directly benefit them. Those assigned to the second group (the control group) either would be administered no treatment or would be administered a treatment that the experimenter did not expect to be as successful as the one administered to subjects in the first group. Thus, the subjects in the first group would be expected to benefit directly, and those in the second group either would not be expected to benefit directly or would not be expected to benefit to the same extent as those in the first group.

Nontherapeutic Clinical Research

While the persons who function as subjects in nontherapeutic clinical research may receive a small sum of money and/or personal satisfaction for doing so, they are unlikely to benefit directly in any substantial way from the experience. And by participating in the research they are risking their mental and/or physical health. In some types of research the risks to their health would be almost nonexistent; in others the risks would be substantial.

It has been argued (Fried, 1974) that there are no special legal doctrines that apply to nontherapeutic clinical research and that those that do apply (particularly with regard to the need for disclosing potential hazards) are the same as those that apply to the selling of products:

> In general, the law imposes a strict duty of disclosure, wherever an individual with a great deal to lose is exposed to a risk or is asked to relinquish rights by someone with considerably greater knowledge [italics mine]. And this is true, whether the relation is one of buyer and seller or involves some public interest. Persons selling cosmetics, automobiles, or pharmaceuticals are required to make full disclosure of all the hazards involved in the products they sell. . . . There is no reason why the case should be any different where a researcher asks an experimental subject to risk his health. (Fried, 1974, p. 27)

Since experimenters would ordinarily have considerably greater knowledge of the potential risks associated with the methodology being used than would their subjects and since their subjects are risking their health by participating in the experiment, experimenters are obliged to make a full disclosure of potential hazards to subjects when seeking their consent to participate. It could be argued that the failure of the experimenter to do so would be more damaging with this type of research if a subject sued for battery than it would be with research having a therapeutic intent.

While it is almost always desirable to be able to document a subject's informed consent to participate in research, there are some types of nontherapeutic studies for which failure to do so ordinarily would result in minimal risks to either investigators or the institutions under whose auspices their research is being conducted. These are studies that involve only slight or remote risks of harm to subjects. The U.S. Department of Health and Human Services, for example, in its "Final Regulations Amending Basic HHS Policy for the Protection of Human Research Subjects" *(Federal Register,* January 26, 1981) classified the following types of research as having no, slight, or only remote risks of harm to subjects:

1. Research conducted in established or commonly accepted educational settings, involving normal educational practices, such as (i) research on regular and special education instructional strategies, or (ii) research on the effectiveness of or the comparison among instructional techniques, curricula, or classroom management methods.
2. Research involving the use of educational tests (cognitive, diagnostic, aptitude, achievement), if information taken from these sources are recorded in such a manner that subjects cannot be identified, directly or through identifiers linked to the subjects.
3. Research involving survey or interview procedures, except where all of the following conditions exist: (i) responses are recorded in such a manner that the human subjects can be identified, directly or through identifiers linked to the subjects, (ii) the subject's responses, if they became known outside the research, could reasonably place the subject at risk of criminal or civil liability or be damaging to the subject's financial standing or employability, and (iii) the research deals with sensitive aspects of the subject's own behavior, such as illegal conduct, drug use, sexual behavior, or the use of alcohol.

   Research involving the observation (including the observation by participants) of public behavior, except where all of the following conditions exist: (i) observations are recorded in such a manner that the human subjects can be identified, directly or through identifiers linked to the subjects, (ii) the observations recorded about the individual, if they become known outside the research, could reasonably place the subject at risk of criminal or civil liability or be damaging to the subject's financial standing or employability, and (iii) the research deals with sensitive aspects of the subject's own behavior such as illegal conduct, drug use, sexual behavior, or use of alcohol.
4. Research involving the collection or study of existing data, documents, pathological specimens, or diagnostic specimens, if these sources are pub-

licly available or if the information is recorded by the investigator in such a manner that subjects cannot be identified, directly or through identifiers linked to the subjects. *(Federal Register,* January 26, 1981, pp. 8371–8372)

How would a person be compensated for harm resulting from his or her participation (as a subject) in a nontherapeutic research study? Such a person probably would have to initiate some type of litigation against the investigator and/or the institution under whose auspices the research was being conducted. A number of authorities on legal-ethical implications of using human subjects in research (e.g., Fried, 1974; Ladimer, 1970) have stated that investigators and their institutions have a moral obligation to voluntarily compensate subjects harmed in nontherapeutic research. Perhaps a special liability insurance could be carried by investigators or their institutions for this purpose.

For further information about legal-ethical aspects of nontherapeutic research, see Freund (1970), Fried (1974), Greenwald, Ryan, and Mulvihill (1982), Metz and Folkins (1985), and the publications of the Office for Protection from Research Risks, National Institutes of Health, Bethesda, Maryland 20205.

Therapeutic Clinical Research

Speech-language pathologists, audiologists, and other clinicians legally are justified only in using accepted therapies unless their clients specifically consent to the use of an experimental therapy. An *accepted therapy,* in this context, is a treatment program that at least some of one's professional peers would regard as appropriate for the particular condition being treated. If a speech-language pathologist treated a stutterer with a therapy program that at least some authorities on stuttering would regard as appropriate, this program would be likely to be classified as *accepted* therapy by the courts. It would not be necessary that all authorities on stuttering regard it as appropriate. The courts recognize that there are often different "schools of thought" on the appropriate therapy for a condition, and, hence, they will classify as accepted almost any therapy advocated by a recognized authority.

So long as the therapy program being used in the research is one that would be classified by the courts as accepted, the legal-ethical considerations (e.g., informed consent) would be essentially the same as for *clinical treatment.*

The further away an experimental therapy program lies from the standard and the accepted, the more acute the need for subjects to be fully informed about risks and *alternative treatment programs,* and the greater the need for the investigator to be able to document the subjects' free and informed consent to participate in research. The investigator's obligation to inform subjects about alternative treatment programs ordinarily does not extend to other alternative programs (Fried, 1974). The information presented about the experimental program should include a statement summarizing research findings and professional opinion relevant to its efficacy.

A situation that may pose a legal-ethical dilemma for an investigator is one in which there are alternative treatment programs that are regarded by other professionals as *effective* for treating the condition the experimental program is intended to treat. Full disclosure requires that the subjects be informed about these alternatives. However, informing potential subjects about such alternatives may cause them to refuse to participate in the experimental program. An investigator may be tempted, therefore, to make a less than full disclosure about alternative treatment programs in order to ensure having an adequate number of subjects for the research. While doing so may increase the probability of having an adequate number of subjects for the research, it also could invalidate the subjects' consent to participate in the research, leaving the investigator vulnerable to several types of litigation, including battery. An investigator when confronted with this situation would be wise to make a full disclosure, including a statement summarizing research and professional opinion relevant to why the experimental therapy *may* be superior to existing accepted alternative treatment programs. An investigator should be able to develop such a statement—otherwise, one could reasonably question whether it would be *ethical* to expose subjects to an experimental treatment program that there is no reason to believe is superior to existing accepted ones. Institutional review boards have a responsibility to determine whether proposed experimental treatment programs have a reasonable chance of satisfying a *real need.*

Mixed Therapeutic and Nontherapeutic Clinical Research

The type of clinical research that tends to have the greatest legal-ethical perplexities associated with it is that which has both therapeutic and nontherapeutic aspects. A speech-language pathologist or audiologist, for example, who was engaged in therapy outcome research would indeed be attempting to ameliorate the client's communicative disorder (which would be the *therapeutic aspect*). The intervention strategy chosen, however, would not be selected *solely* from the perspective of the client's needs. Therapy would be administered in the context of a research program that was intended either to test new procedures or to compare the efficacy of various established procedures (which would be the *nontherapeutic aspect.*) Hence, the treatment that a client received would be dictated, at least partially, by the requirements of the research design. In a study of the relative efficacy of two established procedures, the one the client is administered is likely to be determined by a table of random numbers. And in a study of the efficacy of a new procedure (experimental therapy), the decision whether a particular subject would be given it would be partially a function of the investigator's need for subjects with particular *demographic characteristics* (e.g., age and sex) to meet the requirements of the research design.

If the treatment dictated by a research design is the one that a client would have received anyway, then the presence of a research design ordinarily would not create any special legal-ethical problems. However, if the treatment dictated by a research design is *not* the one that a client ordinarily would have received, then the presence of a research design could indicate legal-ethical problems.

In clinical research having both therapeutic and nontherapeutic aspects, there obviously is a legal obligation to make a full disclosure of *possible benefits and hazards*. This would be necessary even if the therapy that the clients were receiving was not part of a research project. Would it also be necessary to disclose (1) that at least some of the therapy they will be receiving *is part of a research project* and (2) the *nature* of the research project and the experimental design? A speech-language pathologist who was planning to describe the therapy program used with a client in an individual case study in an article published in a professional journal would have to answer that question. Would the client's consent be needed to publish the case study? If it were *impossible* for anyone to recognize the client from the information included in the case study, the answer to this question probably would be no. A client may be recognizable not only from a name or initials but also from specific information about his or her life history, such as the names of schools attended. An investigator would be wise, therefore, to carefully examine the life history data on subjects of case studies and to delete any nonessential information that would make them recognizable. Of course, the client (or the client's guardian) in some instances would be very willing to have a description of the therapy received published, particularly if (1) the client felt treatment was successful, and/or (2) the client was convinced that the information presented could help in the treatment of others with similar conditions.

While clinicians who do not disclose to a client that the therapy is part of a research project or do not describe the *impact* that being part of a research project will have on the therapy the client will be receiving may be relatively safe legally, they may find themselves vulnerable from a *public relations* perspective. Most clients, for example, probably would feel that they had been deceived if they discovered they received the therapy program they did because they were randomly assigned to a particular treatment group. Such a discovery would be likely to adversely affect their relationship with their clinician if they are still in therapy. And the disclosure of such a discovery in the media could severely damage the reputation of both the investigator and the institution under whose auspices the research was conducted. The general public would tend to regard the random assignment of subjects to treatment groups without their knowledge as irresponsible, even if the therapy subjects received had been successful.

DOCUMENTING A PERSON'S INFORMED CONSENT
TO SERVE AS A RESEARCH SUBJECT

An outline of a form for documenting a person's informed consent to serve as a subject in a research project is presented in Figure 14.1. This outline includes the information that ordinarily is necessary for explaining to potential subjects (1) the purpose and value of the study, (2) what they will be asked to do and what will be done to them, and (3) the possible benefits and risks to them. It also provides a means for documenting that subjects were informed that they may withdraw their consent at any time and that they have consented to having information about them published (if they cannot be recognized). In addition, it provides documentation that their consent was given freely (that it was not coerced or forced). Paragraph *g* in Figure 14.1 would be included only if provision had been made for compensating subjects for injuries that they receive (e.g., if the investigator or the institution had liability insurance that covered such injuries). Note that subjects' signatures should be witnessed. Obviously, if the information presented in the form was inaccurate or incomplete, a subject's signature on it might not constitute *informed* consent. Whether it would constitute informed consent would depend on how essential the inaccurate or incomplete information was for alerting subjects to potential risks.

UTILIZATION OF DATA FROM RESEARCH
IN WHICH SUBJECTS WERE ABUSED

Is it ethical to utilize data from research in which subjects were abused, particularly from that in which they were knowingly abused? Perhaps the most extreme, contemporary example of such data would be that gathered in Nazi Germany during World War II which motivated the development of the Nuremberg Code (see Appendix D). Each of us must answer this question for ourself. The following comment by Dr. Tomas Radil-Weiss, a psychiatrist and head of the Section on Neurophysiology of the Czechoslovak Academy of Sciences, who was imprisoned at Auschwitz Concentration Camp when he was 14 years old may be helpful when doing so:

> The second world war ended many years ago. Most of those who survived the stay at the German concentration camp at Auschwitz have already died of the consequences of their imprisonment; those still alive are already in the last third of their life. Is there any point to returning to the experiences of those days? Consideration of the mental hygiene of former prisoners cautions us that perhaps we should not do it. *But consideration of the general interest holds that we are not entitled to ignore any knowledge that can contribute to social development—including medicine and psychology— even if acquired under unspeakably awful conditions* [italics mine]. (Radil-Weiss, 1983, p. 259)

RESPONSIBLE INVESTIGATOR:

TITLE OF PROTOCOL:

TITLE OF CONSENT FORM *(if different from protocol):*

I have been asked to participate in a research study that is investigating *(describe purpose of study).* In participating in this study I agree to *(describe briefly and in lay terms procedures to which subject is consenting).*

I understand that

   a) The possible risks of this procedure include *(list known risks or side effects; if none, so state).* Alternative treatments include *(list alternative treatments and briefly describe advantages and disadvantages of each; if none, so state).*

   b) The possible benefits of this study to me are *(enumerate; if none, so state).*

   c) Any questions I have concerning my participation in this study will be answered by *(list names and degrees of people who will be available to answer questions).*

   d) I may withdraw from the study at any time without prejudice.

   e) The results of this study may be published, but my name or identity will not be revealed and my records will remain confidential unless disclosure of my identity is required by law.

   f) My consent is given voluntarily without being coerced or forced.

   g) In the event of physical injury resulting from the study, medical care and treatment will be available at this institution.

   For eligible veterans, compensation (damages) may be payable under 38USC 351 or, in some circumstances, under the Federal Tort claims Act.

   For non-eligible veterans and non-veterans, compensation would be limited to situations where negligence occurred and would be controlled by the provisions of the Federal Tort Claims Act.

   For clarification of these laws, contact the District Counsel (213) 824-7379.

_____   _____

DATE   PATIENT OR RESPONSIBLE PARTY

                            _____

                            PATIENT'S SOCIAL SECURITY NUMBER

                            _____

                            AUDITOR/WITNESS

                            _____

                            INVESTIGATOR/PHYSICIAN REPRESENTATIVE

FIGURE 14.1   Outline for a consent form for documenting a person's informed consent to serve a subject in a research project (Purtile and Cassel, 1981).

The utilization of such data may allow a little good to come from the suffering of those research subjects who have been abused physically or psychologically, purposefully or through negligence.

EXERCISES AND DISCUSSION TOPICS

1. Read the "Monster" Study (Silverman, 1988). What would be the ethical arguments, both "pro" and "con," for utilizing these data?

2. Is it ethical to do research in which the methodology includes response-contingent punishment (e.g., "time out")? Why?

3. Is it ethical in therapy outcome research either to deprive a client of therapy for a period of time or to use one with him or her that you don't expect to be effective in order to have a baseline or "control" condition? Why?

4. Should a client's informed consent be sought and documented if a therapy being used is "experimental"—ie., if its efficacy has not been established empirically? Why?

15

Conducting and Funding Research in a Clinical Setting

This book has attempted to demonstrate what benefits speech-language pathologists and audiologists would derive from doing clinical research (i.e., functioning as clinician-investigators) and to provide the information that they need to do it. Suppose a speech-language pathologist or audiologist who was employed as a clinician in a school or medical setting wanted to function as a clinician-investigator. How might he or she go about achieving the necessary administrative and financial support? The information presented here should enable him or her to at least partially answer this question.

ACHIEVING ADMINISTRATIVE SUPPORT

It would be difficult (though certainly not impossible) for a speech-language pathologist or audiologist employed in a clinical setting to do clinical research without at least some administrative support. Doing such research obviously requires an investment of time. Since most master's-level speech-language pathologists and audiologists are hired for the purpose of providing clinical services, they may have to convince their supervisor and/or other administrators that it would be likely to benefit the institution (including its administrators) if they were allowed some time for clinical research. The time investment required could be relatively small if their questions could be answered by observations they could make while providing clinical services (e.g., questions dealing with therapy outcome).

Some arguments for your doing clinical research that may be viewed as compelling by administrators at your institution are the following:

1. Your doing it can help you to meet the requirement for accountability. Data concerning the impacts of intervention strategies on your clients can be used for this purpose by various groups, including: (a) administrators at the institution in which the program is located, (b) potential consumers of the services it offers, i.e., the communicatively handicapped and their families, (c) third parties who are paying for these services, e.g., voluntary organizations, governmental agencies, and insurance companies, and (d) the community.
2. Evaluating your clinical programs systematically will provide you with information you need to maximize their effectiveness. If you do not systematically evaluate the impacts of your intervention strategies on your clients, how can you tell if you are achieving their objectives?
3. The presence of an ongoing clinical research program is likely to bring local, state, national, and international recognition to the institution that should help in attracting grants and gifts from individuals, private foundations, and governmental sources.
4. The research you want to do would not be very costly (either in time or money) since you would be gathering the data you need to answer your questions while providing clinical services.

Of course, your administrator would be unlikely to look upon all of these arguments as being equally compelling. You must decide based on your previous experience which ones he or she is most likely to regard as being so. (Incidentally, at least some of the arguments presented in Chapter 2 pertaining to the benefits of functioning as a clinician-investigator could be usable here.)

PREPARING A RESEARCH PROPOSAL

We have considered several arguments that may be helpful when attempting to secure administrative support for research. How should they be communicated to the administrator or administrators whose support you are seeking? In most instances, the best way would probably be as a part of a written proposal, or prospectus, that could be drafted as a *memorandum*. The kinds of information that should be presented include the following:

1. the question(s) you want to answer
2. possible practical implications of the answer(s) for your clients and those of other clinicians
3. why it would be of benefit to your institution for *you* to undertake the project

4. why you believe you are qualified to undertake the project
5. the time and financial investment that would be necessary and the source or sources from which you would seek funding
6. where you would plan to report the results of the project
7. coinvestigators and consultants who would be involved in the project and a statement describing their roles and qualifications for performing them
8. a description of the methodology that would be used to answer each question, including a statement concerning possible dangers to subjects and how you plan to document their informed consent to participate (see Chapter 14)
9. a description of how the data would be analyzed for answering each question

Let us now examine briefly the contribution of each of these kinds of information to a proposal.

Your statement about the question(s) you wish to answer should communicate to an administrator the topic of your proposed research. Since he or she may not be familiar with the technical terminology used by speech-language pathologists or audiologists, this should not be used unless absolutely necessary; those technical terms that are used should be defined. If data have been reported that are relevant to your questions, they should be summarized; you should indicate why additional data are needed to answer each question.

Next, you should indicate why it would be advantageous for you to attempt to answer them in your clinical setting. You should indicate as cogently as you can why answering them would be beneficial to you, your clients, and to your institution. Some of the arguments summarized in Chapter 2 may be applicable here.

Your next task is to demonstrate that you are qualified to make the observations necessary to answer each question. It is particularly important to document the specific training and experience that qualifies you to use the instruments (e.g., tests) by which you plan to make them.

The time and financial investment required to complete the proposed research and the source or sources from which the necessary funding might be obtained should be indicated. You should provide an estimate of the total number of hours or the average number of hours per week it probably would be necessary to spend on the project. And you should include a detailed budget, with justification for each item. Sources (internal, external, or both) from which the necessary funding might be obtained should be specified.

Some information should be included about how you plan to disseminate your questions, answers, and interpretations. If this information is going to be communicated in a written report, specify the journal to which you plan to submit it (unless, of course, the report is intended to be used solely by persons in your institution).

Others (e.g., coinvestigators and consultants) who would be involved in the project should be mentioned. The role of each should be indicated, and there should be a statement about his or her qualifications to perform it.

A detailed description of the methodology that would be used for answering each question should be included. You should describe in as much detail as you would for the "methods" section of a research report (see Chapter 12) who you are going to observe and how you are going to observe them. Any possible ways by which subjects could be harmed by the experimental procedures should be indicated, along with a statement concerning the likelihood of their being so. An investigator has both an ethical and a legal responsibility not to expose subjects to potentially dangerous experimental procedures without their informed consent (see Chapter 14).

The manner in which the data will be analyzed for answering each question should be indicated. It should be clear from the proposal how the data necessary for answering each will be organized for doing so (see Chapters 9 and 10).

The types of information mentioned here should be included in all research proposals. They may not, however, be the only types it is necessary to include. You would be wise before beginning to prepare a proposal to inquire whether the institution in which you are employed has a format, or set of forms, they wish used for this purpose. Many institutions in which clinical speech, language, or hearing programs are located (e.g., Veterans' Administration hospitals) have specific forms for this purpose.

RESEARCH FUNDING

All research projects require the expenditure of some funds. The amount of funding needed to answer some questions is so small that it can often be taken from the operating budget provided by the institution. This would probably be true for many questions relevant to therapy outcome.

If the funding needed for answering your question(s) exceeded that available from your operating budget, you would probably have to apply for some sort of grant. Speech-language pathologists and audiologists have received funding from a variety of sources for their research activities. For purposes of discussion we will divide them into two groups: internal and external (extramural).

Internal grants are awarded by the institution (school system, hospital, rehabilitation center, and so on) with which the person applying is affiliated. Their maximum size tends to be relatively small (i.e., usually less than $2,000). They usually are intended either to support research that only requires a relatively low level of funding (which would include almost all therapy outcome research in speech-language pathology and audiology) or to provide "seed" money for the preliminary ("pilot") research of investigators who plan to apply for extramural funding. These grants are usually easier for beginning investigators to obtain than extramural ones. They also tend to require a less complex application procedure than the latter.

If the funding needed to answer your question(s) exceeds several thousand dollars, you will probably have to apply for an extramural grant. An extramural grant is one from any source other than the institution by which you are employed. Such a source could be a corporation (e.g., IBM), an organization (e.g., the Heart Association or United Cerebral Palsy), a private foundation (e.g., the Ford Foundation), or a governmental agency (e.g., the National Institutes of Health, the Office of Education, or the National Science Foundation). Funds for research in speech-language pathology and audiology have been obtained from all four sources. The federal government, through such agencies as the National Institutes of Health (NIH), the Office of Education (OE), and the National Science Foundation (NSF), has provided more funds for this purpose than any other source. These agencies offer a variety of research support programs, including some for which beginning investigators are eligible.

How do you identify the agencies, corporations, foundations, and organizations that are most likely to fund a particular project? The decision about where to submit a grant proposal is one of the most important in the grantsmanship/grant-seeking process (Gelatt, 1989; Hall, 1988; Sparks, 1989). An excellent proposal is unlikely to get funded if it is submitted to an agency, corporation, foundation, or organization that does not have as a part of its mission supporting the type of research that is being proposed. Also, if there are several appropriate places to which a proposal could be submitted, the odds of being funded may not be the same for all of them—i.e., some may be more competitive than others (Gelatt, 1989).

Information about programs that support research on communication disorders can be acquired from a number of sources, including the following:

- The *Catalog of Federal Domestic Assistance (CFDA)*, a catalog that is published annually by the Government Printing Office, is one of the most valuable reference sources for finding out about federal programs. It contains a number of indexes to help users locate specific programs of interest, determine eligibility, and obtain information about application deadlines. The *Federal Automated Program Retrieval Information System (FAPRIS)* is a computer database version of this catalog.
- The *Foundation Center* is a national clearinghouse for information on foundation and corporate giving. One way that it disseminates such information is through a national network of more than 150 library reference collections. The Center offered its services to the public free of charge when this chapter was written.
- The *Annual Register of Grant Support* is a directory of fellowship and grant support programs of government agencies, foundations, business, professional, and other organizations.

- The *Directory of Biomedical and Health Care Grants* covers funding programs supported by government agencies, private foundations, corporations, and professional organizations.
- The *Federal Grants and Contracts Weekly* lists selected grant and contract programs. A contract program is one in which an agency describes what it wants to have done and invites interested persons to submit proposals for doing it.
- The *Taft Corporate Giving Directory* is a guide to over 500 corporate foundations or direct giving programs.
- The *Sponsored Programs Information Network (SPIN)* is a computer database that contained information about more than 3000 funding opportunities (federal, nonfederal, and corporate) when this chapter was written.
- The *Computer Retrieval of Information on Scientific Projects (CRISP)* database contains information on research programs supported by the U.S. Public Health Service.

After you have identified one or more places to apply for funding, your next task is to prepare a grant proposal. There are several sources from which you may be able to obtain assistance when doing so. One is from persons who have applied for research grants, particularly from those who have been successful. Help from a person whose research has been supported by an organization to which you plan to apply can be particularly valuable.

A second source from which you should be able to get some help is the office of research support at your institution. Many educational and medical facilities that employ speech-language pathologists and audiologists have such an office.

A third source from which help can be sought is publications on grantsmanship. Several very informative ones were published in the February 1989 issue of *Asha* (Catlett, 1989; Gelatt, 1989; "How to Be Sure You Don't Get Funded," 1989; Sparks, 1989). A number of others that can be helpful, particularly when preparing an NIH application, were reprinted in a book entitled *Preparing a Research Grant Application to the National Institutes of Health* (1989).

Almost all extramural funding programs are highly competitive, and their proposal-processing procedures tend to be quite complex and time-consuming (see Lore and Gutter, 1968, and Summers, 1987, for descriptions of such procedures at NIH). More proposals usually are submitted than can be funded. Furthermore, most granting organizations look for evidence of "demonstrated research competence"—i.e., the ability to successfully complete research projects as evidenced by publication. This, of course, would tend to put a beginning investigator at a disadvantage. Such an investigator probably would be wise, therefore, to select as his or her first research projects ones that could be funded internally.

USE OF CONSULTANTS

This book hopefully has provided you with an intuitive understanding of much of the information you need to function as a clinician-investigator. Obviously, the information provided may not be sufficient to bring you to the point where it is unnecessary to have your methodology checked by someone. Many institutions with speech and hearing facilities (including colleges, hospitals, and school systems) employ persons knowledgeable about statistics and research methodology for consultation with members of their staff. As mentioned previously, there may be faculty at local colleges and universities who are competent in this area who would be willing to consult with you.

It is important to contact a consultant, particularly a research design consultant, before you begin data collection. If something is wrong with your design, the data you collect may be worthless. That is, they may not possess an adequate level of validity, reliability, and generality for accurately answering your question(s). It is crucial, therefore, to have your proposal checked before beginning to collect data.

Any recommendations that are made by a consultant, of course, have to be carefully evaluated because they might be inappropriate. They may not result in a design that will yield the data necessary to answer your questions. Or they may not result in the most efficient or practical design for this purpose.

Why might a consultant's recommendations be inappropriate? There are several possible reasons. First, he or she may commit what Kimball (1957) has referred to as an "error of the third kind"—i.e., giving the right answer to the wrong question. Here, the consultant does not understand the question or questions the investigator is attempting to answer. Hence, his or her recommendations are appropriate not for answering these questions but for those he thinks the investigator is trying to answer. A consultant is most likely to make this type of error when he or she is completely unfamiliar with the content area in which the research is being done.

A consultant's recommendations may also be inappropriate because they are not sufficiently practical or efficient. For assessing the impact of a particular therapy, a consultant may recommend using a design in which 40 persons who have a particular communicative disorder are randomly assigned to one of two groups: the members of one group receive the experimental therapy and the members of the other do not. Such a design may not be practical because 40 persons with that communicative disorder may not be available to serve as subjects, and it would not be ethical (or possible) to deprive half of them of the therapy for the duration of the program (see Chapter 14). Even if it were practical to use such a design, it might not be efficient because of the time needed to administer therapy to 20 clients and evaluate its impact on a group of this size. A single subject design using 10 persons, in which each served as his own "control," could well be both more efficient and more practical for collecting the necessary data.

A third reason a consultant's recommendations may be inappropriate is that he or she has made a mistake. Consultants, like all humans, are fallible. A certain percentage of the time their recommendations will be wrong.

What should you do if you feel a consultant's recommendations may be inappropriate? Your best strategy would probably be to seek one or more additional opinions, weigh them (considering the reasons for them), and then make the best decision you can. This, of course, is similar to the situation you sometimes find yourself in when you are forced to make clinical decisions from equivocal or incomplete data.

Our emphasis in this discussion has been on research design consultants. However, most of these comments are relevant to other types of consultants as well.

EXERCISES AND DISCUSSION TOPICS

1. Based upon your clinical experience, formulate an answerable question you probably could answer while employed as a speech-language pathologist or audiologist in a clinical setting that probably would not require an unrealistic time investment or external funding.

2. Write a proposal you could submit to your employer that should motivate him or her to allow you to do the research needed for answering the question you formulated.

3. Describe how you would make the observations needed to answer this question (i.e., formulate a research design for answering it). The material in Chapters 6 through 10 should be helpful.

Appendix A
Computational Formulas, Worked Examples, Exercises, and MINITAB Commands for Selected Descriptive and Inferential Statistics

CONTENTS

NOTE

The calculations required for these statistics can be made with either a calculator or a computer. Programs for making them are available for all mainframes, minicomputers, and microcomputers. These programs require data to be inputted in a particular way, and they can issue commands that cause the calculations specified by a computational formula to be made on all, or part, of it. Unfortunately, all do not use the same set of commands for computing particular statistics.

The commands needed for computing some of the statistics in this appendix with the MINITAB Statistical Software (Ryan, Joiner, and Ryan, 1985) are included. This program, which was developed in 1972 at Pennsylvania State University to help teach introductory courses in statistics, is interactive in nature and relatively easy to learn to use. It is utilized in such courses at more than 1500 colleges and universities, and versions are available for almost all mainframes and minicomputers as well as Macintosh and IBM-compatible microcomputers. It is, to my knowledge, the only interactive statistical software intended for use with students in an introductory course *that can be run on most computers.* For further information about the program, contact Minitab, Inc., 3081 Enterprise Drive, State College, Pennsylvania 16801-2756 (Telephone: 814-238-3280).

A single set of data is used for all statistical analyses in this appendix (see Table A.1). This was done both to permit comparisons between alternative statistical analyses that could be used to answer a question and to permit the data (i.e., numbers being analyzed) to remain in the background. The labels C1 to C8 in Table A.1 stand for Column 1 to Column 8; these labels are used both when inputting these data and analyzing them with the MINITAB program. The statistics dealt with in this appendix are discussed in Chapters 9 and 10.

SOME NOTATION USED IN THIS APPENDIX

SYMBOL	OPERATION(S) NECESSARY TO COMPUTE, OR MEANING
$\Sigma\, X$	Sum (or add) scores on variable labeled X.
$\Sigma\, X^2$	Square scores on variable labeled X and then sum (or add) them.
$(\Sigma\, X)^2$	Sum (or add) scores on variable labeled X and then square this sum.

(*continued* p. 296)

TABLE A.1 **Frequencies per 100 words of interjection of sounds and syllables (I), part-word repetition (PW), word repetition (W), and revision-incomplete phrase (R-IP) produced by 56 second through sixth-grade nonstutterers during their performance of a spontaneous speech task.**

Subject Number	School Grade	I	PW	W	R-IP
		CI	**C2**	**C3**	**C4**
1	2	0.50	1.16	0.50	2.16
2	2	2.13	1.42	0.35	5.67
3	2	1.40	0.00	0.00	5.14
4	2	0.40	1.21	0.40	1.62
5	2	0.31	0.94	0.63	2.52
6	2	0.00	0.35	0.35	1.74
7	2	0.00	0.00	1.28	3.21
8	2	0.47	2.37	0.95	1.90
9	2	0.30	1.80	1.50	4.49
10	2	0.50	1.00	1.33	6.16
11	2	8.53	0.34	2.39	2.73
12	2	1.04	1.04	1.04	1.56
13	2	1.46	0.29	0.44	4.54
14	2	0.36	0.36	0.72	1.08
15	2	1.87	0.00	0.75	2.24
16	3	0.46	1.14	1.60	3.65
17	3	3.78	1.13	2.64	3.02
18	3	2.23	1.49	2.97	4.83
19	3	0.33	0.99	0.99	1.64
20	3	0.49	0.00	0.49	0.49
21	3	1.07	1.43	1.07	6.79
22	3	0.55	4.42	3.31	6.08
23	3	0.84	0.28	0.28	1.68
24	3	0.28	0.41	0.28	3.72
25	3	3.40	1.51	1.89	1.89
26	3	1.80	0.90	0.60	2.40
		C5	**C6**	**C7**	**C8**
27	4	0.44	1.54	0.00	3.30
28	4	0.94	1.57	0.78	2.83
29	4	0.00	2.41	2.78	3.33
30	4	0.33	0.65	0.49	3.41
31	4	0.56	1.29	0.88	5.31
32	4	0.00	0.12	0.12	0.97
33	4	0.43	0.22	0.65	4.13
34	4	0.00	1.21	2.02	4.48
35	4	3.67	0.83	0.83	3.33
36	5	0.84	0.84	0.42	3.38
37	5	0.16	0.82	0.82	8.20
38	5	1.61	0.00	0.36	1.97
39	5	1.76	1.58	3.25	4.55
40	5	0.28	0.14	1.14	1.99
41	5	2.92	0.93	0.80	4.77

(Continued)

TABLE A.1   Continued

42	5	1.72	0.81	1.26	2.80
43	5	0.72	0.21	0.21	1.65
44	5	0.00	0.54	0.27	2.41
45	5	1.82	0.61	1.70	3.64
46	5	0.52	0.34	2.41	4.83
47	6	0.00	0.28	0.28	0.86
48	6	0.00	0.19	0.77	0.96
49	6	1.99	0.00	0.85	3.42
50	6	0.00	0.47	0.47	1.10
51	6	0.00	0.93	0.00	1.39
52	6	0.69	0.00	0.00	1.72
53	6	0.00	0.66	0.99	1.32
54	6	0.73	0.91	0.18	3.09
55	6	0.78	0.26	0.26	1.03
56	6	0.30	0.41	0.51	2.03

$\overline{X}$	Sum (or add) scores on variable labeled X and then divide total by number of scores summed.
$\overline{X}^2$	Compute mean of variable labeled X (as indicated above) and square it.
ΣY	Sum (or add) scores on variable labeled Y.
ΣY^2	Square scores on variable labeled Y and then sum (or add) them.
$(\Sigma Y)^2$	Sum (or add) scores on variable labeled Y and then square this sum.
$\overline{Y}$	Sum (or add) scores on variable labeled Y and then divide total by number of scores summed.
$\overline{Y}^2$	Compute mean of variable labeled Y (as indicated above) and square it.
$\Sigma X Y$	Multiply each individual's X-score by his Y-score and then sum (or add) the results of these multiplications.
N	The number of individuals in the sample.
$\sqrt{}$	Compute square root.
$\vert\ \vert$	Compute absolute value.

(Other notation is defined when used.)

DESCRIPTIVE STATISTICS: MEASURES OF CENTRAL TENDENCY

1. Mean ($\overline{X}$)

QUESTION: How many instances of interjection per 100 words did the *average* child produce during his performance of the spontaneous speech task?

$$\overline{X} = \frac{\Sigma X}{N} = \frac{57.71}{56} = 1.03$$

ANSWER: The average child produced 1.03 instances of interjection per 100 words during his performance of the spontaneous task?

QUESTION: How many instances of part-word repetition per 100 words did the *average* child produce during his performance of the spontaneous speech task?

$$\overline{X} = \frac{\Sigma X}{N} = \frac{46.75}{56} = 0.83$$

ANSWER: The average child produced 0.83 instances of part-word repetition per 100 words during his performance of the spontaneous speech task.

EXERCISE: Determine the mean numbers of word repetitions and revisions-
(Number 1) incomplete phrases per 100 words that were produced by these 56 children. (Your answers should be approximately 0.97 and 3.06 for word repetition and revision-incomplete phrase, respectively.)

2. Median (Mdn)

QUESTION: How many instances of interjection per 100 words did the *typical* child produce during his performance of the spontaneous speech task?
The first step in computing the median is to order the 56 interjection frequencies from lowest to highest.

0.00	0.30	0.52	1.61
0.00	0.30	0.55	1.72
0.00	0.31	0.56	1.76
0.00	0.33	0.69	1.80
0.00	0.33	0.72	1.82
0.00	0.36	0.73	1.87
0.00	0.40	0.78	1.99
0.00	0.43	0.84	2.13
0.00	0.44	0.84	2.23
0.00	0.46	0.94	2.92
0.00	0.47	1.04	3.40
0.16	0.49	1.07	3.67
0.28	0.50	1.40	3.78
0.28	0.50	1.46	8.53

Since there is an *even* number of scores, the median score would be midway between the N/2 score (0.50) and N/2 + 1 score (0.52). The median interjection frequency, therefore, would be 0.51. (If there had been an *odd* number of scores, the median score would have been the middle one.)

ANSWER: The typical child produced 0.51 instances of interjection per 100 words during his performance of the spontaneous speech task.

REMARK: Note that the mean interjection frequency (1.03) is approximately twice as high as the median interjection frequency (0.51). This discrepancy is primarily due to five children who had relatively high interjection frequencies, i.e., frequencies greater than 2.5 per 100 words. A few persons who have relatively high (or relatively low) scores on a task can substantially influence the mean score on that task.

QUESTION: How many instances of part-word repetition per 100 words did the typical child produce during the performance of the spontaneous speech task?

The first step in computing the median is to order the 56 part-word repetition frequencies from lowest to highest.

0.00	0.28	0.82	1.21
0.00	0.29	0.83	1.21
0.00	0.34	0.84	1.29
0.00	0.34	0.90	1.42
0.00	0.35	0.91	1.43
0.00	0.36	0.93	1.49
0.00	0.41	0.93	1.51
0.12	0.41	0.94	1.54
0.14	0.47	0.99	1.57
0.19	0.54	1.00	1.58
0.21	0.61	1.04	1.80
0.22	0.65	1.13	2.37
0.26	0.66	1.14	2.41
0.28	0.81	1.16	4.42

Since there is an even number of scores, the median score would be midway between the $N/2$ score (0.81) and $N/2 + 1$ score (0.82). The median part-word repetition frequency, therefore, would be 0.815.

ANSWER: The typical child produced 0.815 instances of part-word repetition per 100 words during his performance of the spontaneous speech task.

REMARK: Note that the mean part-word repetition frequency (0.83) is approximately the same as the median part-word repetition frequency (0.815). The lack of discrepancy is primarily due to the fact that only one child had a relatively high part-word repetition frequency (i.e., greater than 2.5 per 100 words).

EXERCISE: Determine the median numbers of word repetitions and revisions-
(Number 2) incomplete phrases per 100 words that were produced by these 56 children. (Your answers should be approximately 0.76 and 2.82 for word repetition and revision-incomplete phrase, respectively.)

3. Mode

QUESTION: What frequency of interjection per 100 words was most typical (i.e., occurred most often) during the children's performance of the spontaneous speech task?

Since the mode is the most frequently occurring score, the

modal interjection frequency per 100 words would be 0.00. (Note that in the frequency distribution on p. 297, 0.00 occurs 11 times. No other frequency occurred this often.)

ANSWER: The frequency of interjection per 100 words that was most typical during the children's performance of the spontaneous speech task was 0.00.

QUESTION: What frequency of part-word repetition per 100 words was most typical (i.e., occurred most often) during the children's performance of the spontaneous speech task?

Since the mode is the most frequently occurring score, the modal part-word repetition frequency per 100 words would be 0.00. (Note that in the frequency distribution on p. 298, 0.00 occurs seven times. No other frequency occurred this often.)

ANSWER: The frequency of part-word repetition per 100 words that was most typical during the children's performance of the spontaneous speech task was 0.00.

EXERCISE: Determine the modal numbers of word repetitions and revisions-
(Number 3)   incomplete phrases per 100 words that were produced by these 56 children. (Your answers should be 0.00 and 3.33, 4.83 for word repetition and revision-incomplete phrase, respectively.)

DESCRIPTIVE STATISTICS: MEASURES OF VARIABILITY

1. Range

QUESTION: What was the range of interjection frequencies produced by these children during their performance of the spontaneous speech task?

The range is the difference between the largest score in the data and the smallest score in the data. The interjection frequencies for the 56 children range from 0.00 to 8.53 (see p. 297). The range of interjection frequencies would be 8.53, since $8.53 - 0.00 = 8.53$.

ANSWER: The interjection frequencies produced by these children during their performance of the spontaneous speech task ranged from 0.00 to 8.53. The difference between the highest and lowest frequencies produced by these children was 8.53 per 100 words.

QUESTION: What was the range of part-word repetition frequencies produced by these children during their performance of the spontaneous speech task?

The part-word repetition frequencies for the 56 children range from 0.00 to 4.42 (see p. 298). The range of part-word repetition frequencies would be 4.42, since $4.42 - 0.00 = 4.42$.

ANSWER: The part-word repetition frequencies produced by these children during their performance of the spontaneous speech task ranged from 0.00 to 4.42. The difference between the highest and lowest frequencies produced by these children was 4.42 per 100 words.

EXERCISE: Determine the ranges of word repetition frequencies and revision-
(Number 4) incomplete phrase frequencies for these 56 children. (Your answers
should be 3.31 and 7.71 for word repetition and revision-incomplete
phrase, respectively.)

2. Interquartile Range

QUESTION: Within what range of interjection frequencies did the middle 50 percent of children fall during their performance of the spontaneous
speech task?

The interquartile range (Q) is the differences between the third
quartile (Q_3)—i.e., the score below which 75 percent of the scores fall—
and the first quartile (Q_1)—i.e., the score below which 25 percent of
the scores fall. For the interjection frequencies

$$Q = Q_3 - Q_1 = 1.535 - 0.29 = 1.245$$

Q_1 and Q_3 values were determined from the frequency distribution on
p. 297.

ANSWER: The interjection frequencies for the middle 50 percent of the children
differed from each other by a maximum of 1.245 instances per 100
words.

QUESTION: Within what range of part-word repetition frequencies did the middle
50 percent of children fall during their performance of the spontaneous speech task?

The interquartile range for the part-word repetition frequencies
(based on Q_1 and Q_3 values derived from the frequency distribution on
p. 298) would be:

$$Q = Q_3 - Q_1 = 1.185 - 0.28 = 0.905$$

ANSWER: The part-word repetition frequencies for the middle 50 percent of the
children differed from each other by a maximum of 0.905 instances
per 100 words.

EXERCISE: Determine the interquartile ranges of word repetition frequencies and
(Number 5) revision-incomplete phrase frequencies for these 56 children. (Your answers should be approximately 0.92 and 2.61 for word repetition and
revision-incomplete phrase, respectively.)

3. Standard Deviation (S)

QUESTION: How different were the children's interjection frequencies from each
other during their performance of the spontaneous speech task?

The standard deviation is a measure of how different various
scores are from each other. The larger the standard deviation, the more
different they would be. The standard deviation of the children's interjection frequencies is:

$$S = \sqrt{\frac{\Sigma X^2}{N} - \overline{X}^2} = \sqrt{\frac{166.92}{56} - (1.03)^2} = \sqrt{1.92} = 1.39$$

ANSWER: The children's interjection frequencies were quite different from each other judging by the fact that the standard deviation (1.39) was larger than the mean (1.03).

QUESTION: How different were the children's part-word repetition frequencies from each other during their performance of the spontaneous speech task?

The standard deviation of the children's part-word repetition frequencies is:

$$S = \sqrt{\frac{\Sigma X^2}{N} - \overline{X}^2} = \sqrt{\frac{71.68}{56} - (0.83)^2} = \sqrt{0.59} = 0.77$$

ANSWER: The children's part-word repetition frequencies differed from each other to a considerable extent, judging by the fact that the standard deviation (0.77) was almost as large as the mean (0.83). However, they did not differ as much from each other as their interjection frequencies, since their standard deviation was smaller.

EXERCISE: Determine the standard deviation of the children's word repetition fre-
(Number 6) quencies and revision-incomplete phrase frequencies. (Your answers should be approximately 0.85 and 1.66 for word repetition and revision-incomplete phrase, respectively.)

DESCRIPTIVE STATISTICS: MEASURES OF ASSOCIATION

1. Contingency Coefficient (C)

QUESTION: Were the children who produced the highest frequencies of interjection per 100 words on the spontaneous speech task the same ones who produced the highest frequencies of part-word repetition per 100 words on this task, and vice versa?

The first step in computing the contingency coefficient is to assign each of the 56 children to one of the four cells of a 2 × 2 table:

INTERJECTION

	Below Median	Above Median
Above Median	13 (a)	15 (b)
Below Median	15 (c)	13 (d)

PART-WORD REPETITION

If a child's interjection frequency was below the median (i.e., less than 0.51) and his part-word repetition frequency was above the median (i.e., greater than 0.815), he was assigned to cell a. If his interjection frequency was above the median (i.e., greater than 0.51) and his part-word repetition frequency also was above the median (i.e., greater than 0.815), he was assigned to cell b. If both his interjection and part-word repetition frequencies were below their respective medians, he was assigned to cell c. And if his interjection frequency was above the median and his part-word repetition frequency was below the median, he was assigned to cell d.

The next step is to compute the value of chi square (x^2) for the frequencies in the table. The value of chi square that was computed for this table (see p. 306) is 0.07. (Note that X^2 has a different meaning here than it has had previously.) The contingency coefficient for this table would be:

$$C = \sqrt{\frac{x^2}{N + x^2}} = \sqrt{\frac{0.07}{56 + 0.07}} = \sqrt{0.0012} = .035$$

Since the possible values of the contingency coefficient vary between 0.00 and a number somewhat less than 1.00, and the closer the value is to 0.00 the weaker the association between the two variables, the degree of association for these children between level of interjection production and level of part word repetition production would appear to be quite weak.

ANSWER: There was little, if any, tendency for the children who produced the highest frequencies of interjection on the spontaneous speech task to be the same children who produced the highest frequencies of part-word repetition on this task, and vice versa.

EXERCISE: Determine whether the children who produced the highest frequen-
(Number 7) cies of word repetition per 100 words on the spontaneous speech task were the same ones who produced the highest frequencies of revision-incomplete phrase per 100 words on this task, and vice versa, through the use of a contingency coefficient. (The value of the contingency coefficient you compute should be approximately 0.31.)

2. Phi Coefficient (Φ)

QUESTION: Were the children who produced the highest frequencies of interjection per 100 words on the spontaneous speech task the same ones who produced the highest frequencies of part-word repetition per 100 words on this task, and vice versa?

The first step in computing the phi coefficient is to assign each of the 56 children to one of the four cells of a 2 × 2 table in the same manner as for the contingency coefficient (see p. 301). The next step is to compute the value of phi (Φ) for the frequencies in the table (see p. 301) through the use of the following formula:

$$\Phi = \frac{(bc - ad)}{\sqrt{(a + b)(c + d)(a + c)(b + d)}}$$

$$= \frac{(15)(15) - (13)(13)}{\sqrt{(13 + 15)(15 + 13)(13 + 15)(15 + 13)}} = \frac{56}{\sqrt{614656}}$$

$$= \frac{56}{784} = 0.071$$

Since the possible values of the phi coefficient range from -1.00 to $+1.00$, and the closer the value is to 0.00 the weaker the association between the two variables, the degree of association for these children between level of interjection production and level of part-word repetition production would appear to be quite weak.

ANSWER: There was little, if any, tendency for the children who produced the highest frequencies of interjection on the spontaneous speech task to be the same children who produced the highest frequencies of part-word repetition on this task, and vice versa.

REMARKS: The values of the contingency coefficient and phi coefficient computed for this table are slightly different due to differences in the computational procedures involved. The phi coefficient only can be used for 2×2 tables. The contingency coefficient can be used as a measure of association for larger tables as well. The magnitude of the phi coefficient is simpler to interpret than that of the contingency coefficient because the highest possible value is always the same, i.e., 1.00.

EXERCISE: Determine whether the children who produced the highest frequen-
(Number 8) cies of word repetition per 100 words on the spontaneous speech task were the same ones who produced the highest frequencies of revision-incomplete phrase per 100 words on this task, and vice versa, through the use of a phi coefficient. (The value of the phi coefficient you compute should be approximately 0.36.)

3. Spearman Rank-Order Coefficient (r_s)

QUESTION: How similar was the ordering of the second graders with regard to their interjection frequencies and part-word repetition frequencies during their performance of the spontaneous speech task?

The first step in computing a Spearman rank-order correlation coefficient between the interjection frequencies and part-word repetition frequencies of the 15 second graders (see p. 295) is to determine each child's rank for interjection frequency and each child's rank for part-word repetition frequency. The child who had the lowest frequency of part-word repetition would be assigned the rank 1; the one who had the second lowest, the rank 2; the one who had the third lowest, the rank 3; and so on. If more than one child had the same frequency, each would be assigned the mean of the tied ranks. The ranks assigned to the 15 children for their interjection frequencies and part-word repetition frequencies are indicated in the table that follows. Also included in the table is the difference between each child's two ranks (d_i) and this difference squared (d_i^2). The sum of the squared differences between ranks for the 15 children is used for computing the Spearman rank-order coefficient (r_s).

Subject Number	Rank		d_i	d_i^2
	I	*PW*		
1	8.5	11.0	− 2.5	6.25
2	14.0	13.0	1.0	1.00
3	11.0	2.0	9.0	81.00
4	6.0	12.0	− 6.0	36.00
5	4.0	8.0	4.0	16.00
6	1.5	6.0	− 4.5	20.25
7	1.5	2.0	− 0.5	0.25
8	7.0	15.0	− 8.0	64.00
9	3.0	14.0	− 11.0	121.00
10	8.5	9.0	− 0.5	0.25
11	15.0	5.0	10.0	100.00
12	10.0	10.0	0.0	0.00
13	12.0	4.0	8.0	64.00
14	5.0	7.0	− 2.0	4.00
15	13.0	2.0	11.0	121.00
				$\Sigma d_i^2 = 635.00$

The value of r_s for these data would be:

$$r_s = 1 - \frac{6\Sigma\, d_i^2}{N^3 - N} = 1 - \frac{(6)\,(635)}{(15)^3 - 15}$$

$$= 1 - \frac{3810}{3375 - 15} = 1 - 1.13 = -0.13$$

Since the possible values range from −1.00 to +1.00, and the closer the value is to 0.00 the weaker the association between the two variables, the degree of association for these children between level of interjection production and level of part-word repetition production would appear to be quite weak.

ANSWER: There was little, if any, similarity in the ordering of the second graders with regard to their interjection frequencies and part-word repetition frequencies during their performance of the spontaneous speech task.

EXERCISE: Determine the degree of similarity of the ordering of the third graders
(Number 9) with regard to their interjection frequencies and part-word repetition frequencies during their performance of the spontaneous speech task through the use of r_s. (The value of r_s you compute should be approximately 0.40.)

4. Pearson Product-Moment Correlation Coefficient (r)

QUESTION: Were the levels of the children's interjection frequencies related to those of their part-word repetition frequencies during their performances of the spontaneous speech task?

The first step in computing a Pearson product-moment correlation coefficient between the interjection frequencies and part-word repetition frequencies of the 56 children (see Table A.1) is to compute the following sums:

Σ X = sum of the 56 interjection frequencies = 57.71
Σ Y = sum of the 56 part-word repetition frequencies
   = 46.75
Σ X^2 = sum of the squares of the 56 interjection frequencies
   = 166.92
Σ Y^2 = sum of the squares of the 56 part-word repetition frequencies
   = 71.68
Σ X Y = sum of the products of the 56 pairs of frequencies
   = 47.00

The Pearson product-moment correlation coefficient for these data would be:

$$r = \frac{N\Sigma XY - (\Sigma X)(\Sigma Y)}{\sqrt{[N\Sigma X^2 - (\Sigma X)^2][N\Sigma Y^2 - (\Sigma Y)^2]}}$$

$$= \frac{(56)(47.00) - (57.71)(46.75)}{\sqrt{[(56)(166.92) - (57.71)^2][(56)(71.68) - (46.75)^2]}}$$

$$= \frac{2632.00 - 2697.94}{\sqrt{[9347.52 - 3330.44][4014.08 - 2185.56]}}$$

$$= \frac{-65.94}{\sqrt{11,002,351}} = \frac{-65.94}{3316.98}$$

$$= -0.02$$

Since the possible values of r range from -1.00 to $+1.00$, and the closer the value is to 0.00 the weaker the association between the two variables, there would appear to be little, if any, association between these children's interjection and part-word repetition frequencies.

ANSWER: There was little or no relationship between the children's interjection frequency levels and part-word repetition frequency levels during their performance of the spontaneous speech task.

EXERCISE: Determine the degree of relationship between the children's word
(Number 10) repetition frequencies and revision-incomplete phrase frequencies through the use of r. (The value of r you compute should be approximately 0.37.)

INFERENTIAL STATISTICAL TESTS: NOMINAL DATA

1. Chi Square Test (χ^2)

QUESTION: Was there a tendency for the children who had interjection frequencies above the median for the group also to have part-word repetition frequencies above the median for the group, or vice versa?

The first step in performing a chi square test is selecting an *alpha* level, or a maximum acceptable probability for a *Type I* error (i.e., concluding that the children who had interjection frequencies that were above the median for the group also tended to have part-word repetition frequencies that were above the median for the group, or vice versa, when there was no such tendency). A 0.05 alpha level will be used for this test. Since to answer the question it would be necessary to detect both positive and negative relationships between interjection level and part-word repetition level, the region of rejection for the test will be *two-tailed.*

The next step is to compute the value of chi square. Each of the 56 children is assigned to one of the four cells in a 2 × 2 table in the same manner as for the contingency coefficient (see p. 301). The value of chi square would be computed from this table as follows:

$$\chi^2 = \frac{N\left(|ad - bc| - \dfrac{N}{2}\right)^2}{(a + b)(c + d)(a + c)(b + d)}$$

$$= \frac{56\left(|(13)(13) - (15)(15)| - \dfrac{56}{2}\right)^2}{(13 + 15)(15 + 13)(13 + 15)(15 + 13)}$$

$$= \frac{56(|169 - 225| - 28)^2}{(28)(28)(28)(28)} = \frac{56(28)^2}{614,656}$$

$$= \frac{43,904}{614,656} = 0.07$$

To determine whether the value of chi square computed is large enough for the null hypothesis to be rejected, the value of chi square required for rejection is located in Table A.2. The degrees of freedom (*df*) here would be 1 (i.e., the number of rows minus one times the number of columns minus one). The value of chi square required for rejection at the 0.05 alpha level when *df* = 1 is 3.84. Since the value computed is smaller than this, i.e., 0.07, the null hypothesis would not be rejected.

ANSWER: There was no tendency for the children who had interjection frequencies above the median for the group also to have part-word repetition frequencies above the median for the group, or vice versa (chi square test; alpha = 0.05).

REMARKS: This application of the chi square test illustrates that it is not limited to nominal data; it can be used with ordinal, interval, and ratio data as well. The chi square formula that was used is a special one for 2 × 2 tables when *N* is larger than 40. The chi square formulas for other tables can be found in most education and psychology statistics texts.

EXERCISE: Determine whether there was a tendency for the children who had
(Number 11) word repetition frequencies above the median for the group also to

TABLE A.2.   Table of critical values of chi square.[a]

df	Probability under H_0 that $\chi^2 \geq$ chi square													
	.99	.98	.95	.90	.80	.70	.50	.30	.20	.10	.05	.02	.01	.001
1	.00016	.00063	.0039	.016	.064	.15	.46	1.07	1.64	2.71	3.84	5.41	6.64	10.83
2	.02	.04	.10	.21	.45	.71	1.39	2.41	3.22	4.60	5.99	7.82	9.21	13.82
3	.12	.18	.35	.58	1.00	1.42	2.37	3.66	4.64	6.25	7.82	9.84	11.34	16.27
4	.30	.43	.71	1.06	1.65	2.20	3.36	4.88	5.99	7.78	9.49	11.67	13.28	18.46
5	.55	.75	1.14	1.61	2.34	3.00	4.35	6.06	7.29	9.24	11.07	13.39	15.09	20.52
6	.87	1.13	1.64	2.20	3.07	3.83	5.35	7.23	8.56	10.64	12.59	15.03	16.81	22.46
7	1.24	1.56	2.17	2.83	3.82	4.67	6.35	8.38	9.80	12.02	14.07	16.62	18.48	24.32
8	1.65	2.03	2.73	3.49	4.59	5.53	7.34	9.52	11.03	13.36	15.51	18.17	20.09	26.12
9	2.09	2.53	3.32	4.17	5.38	6.39	8.34	10.66	12.24	14.68	16.92	19.68	21.67	27.88
10	2.56	3.06	3.94	4.86	6.18	7.27	9.34	11.78	13.44	15.99	18.31	21.16	23.21	29.59
11	3.05	3.61	4.58	5.58	6.99	8.15	10.34	12.90	14.63	17.28	19.68	22.62	24.72	31.26
12	3.57	4.18	5.23	6.30	7.81	9.03	11.34	14.01	15.81	18.55	21.03	24.05	26.22	32.91
13	4.11	4.76	5.89	7.04	8.63	9.93	12.34	15.12	16.98	19.81	22.36	25.47	27.69	34.53
14	4.66	5.37	6.57	7.79	9.47	10.82	13.34	16.22	18.15	21.06	23.68	26.87	29.14	36.12
15	5.23	5.98	7.26	8.55	10.31	11.72	14.34	17.32	19.31	22.31	25.00	28.26	30.58	37.70
16	5.81	6.61	7.96	9.31	11.15	12.62	15.34	18.42	20.46	23.54	26.30	29.63	32.00	39.29
17	6.41	7.26	8.67	10.08	12.00	13.53	16.34	19.51	21.62	24.77	27.59	31.00	33.41	40.75
18	7.02	7.91	9.39	10.86	12.86	14.44	17.34	20.60	22.76	25.99	28.87	32.35	34.80	42.31
19	7.63	8.57	10.12	11.65	13.72	15.35	18.34	21.69	23.90	27.20	30.14	33.69	36.19	43.82
20	8.26	9.24	10.85	12.44	14.58	16.27	19.34	22.78	25.04	28.41	31.41	35.02	37.57	45.32
21	8.90	9.92	11.59	13.24	15.44	17.18	20.34	23.86	26.17	29.62	32.67	36.34	38.93	46.80
22	9.54	10.60	12.34	14.04	16.31	18.10	21.24	24.94	27.30	30.81	33.92	37.66	40.29	48.27
23	10.20	11.29	13.09	14.85	17.19	19.02	22.34	26.02	28.43	32.01	35.17	38.97	41.64	49.73
24	10.86	11.99	13.85	15.66	18.06	19.94	23.34	27.10	29.55	33.20	36.42	40.27	42.98	51.18
25	11.52	12.70	14.61	16.47	18.94	20.87	24.34	28.17	30.68	34.38	37.65	41.57	44.31	52.62
26	12.20	13.41	15.38	17.29	19.82	21.79	25.34	29.25	31.80	35.56	38.88	42.86	45.64	54.05
27	12.88	14.12	16.15	18.11	20.70	22.72	26.34	30.32	32.91	36.74	40.11	44.14	46.96	55.48
28	13.56	14.85	16.93	18.94	21.59	23.65	27.34	31.39	34.03	37.92	41.34	45.42	48.28	56.89
29	14.26	15.57	17.71	19.77	22.48	24.58	28.34	32.46	35.14	39.09	42.56	46.69	49.59	58.30
30	14.95	16.31	18.49	20.60	23.36	25.51	29.34	33.53	36.25	40.26	43.77	47.96	50.89	59.70

[a]*Adapted from Table IV of Fisher and Yates:* Statistical Tables for Biological, Agricultural, and Medical Research *(6th edition). Copyright 1974 by Longman Group, Ltd. With permission of Longman Group, Ltd.*

have revision-incomplete phrase frequencies above the median for the group, or vice versa, through the use of the chi square test. (The value of chi square you compute should be approximately 5.78.)

INFERENTIAL STATISTICAL TESTS: ORDINAL DATA

1. Sign Test

QUESTION: Did the second graders tend to produce higher frequencies of interjection than of part-word repetition?

The first step in performing a sign test is selecting an *alpha* level, or a maximum acceptable probability for a *Type I* error (i.e., concluding there was a tendency for the second graders to produce higher frequencies of interjection than of part-word repetition when there was no such tendency). A 0.05 alpha level will be used for this test. Since to answer the question it only would be necessary to detect a difference between interjection frequency and part-word repetition frequency in one direction, the region of rejection for the test will be *one-tailed*.

The next step is to compute the value for the sign test. Each of the 15 second graders is assigned a + or a −, depending on whether his interjection frequency or part-word repetition frequency is higher. If his interjection frequency is higher than his part-word repetition frequency, he is assigned a +; if his part-word repetition frequency is higher than his interjection frequency, he is assigned a −. If his interjection and part-word repetition frequencies are the same, he is assigned a 0. The sign assignments for the 15 children are as follows:

Subject	Sign	Subject	Sign
1	−	9	−
2	+	10	−
3	+	11	+
4	−	12	0
5	−	13	+
6	−	14	0
7	0	15	+
8	−		

The number of subjects for whom the two frequencies are not the same (N), and the number of times the sign occurs which occurs *least* often (x), are determined for this distribution. The values of N and x are 12 and 5, respectively. Based on the binomial distribution (see Table A.3) when $N = 12$, the probability of five pluses (x) occurring by chance is 0.387. Since this value is larger than 0.05, the null hypothesis would not be rejected.

ANSWER: The second graders did not exhibit a tendency to produce higher frequencies of interjection than of part-word repetition (sign test; alpha = 0.05).

REMARK: This procedure can be used to compute the probability value for the sign test when the number of subjects for whom the two frequencies are not the same (N) is 25 or fewer. When the value of N exceeds 25, the procedure used to answer the next question is appropriate.

QUESTION: Did the second, third, and fourth graders tend to produce higher frequencies of interjection than of part-word repetition?

The alpha level that will be used for this sign test is 0.05. The region of rejection will be *one-tailed* for the same reason as indicated for the previous question.

Next, each of the 35 second, third, and fourth graders is assigned a sign in the same manner as for the previous question. The sign assignments for these children are as follows:

Subject	Sign	Subject	Sign
1	−	19	−
2	+	20	+
3	+	21	−
4	−	22	−
5	−	23	+
6	−	24	−
7	0	25	+
8	−	26	+
9	−	27	−
10	−	28	−
11	+	29	−
12	0	30	−
13	+	31	−
14	0	32	−
15	+	33	+
16	−	34	−
17	+	35	+
18	+		

The values of N and x for this distribution (which were determined in the same manner as for the previous question) are 32 and 13, respectively. The probability of 13 pluses (x) occurring by chance when $N = 32$ can be determined by means of the following formula (which is based on the "normal curve"):

$$Z = \frac{(x \pm 0.5) - \frac{1}{2}N}{\frac{1}{2}\sqrt{N}} \quad \text{where } x + 0.5 \text{ is used when } x < \tfrac{1}{2}N,$$
$$\text{and } x - 0.5 \text{ is used when } x > \tfrac{1}{2}N.$$

$$= \frac{(13 + 0.5) - \frac{1}{2}(32)}{\frac{1}{2}\sqrt{32}}$$

$$= \frac{13.5 - 16.0}{\frac{1}{2}(5.66)} = \frac{-2.5}{2.83} = -0.88$$

Based on the normal distribution (see Table A.4) the probability of this outcome occurring by chance is 0.189. Since this value is larger than 0.05, the null hypothesis would not be rejected.

ANSWER: The second, third, and fourth graders did not exhibit a tendency to produce higher frequencies of interjection than of part-word repetition (sign test; alpha = 0.05).

EXERCISE: Determine whether the second and third graders exhibited a tendency
(Number 12) to produce higher frequencies of revision-incomplete phrase than of word repetition through the use of *both* sign test computational procedures. (The probability values you compute by the "small" sample and the "large" sample computational procedures should be approximately 0.001 and 0.00003, respectively.)

TABLE A.3.   Table of probabilities associated with values as small as observed values of x in the sign test.[a]

Given in the body of this table are one-tailed probabilities under H_0 for the binomial test when $P = Q = \frac{1}{2}$. To save space, decimal points are omitted in the p's.

N \ x	0	1	2	3	4	5	6	7	8	9	10	11	12	13	14	15
5	031	188	500	812	969	†										
6	016	109	344	656	891	984	†									
7	008	062	227	500	773	938	992	†								
8	004	035	145	363	637	855	965	996	†							
9	002	020	090	254	500	746	910	980	998	†						
10	001	011	055	172	377	623	828	945	989	999	†					
11		006	033	113	274	500	726	887	967	994	†	†				
12		003	019	073	194	387	613	806	927	981	997	†	†			
13		002	011	046	133	291	500	709	867	954	989	998	†	†		
14		001	006	029	090	212	395	605	788	910	971	994	999	†	†	
15			004	018	059	151	304	500	696	849	941	982	996	†	†	†
16			002	011	038	105	227	402	598	773	895	962	989	998	†	†
17			001	006	025	072	166	315	500	685	834	928	975	994	999	†
18			001	004	015	048	119	240	407	593	760	881	952	985	996	999
19				002	010	032	084	180	324	500	676	820	916	968	990	998
20				001	006	021	058	132	252	412	588	748	868	942	979	994
21				001	004	013	039	095	192	332	500	668	808	905	961	987
22					002	008	026	067	143	262	416	584	738	857	933	974
23					001	005	017	047	105	202	339	500	661	798	895	953
24					001	003	011	032	076	154	271	419	581	729	846	924
25						002	007	022	054	115	212	345	500	655	788	885

†1.0 or approximately 1.0

[a]*Adapted from Table IV, B, of Walker and Lev. 1953.* Statistical Inference. *New York: Holt,* p. 458.

2. Mann-Whitney U Test

QUESTION: Did the typical (i.e., median) second or third grader have a higher frequency of interjection than did the typical fourth, fifth, or sixth grader?

The first step in performing a Mann-Whitney U Test is selecting an *alpha* level, or a maximum acceptable probability for a *Type I* error (i.e., concluding the median second or third grader had a higher frequency of interjection than did the median fourth, fifth, or sixth grader when there was no such difference). A 0.05 alpha level will be used for this test. Since to answer the question it only would be necessary to detect a difference between the two groups in one direction, the region of rejection for the test will be *one-tailed*.

The next step is to compute the value for the Mann-Whitney U Test. The 56 children are ordered on the basis of their interjection frequencies, and the rank is assigned to each child that designates his

TABLE A.4. Table of probabilities associated with values as extreme as observed values of z in the normal distribution.[a]

z	.00	.01	.02	.03	.04	.05	.06	.07	.08	.09
.0	.5000	.4960	.4920	.4880	.4840	.4801	.4761	.4721	.4681	4641
.1	.4602	.4562	.4522	.4483	.4443	.4404	.4364	.4325	.4286	.4247
.2	.4207	.4168	.4129	.4090	.4052	.4013	.3974	.3936	.3897	.3859
.3	.3821	.3783	.3745	.3707	.3669	.3632	.3594	.3557	.3520	.3483
.4	.3446	.3409	.3372	.3336	.3300	.3264	.3228	.3192	.3156	.3121
.5	.3085	.3050	.3015	.2981	.2946	.2912	.2877	.2843	.2810	.2776
.6	.2743	.2709	.2676	.2643	.2611	.2578	.2546	.2514	.2483	.2451
.7	.2420	.2389	.2358	.2327	.2296	.2266	.2236	.2206	.2177	.2148
.8	.2119	.2090	.2061	.2033	.2005	.1977	.1949	.1922	.1894	.1867
.9	.1841	.1814	.1788	.1762	.1736	.1711	.1685	.1660	.1635	.1611
1.0	.1587	.1562	.1539	.1515	.1492	.1469	.1446	.1423	.1401	.1379
1.1	.1357	.1335	.1314	.1292	.1271	.1251	.1230	.1210	.1190	.1170
1.2	.1151	.1131	.1112	.1093	.1075	.1056	.1038	.1020	.1003	.0985
1.3	.0968	.0951	.0934	.0918	.0901	.0885	.0869	.0853	.0838	.0823
1.4	.0808	.0793	.0778	.0764	.0749	.0735	.0721	.0708	.0694	.0681
1.5	.0668	.0655	.0643	.0630	.0618	.0606	.0594	.0582	.0571	.0559
1.6	.0548	.0537	.0526	.0516	.0505	.0495	.0485	.0475	.0465	.0455
1.7	.0446	.0436	.0427	.0418	.0409	.0401	.0392	.0384	.0375	.0367
1.8	.0359	.0351	.0344	.0336	.0329	.0322	.0314	.0307	.0301	.0294
1.9	.0287	.0281	.0274	.0268	.0262	.0256	.0250	.0244	.0239	.0233
2.0	.0228	.0222	.0217	.0212	.0207	.0202	.0197	.0192	.0188	.0183
2.1	.0179	.0174	.0170	.0166	.0162	.0158	.0154	.0150	.0146	.0143
2.2	.0139	.0136	.0132	.0129	.0125	.0122	.0119	.0116	.0113	.0110
2.3	.0107	.0104	.0102	.0099	.0096	.0094	.0091	.0089	.0087	.0084
2.4	.0082	.0080	.0078	.0075	.0073	.0071	.0069	.0068	.0066	.0064
2.5	.0062	.0060	.0059	.0057	.0055	.0054	.0052	.0051	.0049	.0048
2.6	.0047	.0045	.0044	.0043	.0041	.0040	.0039	.0038	.0037	.0036
2.7	.0035	.0034	.0033	.0032	.0031	.0030	.0029	.0028	.0027	.0026
2.8	.0026	.0025	.0024	.0023	.0023	.0022	.0021	.0021	.0020	.0019
2.9	.0019	.0018	.0018	.0017	.0016	.0016	.0015	.0015	.0014	.0014
3.0	.0013	.0013	.0013	.0012	.0012	.0011	.0011	.0011	.0010	.0010
3.1	.0010	.0009	.0009	.0009	.0008	.0008	.0008	.0008	.0007	.0007
3.2	.0007									
3.3	.0005									
3.4	.0003									
3.5	.00023									
3.6	.00016									
3.7	.00011									
3.8	.00007									
3.9	.00005									
4.0	.00003									

[a]*Adapted from Table A of Siegel.* Nonparametric Statistics for the Behavioral Sciences. *Copyright 1956 by McGraw-Hill Inc. With permission of McGraw-Hill Book Company.*

place in the ordering. The child who had the lowest interjection frequency would be assigned the rank 1; the one who had the second lowest, the rank 2; the one who had the third lowest, the rank 3; and so on. If more than one child had the same frequency, each would be assigned the mean of the tied ranks. The ranks assigned to the children are indicated as follows:

2nd and 3rd Graders		4th, 5th, and 6th Graders	
Frequency	Rank	Frequency	Rank
0.00	6.0	0.00	6.0
0.00	6.0	0.00	6.0
0.28	13.5	0.00	6.0
0.30	15.5	0.00	6.0
0.31	17.0	0.00	6.0
0.33	18.5	0.00	6.0
0.36	20.0	0.00	6.0
0.40	21.0	0.00	6.0
0.46	24.0	0.00	6.0
0.47	25.0	0.16	12.0
0.49	26.0	0.28	13.5
0.50	27.5	0.30	15.5
0.50	27.5	0.33	18.5
0.55	30.0	0.43	22.0
0.84	36.5	0.44	23.0
1.04	39.0	0.52	29.0
1.07	40.0	0.56	31.0
1.40	41.0	0.69	32.0
1.46	42.0	0.72	33.0
1.80	46.0	0.73	34.0
1.87	48.0	0.78	35.0
2.13	50.0	0.84	36.5
2.23	51.0	0.94	38.0
3.40	53.0	1.61	43.0
3.78	55.0	1.72	44.0
8.53	56.0	1.76	45.0
		1.82	47.0
		1.99	49.0
		2.92	52.0
		3.67	54.0
$R_1 = \overline{835.0}$		$R_2 = \overline{761.0}$	
$n_1 = 26$		$n_2 = 30$	

Next, two estimates of U are computed from the sums of the ranks of the second and third graders (R_1) and of the fourth, fifth, and sixth graders (R_2). In these formulas, n_1 refers to the number of second and third graders and n_2 to the number of fourth, fifth, and sixth graders.

$$U = n_1 n_2 + \frac{n_1(n_1 + 1)}{2} - R_1$$
$$= (26)(30) + \frac{26(26 + 1)}{2} - 835.0$$
$$= 780.0 + 351.0 - 835.0 = 296.0$$

$$U = n_1n_2 + \frac{n_2(n_2 + 1)}{2} - R_2$$

$$= (26)(30) + \frac{30(30 + 1)}{2} - 761.0$$

$$= 780.0 + 465.0 - 761.0 = 484.0$$

The *lowest* estimate of U then is used to compute the value of Z, the test statistic.

$$Z = \frac{U - \dfrac{n_1n_2}{2}}{\sqrt{\dfrac{(n_1)\,(n_2)\,(n_1 + n_2 + 1)}{12}}}$$

$$= \frac{296 - \dfrac{(26)\,(30)}{2}}{\sqrt{\dfrac{(26)\,(30)\,(26 + 30 + 1)}{12}}}$$

$$= \frac{296 - 390}{\sqrt{3705}} = \frac{-94}{60.87} = -1.54$$

Based on the normal distribution (see Table A.4), the probability of this outcome occurring by chance is 0.062. Since this value is larger than 0.05, the null hypothesis would not be rejected.

ANSWER: The typical second or third grader did not have a higher frequency of interjection than the typical fourth, fifth, or sixth grader (Mann-Whitney U Test; alpha = 0.05).

REMARK: This computational procedure is appropriate when the number of subjects in the larger groups is more than 20. Appropriate computational procedures when this number is 20 or smaller can be found in several education and psychology statistical texts, including that of Siegel (1956, 1988).

EXERCISE: Determine whether the typical (i.e., median) second or third grader
(Number 13) had a higher frequency of part-word repetition than did the typical fourth, fifth, or sixth grader through the use of the Mann-Whitney U Test. (The value you compute for Z should be approximately -1.40.)

3. Friedman Two-Way Analysis of Variance (x_r^2)

QUESTION: Did the second graders tend to produce higher frequencies of some of the four disfluency types (i.e., interjection, part-word repetition, word repetition, and revision-incomplete phrase) than of others?

The first step in performing a Friedman Two-Way Analysis of Variance is selecting an *alpha* level, or a maximum acceptable probability for a *Type I* error (i.e., concluding there was a tendency for the second graders to produce higher frequencies of some of the disfluency types than of others when there was no such tendency). A 0.05 alpha level will be used for this test.

The next step is to compute the value of χ_r^2. Each second grader's disfluency frequencies for interjection, part-word repetition, word repetition, and revision-incomplete phrase are ordered from lowest to highest. The rank is then assigned to each that designates its position in the ordering (1 is assigned to the lowest frequency, 2 to the second lowest frequency, and so on). If more than one disfluency type has the same frequency, each is assigned the mean of the tied ranks. The ranks assigned to the 15 second graders which were based on the frequencies of the four disfluency types they produced (see page 295) are as follows:

Subject Number	I	PW	W	R-IP
1	1.5	3.0	1.5	4.0
2	3.0	2.0	1.0	4.0
3	3.0	1.5	1.5	4.0
4	1.5	3.0	1.5	4.0
5	1.0	3.0	2.0	4.0
6	1.0	2.5	2.5	4.0
7	1.5	1.5	3.0	4.0
8	1.0	4.0	2.0	3.0
9	1.0	3.0	2.0	4.0
10	1.0	2.0	3.0	4.0
11	4.0	1.0	2.0	3.0
12	2.0	2.0	2.0	4.0
13	3.0	1.0	2.0	4.0
14	1.5	1.5	3.0	4.0
15	3.0	1.0	2.0	4.0
$R_j =$	29.0	32.0	31.0	58.0

The formula for computing the value of χ_r^2 is:

$$\chi_r^2 = \frac{12}{Nk(k+1)} \sum_{i=1}^{k} (R_j)^2 - 3N(k+1)$$

where

R_j = a column sum (i.e., total)

N = number of rows

k = number of columns

The value of χ_r^2 for these data is:

$$\chi_r^2 = \frac{12}{(15)(4)(4+1)} [(29)^2 + (32)^2 + (31)^2 + (58)^2] - (3)(15)(4+1)$$

$$= \frac{12}{300} (6190) - 225$$

$$= 247.6 - 225.0 = 22.6$$

To determine whether this value of χ_r^2 is large enough for the null hypothesis to be rejected, the value of chi square required for rejection is located in Table A.2. The degrees of freedom (df) here would be 3 (i.e., the number of columns minus one). The value of chi square required for rejection at the 0.05 alpha level when (df) = 3 is 7.82. Since the value computed is larger than this, i.e., 22.6, the null hypothesis would be rejected.

ANSWER: The second graders tended to produce higher frequencies of some of the disfluency types than of others (Friedman Two-Way Analysis of Variance; alpha = 0.05).

EXERCISE: Determine whether the third graders tended to produce higher fre-
(Number 14) quencies of some of the four disfluency types than the others through the use of the Friedman Two-Way Analysis of Variance. (The value of χ_r^2 you compute should be approximately 12.74.)

2. Kruskal-Wallis One-Way Analysis of Variance (H)

QUESTION: Was there a tendency for the amount of part-word repetition produced by the children to vary as a function of grade level?

The first step in performing a Kruskal-Wallis One-Way Analysis of Variance is selecting an *alpha* level, or a maximum acceptable probability for a *Type I* error (i.e., concluding there was a tendency for the amount of part word repetition produced by the children to vary as a function of grade level when there was no such tendency). A 0.05 alpha level will be used for this test.

The next step is to compute the value of H. First, the 56 children are ordered on the basis of their part-word repetition frequency. The rank is then assigned to each that designated his position in the ordering (1 is assigned to the child with the lowest frequency, 2 to the one with the second lowest frequency, and so on). If more than one child has the same frequency, each is assigned the mean of the tied ranks. The ranks assigned to the children in each grade are as follows:

	2nd Grade	3rd Grade	4th Grade	5th Grade	6th Grade
	4.0	4.0	8.0	4.0	4.0
	4.0	14.5	12.0	9.0	4.0
	4.0	21.5	26.0	11.0	10.0
	16.0	32.0	30.0	17.5	13.0
	17.5	37.0	43.5	24.0	14.5
	19.0	40.0	45.0	25.0	21.5
	20.0	41.0	50.0	28.0	23.0
	36.0	47.0	51.0	29.0	27.0
	38.0	48.0	55.0	31.0	33.0
	39.0	49.0		34.5	34.5
	42.0	56.0		52.0	
	43.5				
	46.0				
	53.0				
	54.0				
R_j =	436.0	390.0	320.5	265.0	184.5

The formula for computing the value of H is:

$$H = \frac{12}{N(N+1)} \sum_{i=1}^{k} \frac{R_i^2}{n_i} - 3(N+1)$$

where

R_i = a column sum (i.e., total)
N = the number of subjects
n_i = the number of subjects in a column

The value of H for these data is:

$$H = \frac{12}{56(56+1)} \left[\frac{(436)^2}{15} + \frac{(390)^2}{11} + \frac{(320.5)^2}{9} + \frac{(265)^2}{11} + \frac{(184.5)^2}{10} \right]$$
$$- 3(56+1)$$

$$= \frac{12}{3192} [12,673.07 + 13,827.27 + 11,413.36 + 6384.09 + 3404.02]$$
$$- 171$$

$$= 0.004[47,701.81] - 171$$

$$= 190.81 - 171 = 19.81$$

To determine whether this value of H is large enough for the null hypothesis to be rejected, the value of H required for rejection is located in Table A.2. (H is distributed as chi square, provided that the number of groups is greater than 3 and that there are more than 5 subjects in each of the groups.) The degrees of freedom (df) here would be 4 (i.e., the number of columns minus one). The value of chi square required for rejection at the 0.05 alpha level when df = 4 is 9.49. Since the value of H computed is larger than this, i.e., 19.81, the null hypothesis would be rejected.

ANSWER: There was a tendency for the amount of part-word repetition produced by the children to vary as a function of grade level (Kruskal-Wallis One-Way Analysis of Variance; alpha = 0.05).

REMARK: If 0.003759 had not been rounded to 0.004, the value of H would have been 8.31, and the null hypothesis would not have been rejected.

EXERCISE: Determine whether there was a tendency for the amount of word repe-
(Number 15) tition produced by the children to vary as a function of grade level through the use of the Kruskal-Wallis One-Way Analysis of Variance. (The value of H you compute should be approximately 19.14 if 0.003759 is rounded to 0.004.)

INFERENTIAL STATISTICAL TESTS: INTERVAL AND RATIO DATA

1. *t*-Test for Related Measures (*t*)

QUESTION: Did the children on the average tend to produce higher frequencies of interjection than of part-word repetition?

The first step in performing a *t*-test for related measures is selecting an *alpha* level, or a maximum acceptable probability for a *Type I* error (i.e., concluding that the children on the average tended to produce higher frequencies of interjection than of part-word repetition when there was no such tendency). A 0.05 alpha level will be used for this test. Since to answer the question it only would be necessary to detect a difference between interjection frequency and part-word repetition frequency in one direction, the region of rejection for the test will be *one-tailed*.

The next step is to compute the value for *t*. Each child's part-word repetition frequency is subtracted from his interjection frequency (see Table A.1). If his part-word repetition frequency is smaller than his interjection frequency, this difference is assigned a + sign. If his part-word repetition frequency is larger than his interjection frequency, this difference is assigned a − sign. The difference frequencies for the 56 children are as follows:

Subject	Difference (D)	Subject	Difference (D)
1	− 0.66	29	− 2.41
2	+ 0.71	30	− 0.32
3	+ 1.40	31	− 0.73
4	− 0.81	32	− 0.12
5	− 0.63	33	+ 0.21
6	− 0.35	34	− 1.21
7	0.00	35	+ 2.84
8	− 1.90	36	0.00
9	− 1.50	37	− 0.66
10	− 0.50	38	+ 1.61
11	+ 8.19	39	+ 0.18
12	0.00	40	+ 0.14
13	+ 1.17	41	+ 1.99
14	0.00	42	+ 0.91
15	+ 1.87	43	+ 0.51
16	− 0.68	44	− 0.54
17	+ 2.65	45	+ 1.21
18	+ 0.74	46	+ 0.18
19	− 0.66	47	− 0.28
20	+ 0.49	48	− 0.19
21	− 0.36	49	+ 1.99
22	− 3.87	50	− 0.47
23	+ 0.56	51	− 0.93
24	− 0.13	52	+ 0.69
25	+ 1.89	53	− 0.66
26	+ 0.90	54	− 0.18
27	− 1.10	55	+ 0.52
28	− 0.63	56	− 0.11

The following are computed from these difference frequencies:

ΣD = the algebraic difference between the sum of the differences which have plus signs and the sum of the differences which have minus signs = 33.55 (i.e., plus sum) − 22.59 (i.e., minus sum) = 10.96.

$\overline{D}$ = the mean of the algebraic sum of the differences = 10.96/56
  = 0.196

ΣD^2 = the sum of the squared difference frequencies = 144.596

The value of t here is:

$$t = \frac{\overline{D}\sqrt{N-1}}{\sqrt{\dfrac{\Sigma D^2}{N} - \overline{D}^2}}$$

$$= \frac{0.196\sqrt{56-1}}{\sqrt{\dfrac{144.596}{56} - (0.196)^2}}$$

$$= \frac{0.196\,(7.416)}{\sqrt{2.582 - 0.038}} = \frac{1.454}{1.579}$$

$$= 0.92$$

To determine whether this value of t is large enough for the null hypothesis to be rejected, the value of t required for rejection is located in Table A.5. The degrees of freedom (df) here would be 55 (i.e., the number of subjects minus one). The value of t required for rejection at the 0.05 alpha level when df = 55 is 1.67. Since the value computed—i.e., 0.92—is smaller than this, the null hypothesis would not be rejected.

ANSWER: The children on the average did not tend to produce higher frequencies of interjection than of part-word repetition (t-test for related measures; alpha = 0.05).

EXERCISE: Determine whether the children on the average exhibited a tendency
(Number 16) to produce higher frequencies of revision-incomplete phrase than of word repetition through the use of the t-test for related measures. (The value of t you compute should be approximately 9.88.)

2. t-Test for Independent Measures (t)

QUESTION: Did the second and third graders tend to produce higher frequencies of interjection on the average than the fourth, fifth, and sixth graders?
  The first step in performing a t-test for independent measures is selecting an *alpha* level, or a maximum acceptable probability for a *Type I* error (i.e., concluding that the second and third graders tend to produce higher frequencies of interjection on the average than the fourth, fifth, and sixth graders when there was no such tendency). A 0.05 alpha level will be used for this test. Since to answer the question it only would be necessary to detect a difference between second and third graders and fourth, fifth, and sixth graders in one direction, the region of rejection for the test will be *one-tailed*.

TABLE A.5.   Table of critical values of *t*.

df	\<span\>Level of significance for one-tailed test\</span\>					
	.10	.05	.025	.01	.005	.0005
	Level of significance for two-tailed test					
	.20	.10	.05	.02	.01	.001
1	3.078	6.314	12.706	31.821	63.657	636.619
2	1.886	2.920	4.303	6.965	9.925	31.598
3	1.638	2.353	3.182	4.541	5.841	12.941
4	1.533	2.132	2.776	3.747	4.604	8.610
5	1.476	2.015	2.571	3.365	4.032	6.859
6	1.440	1.943	2.447	3.143	3.707	5.959
7	1.415	1.895	2.365	2.998	3.499	5.405
8	1.397	1.860	2.306	2.896	3.355	5.041
9	1.383	1.833	2.262	2.821	3.250	4.781
10	1.372	1.812	2.228	2.764	3.169	4.587.
11	1.363	1.796	2.201	2.718	3.106	4.437
12	1.356	1.782	2.179	2.681	3.055	4.318
13	1.350	1.771	2.160	2.650	3.012	4.221
14	1.345	1.761	2.145	2.624	2.977	4.140
15	1.341	1.753	2.131	2.602	2.947	4.073
16	1.337	1.746	2.120	2.583	2.921	4.015
17	1.333	1.740	2.110	2.567	2.898	3.965
18	1.330	1.734	2.101	2.552	2.878	3.922
19	1.328	1.729	2.093	2.539	2.861	3.883
20	1.325	1.725	2.086	2.528	2.845	3.850
21	1.323	1.721	2.080	2.518	2.831	3.819
22	1.321	1.717	2.074	2.508	2.819	3.792
23	1.319	1.714	2.069	2.500	2.807	3.767
24	1.318	1.711	2.064	2.492	2.797	3.745
25	1.316	1.708	2.060	2.485	2.787	3.725
26	1.315	1.706	2.056	2.479	2.779	3.707
27	1.314	1.703	2.052	2.473	2.771	3.690
28	1.313	1.701	2.048	2.467	2.763	3.674
29	1.311	1.699	2.045	2.462	2.756	3.659
30	1.310	1.697	2.042	2.457	2.750	3.646
40	1.303	1.684	2.021	2.423	2.704	3.551
60	1.296	1.671	2.000	2.390	2.660	3.460
120	1.289	1.658	1.980	2.358	2.617	3.373
∞	1.282	1.645	1.960	2.326	2.576	3.291

Adapted from Table III of Fisher and Yates. Statistical Tables for Biological, Agricultural, and Medical Research *(6th edition). Copyright 1974 by Longman Group, Ltd. With permission of Longman Group, Ltd.*

The next step is to compute the value for t. The following values are computed from the interjection frequencies in Table A.1 for each group of children:

2ND AND 3RD GRADE   **4TH, 5TH, AND 6TH GRADE**

$$n_1 = 26 \qquad\qquad n_2 = 30$$
$$\Sigma X_1 = 34.50 \qquad\qquad \Sigma X_2 = 23.21$$
$$\overline{X}_1 = 1.33 \qquad\qquad \overline{X}_2 = 0.77$$
$$\Sigma X_1^2 = 124.02 \qquad\qquad \Sigma X_2^2 = 42.91$$

$$S_1^2 = \frac{\Sigma X_1^2}{N_1} - \overline{X}_1^2 \qquad\qquad S_2^2 = \frac{\Sigma X_2^2}{N_2} - \overline{X}_2^2$$

$$= \frac{124.02}{26} - (1.33)^2 \qquad\qquad = \frac{42.91}{30} - (0.77)^2$$

$$= 4.77 - 1.77 = 3.00 \qquad\qquad = 1.43 - 0.59 = 0.84$$

The value of t here would be:

$$t = \frac{\overline{X}_1 - \overline{X}_2}{\sqrt{\dfrac{n_1 S_1^2 + n_2 S_2^2}{n_1 + n_2 - 2}\left(\dfrac{1}{n_1} + \dfrac{1}{n_2}\right)}}$$

$$= \frac{1.33 - 0.77}{\sqrt{\dfrac{(26)(3.00) + (30)(0.84)}{26 + 30 - 2}\left(\dfrac{1}{26} + \dfrac{1}{30}\right)}}$$

$$= \frac{0.56}{\sqrt{\dfrac{103.2}{54}(0.07)}}$$

$$= \frac{0.56}{\sqrt{0.1337777}} = \frac{0.56}{0.37}$$

$$= 1.51$$

To determine whether this value of t is large enough for the null hypothesis to be rejected, the value of t required for rejection is located in Table A.5. The degrees of freedom (df) here would be 54 (i.e., the number of subjects minus two). The value of t required for rejection at the 0.05 alpha level when $df = 54$ is 1.67. Since the value computed—i.e., 1.51—is smaller than this, the null hypothesis would not be rejected.

ANSWER: The second and third graders did not tend to produce higher frequencies of interjection on the average than the fourth, fifth, and sixth graders (t-test for independent measures; alpha $= 0.05$).

EXERCISE: Determine whether the second and third graders tended to produce
(Number 17) higher frequencies of part-word repetition on the average than the
fourth, fifth, and sixth graders through the use of the *t*-test for independent measures. (The value of *t* you compute should be approximately
1.52.)

3. *t*-Test for the Significance of Pearson Product-Moment Correlation Coefficients

QUESTION: Was there any relationship between the children's interjection frequencies and part-word repetition frequencies during their performances of the spontaneous speech task?

The first step in performing a *t*-test for the significance of the
Pearson product-moment correlation coefficient (*r*) is selecting an *alpha*
level, or a maximum acceptable probability for a *Type I* error (i.e., concluding there was a relationship between the children's interjection
frequencies and part-word repetition frequencies when there was no
such relationship). A 0.05 alpha level will be used for this test. Since to
answer this question it would be necessary to detect both positive and
negative relationships between interjection frequency and part-word
repetition frequency, the region of rejection for the test will be *two-
tailed.*

The next step is to compute the value of *t*. The Pearson product-
moment correlation coefficient for the relationship between interjection frequency and part-word repetition frequency for the 56 children
is −0.02 (see p. 295). The value of *t* here would be:

$$t = \frac{r}{\sqrt{1 - r^2}} \sqrt{N - 2}$$

$$= \frac{-0.02}{\sqrt{1 - (-0.02)^2}} \sqrt{56 - 2}$$

$$= \frac{-0.02}{\sqrt{1 - 0.0004}} \sqrt{54}$$

$$= \frac{-0.02}{0.9998} 7.3485 = (-0.0200)(7.3485)$$

$$= -0.1470$$

To determine whether this value of *t* is large enough for the null hypothesis to be rejected, the value of *t* required for rejection is located
in Table A.5. The degrees of freedom (*df*) here would be 54 (i.e., the
number of subjects minus two). The value of *t* required for rejection
at the 0.05 alpha level, when *df* = 54 and the region of rejection is
two-tailed, is 2.00. Since the value computed, i.e., −0.147, is smaller
than this, the null hypothesis would not be rejected.

ANSWER: There was no relationship between the children's interjection frequencies and part-word repetition frequencies during their performances of

the spontaneous speech task (*t*-test for the significance of a Pearson product-moment correlation coefficient; alpha = 0.05).

EXERCISE: Determine whether there was any relationship between the children's
(Number 18) word repetition frequencies and revision-incomplete phrase frequencies during their performances of the spontaneous speech task through the use of the *t*-test for the significance of Pearson product-moment correlation coefficients. (The value of *t* you compute should be approximately 3.02.)

4. One-Way Analysis of Variance (*F*-Test) for Dependent Measures

QUESTION: Did the second graders on the average tend to produce higher frequencies of some of the four disfluency types (i.e., interjection, part-word repetition, word repetition, and revision-incomplete phrase) than of others?

The first step in performing a one-way analysis of variance for dependent measures (*F*) is selecting an *alpha* level, or a maximum acceptable probability for a *Type I* error (i.e., concluding there was a tendency for the second graders on the average to produce higher frequencies of some of the four disfluency types than of others when there was no such tendency). A 0.05 alpha level will be used for this test.

The next step is to compute the value of *F*. The sum of each second grader's four disfluency frequencies (*T*) and the square of the sum of his four disfluency frequencies divided by the number of disfluency frequencies summed ($T^2/4$) based on Table A.1 are as follows:

Subject	T_r	$T_r^2/4$
1	4.32	4.666
2	9.57	22.896
3	6.54	10.693
4	3.63	3.294
5	4.40	4.840
6	2.44	1.488
7	4.49	5.040
8	5.69	8.094
9	8.09	16.362
10	8.99	20.205
11	13.99	48.930
12	4.68	5.476
13	6.73	11.323
14	2.52	1.588
15	4.86	5.905
	$T = 90.94$	$170.800 = \Sigma\ T_r^2/4$

The following computations are then made from the frequencies in each column—i.e., the disfluency frequencies of each of the four types produced by the 15 second graders.

Measure	I	PW	W	R-IP	
T_c	19.27	12.28	12.63	46.76	$T = 90.34$
$\overline{X}_c$	1.285	0.819	0.842	3.117	
$T_c^2 /15$	24.756	10.053	10.634	145.766	$\Sigma\, T_c^2 /15 = 191.209$
$\Sigma\, X^2$	87.164	17.100	15.680	183.938	$\Sigma\Sigma\, X^2 = 303.782$

Next, *four* sum of square (SS) values are computed from these row and column data analyses. The first is the sum of squares (SS) for columns (*c*), or disfluency types.

$$SS_c = \frac{\Sigma\, T_c^2}{r} - \frac{T^2}{cr}$$

$$= 191.209 - \frac{(90.94)^2}{(4)(15)}$$

$$= 191.209 - 137.835 = 53.374$$

The second is the sum of squares (SS) for rows (*r*), or subjects.

$$SS_r = \frac{\Sigma\, T_r^2}{c} - \frac{T^2}{cr}$$

$$= 170.800 - \frac{(90.94)^2}{(4)(15)}$$

$$= 170.800 - 137.835 = 32.965$$

The third is the total (*T*) sum of squares.

$$SS_T = \Sigma\Sigma\, X^2 - \frac{T^2}{cr} = 303.782 - \frac{(90.94)^2}{(4)(15)}$$

$$= 303.782 - 137.835 = 165.947$$

The fourth is the residual sum of squares, labeled SS_{cr}, which is assumed to represent random measurement error.

$$SS_{cr} = SS_T - SS_c - SS_r = 165.947 - 53.374 - 32.965$$
$$= 79.608$$

The value of *F* can be computed by means of the following formula:

$$F = \frac{SS_c/c - 1}{SS_{cr}/(c - 1)(r - 1)}$$

where $c - 1$ is the degrees of freedom for SS_c and $(c - 1)(r - 1)$ is the degrees of freedom for SS_{cr}. The first is df_1 and the second df_2 (see Table A.6).

TABLE A.6.   Percent points in the distribution of F.[a]

df_2	df_1	1	2	3	4	5	6	8	12	24	∞
1	0.1%	405284	500000	540379	562500	576405	585937	598144	610667	623497	636619
	0.5%	16211	20000	21615	22500	23056	23437	23925	24426	24940	25465
	1%	4052	4999	5403	5625	5764	5859	5981	6106	6234	6366
	2.5%	647.79	799.50	864.16	899.58	921.85	937.11	956.66	976.71	997.25	1018.30
	5%	161.45	199.50	215.71	224.58	230.16	233.99	238.88	243.91	249.05	254.32
	10%	39.86	49.50	53.59	55.83	57.24	58.20	59.44	60.70	62.00	63.33
	20%	9.47	12.00	13.06	13.73	14.01	14.26	14.59	14.90	15.24	15.58
2	0.1	998.5	999.0	999.2	999.2	999.3	999.3	999.4	999.4	999.5	999.5
	0.5	198.50	199.00	199.17	199.25	199.30	199.33	199.37	199.42	199.46	199.51
	1	98.49	99.00	99.17	99.25	99.30	99.33	99.36	99.42	99.46	99.50
	2.5	38.51	39.00	39.17	39.25	39.30	39.33	39.37	39.42	39.46	39.50
	5	18.51	19.00	19.16	19.25	19.30	19.33	19.37	19.41	19.45	19.50
	10	8.53	9.00	9.16	9.24	9.29	9.33	9.37	9.41	9.45	9.49
	20	3.56	4.00	4.16	4.24	4.28	4.32	4.36	4.40	4.44	4.48
3	0.1	167.5	148.5	141.1	137.1	134.6	132.8	130.6	128.3	125.9	123.5
	0.5	55.55	49.80	47.47	46.20	45.39	44.84	44.13	43.39	42.62	41.83
	1	34.12	30.81	29.46	28.71	28.24	27.91	27.49	27.05	26.60	26.12
	2.5	17.44	16.04	15.44	15.10	14.89	14.74	14.54	14.34	14.12	13.90
	5	10.13	9.55	9.28	9.12	9.01	8.94	8.84	8.74	8.64	8.53
	10	5.54	5.46	5.39	5.34	5.31	5.28	5.25	5.22	5.18	5.13
	20	2.68	2.89	2.94	2.96	2.97	2.97	2.98	2.98	2.98	2.98
4	0.1	74.14	61.25	56.18	53.44	51.71	50.53	49.00	47.41	45.77	44.05
	0.5	31.33	26.28	24.26	23.16	22.46	21.98	21.35	20.71	20.03	19.33
	1	21.20	18.00	16.69	15.98	15.52	15.21	14.80	14.37	13.93	13.46
	2.5	12.22	10.65	9.98	9.60	9.36	9.20	8.98	8.75	8.51	8.26
	5	7.71	6.94	6.59	6.39	6.26	6.16	6.04	5.91	5.77	5.63
	10	4.54	4.32	4.19	4.11	4.05	4.01	3.95	3.90	3.83	3.76
	20	2.35	2.47	2.48	2.48	2.48	2.47	2.47	2.46	2.44	2.43
5	0.1	47.04	36.61	33.20	31.09	29.75	28.84	27.64	26.42	25.14	23.78
	0.5	22.79	18.31	16.53	15.56	14.94	14.51	13.96	13.38	12.78	12.14
	1	16.26	13.27	12.06	11.39	10.97	10.67	10.29	9.89	9.47	9.02
	2.5	10.01	8.43	7.76	7.39	7.15	6.98	6.76	6.52	6.28	6.02
	5	6.61	5.79	5.41	5.19	5.05	4.95	4.82	4.68	4.53	4.36
	10	4.06	3.78	3.62	3.52	3.45	3.40	3.34	3.27	3.19	3.10
	20	2.18	2.26	2.25	2.24	2.23	2.22	2.20	2.18	2.16	2.13
6	0.1	35.51	27.00	23.70	21.90	20.81	20.03	19.03	17.99	16.89	15.75
	0.5	18.64	14.54	12.92	12.03	11.46	11.07	10.57	10.03	9.47	8.88
	1	13.74	10.92	9.78	9.15	8.75	8.47	8.10	7.72	7.31	6.88
	2.5	8.81	7.26	6.60	6.23	5.99	5.82	5.60	5.37	5.12	4.85
	5	5.99	5.14	4.76	4.53	4.39	4.28	4.15	4.00	3.84	3.67
	10	3.78	3.46	3.29	3.18	3.11	3.05	2.98	2.90	2.82	2.72
	20	2.07	2.13	2.11	2.09	2.08	2.06	2.04	2.02	1.99	1.95
7	0.1	29.22	21.69	18.77	17.19	16.21	15.52	14.63	13.71	12.73	11.69
	0.5	16.24	12.40	10.88	10.05	9.52	9.16	8.68	8.18	7.65	7.08
	1	12.25	9.55	8.45	7.85	7.46	7.19	6.84	6.47	6.07	5.65
	2.5	8.07	6.54	5.89	5.52	5.29	5.12	4.90	4.67	4.42	4.14
	5	5.59	4.74	4.35	4.12	3.97	3.87	3.73	3.57	3.41	3.23
	10	3.59	3.26	3.07	2.96	2.88	2.83	2.75	2.67	2.58	2.47
	20	2.00	2.04	2.02	1.99	1.97	1.96	1.93	1.91	1.87	1.83
8	0.1	25.42	18.49	15.83	14.39	13.49	12.86	12.04	11.19	10.30	9.34
	0.5	14.69	11.04	9.60	8.81	8.30	7.95	7.50	7.01	6.50	5.95
	1	11.26	8.65	7.59	7.01	6.63	6.37	6.03	5.67	5.28	4.86
	2.5	7.57	6.06	5.42	5.05	4.82	4.65	4.43	4.20	3.95	3.6⁻
	5	5.32	4.46	4.07	3.84	3.69	3.58	3.44	3.28	3.12	2 93
	10	3.46	3.11	2.92	2.81	2.73	2.67	2.59	2.50	2.40	2.2⁻
	20	1.95	1.98	1.95	1.92	1.90	1.88	1.86	1.83	1.79	1.74
9	0.1	22.86	16.39	13.90	12.56	11.71	11.13	10.37	9.57	8.72	7.81
	0.5	13.61	10.11	8.72	7.96	7.47	7.13	6.69	6.23	5.73	5.19
	1	10.56	8.02	6.99	6.42	6.03	5.80	5.47	5.11	4.73	4.31
	2.5	7.21	5.71	5.08	4.72	4.48	4.32	4.10	3.87	3.61	3.33
	5	5.12	4.26	3.86	3.63	3.48	3.37	3.23	3.07	2.90	2.71
	10	3.36	3.01	2.81	2.69	2.61	2.55	2.47	2.38	2.28	2.16
	20	1.91	1.94	1.90	1.87	1.85	1.83	1.80	1.76	1.72	1.67

[a]*Adapted from Table V of Fisher and Yates:* Statistical Tables for Biological, Agricultural, and Medical Research *(6th edition). Copyright 1974 by Longman Group, Ltd. With permission of Longman Group, Ltd. The 0.5% and 2.5% points are reprinted by permission of the Biometrika Trustees from* Biometrika, *volume 33 (April, 1943), pp. 73–78.*

(Continued)

TABLE A.6. Continued

df₁ df₂		1	2	3	4	5	6	8	12	24	∞
10	0.1%	21.04	14.91	12.55	11.28	10.48	9.92	9.20	8.45	7.64	6.76
	0.5%	12.83	9.43	8.08	7.34	6.87	6.54	6.12	5.66	5.17	4.64
	1 %	10.04	7.56	6.55	5.99	5.64	5.39	5.06	4.71	4.33	3.91
	2.5%	6.94	5.46	4.83	4.47	4.24	4.07	3.85	3.62	3.37	3.08
	5 %	4.96	4.10	3.71	3.48	3.33	3.22	3.07	2.91	2.74	2.54
	10 %	3.28	2.92	2.73	2.61	2.52	2.46	2.38	2.28	2.18	2.06
	20 %	1.88	1.90	1.86	1.83	1.80	1.78	1.75	1.72	1.67	1.62
11	0.1	19.69	13.81	11.56	10.35	9.58	9.05	8.35	7.63	6.85	6.00
	0.5	12.23	8.91	7.60	6.88	6.42	6.10	5.68	5.24	4.76	4.23
	1	9.65	7.20	6.22	5.67	5.32	5.07	4.74	4.40	4.02	3.60
	2.5	6.72	5.26	4.63	4.28	4.04	3.88	3.66	3.43	3.17	2.88
	5	4.84	3.98	3.59	3.36	3.20	3.09	2.95	2.79	2.61	2.40
	10	3.23	2.86	2.66	2.54	2.45	2.39	2.30	2.21	2.10	1.97
	20	1.86	1.87	1.83	1.80	1.77	1.75	1.72	1.68	1.63	1.57
12	0.1	18.64	12.97	10.80	9.63	8.89	8.38	7.71	7.00	6.25	5.42
	0.5	11.75	8.51	7.23	6.52	6.07	5.76	5.35	4.91	4.43	3.90
	1	9.33	6.93	5.95	5.41	5.06	4.82	4.50	4.16	3.78	3.36
	2.5	6.55	5.10	4.47	4.12	3.89	3.73	3.51	3.28	3.02	2.72
	5	4.75	3.88	3.49	3.26	3.11	3.00	2.85	2.69	2.50	2.30
	10	3.18	2.81	2.61	2.48	2.39	2.33	2.24	2.15	2.04	1.90
	20	1.84	1.85	1.80	1.77	1.74	1.72	1.69	1.65	1.60	1.54
13	0.1	17.81	12.31	10.21	9.07	8.35	7.86	7.21	6.52	5.78	4.97
	0.5	11.37	8.19	6.93	6.23	5.79	5.48	5.08	4.64	4.17	3.65
	1	9.07	6.70	5.74	5.20	4.86	4.62	4.30	3.96	3.59	3.16
	2.5	6.41	4.97	4.35	4.00	3.77	3.60	3.39	3.15	2.89	2.60
	5	4.67	3.80	3.41	3.18	3.02	2.92	2.77	2.60	2.42	2.21
	10	3.14	2.76	2.56	2.43	2.35	2.28	2.20	2.10	1.98	1.85
	20	1.82	1.83	1.78	1.75	1.72	1.69	1.66	1.62	1.57	1.51
14	0.1	17.14	11.78	9.73	8.62	7.92	7.43	6.80	6.13	5.41	4.60
	0.5	11.06	7.92	6.68	6.00	5.56	5.26	4.86	4.43	3.96	3.44
	1	8.86	6.51	5.56	5.03	4.69	4.46	4.14	3.80	3.43	3.00
	2.5	6.30	4.86	4.24	3.89	3.66	3.50	3.29	3.05	2.79	2.49
	5	4.60	3.74	3.34	3.11	2.96	2.85	2.70	2.53	2.35	2.13
	10	3.10	2.73	2.52	2.39	2.31	2.24	2.15	2.05	1.94	1.80
	20	1.81	1.81	1.76	1.73	1.70	1.67	1.64	1.60	1.55	1.48
15	0.1	16.59	11.34	9.34	8.25	7.57	7.09	6.47	5.81	5.10	4.31
	0.5	10.80	7.70	6.48	5.80	5.37	5.07	4.67	4.25	3.79	3.26
	1	8.68	6.36	5.42	4.89	4.56	4.32	4.00	3.67	3.29	2.87
	2.5	6.20	4.77	4.15	3.80	3.58	3.41	3.20	2.96	2.70	2.40
	5	4.54	3.68	3.29	3.06	2.90	2.79	2.64	2.48	2.29	2.07
	10	3.07	2.70	2.49	2.36	2.27	2.21	2.12	2.02	1.90	1.76
	20	1.80	1.79	1.75	1.71	1.68	1.66	1.62	1.58	1.53	1.46
16	0.1	16.12	10.97	9.00	7.94	7.27	6.81	6.19	5.55	4.85	4.06
	0.5	10.58	7.51	6.30	5.64	5.21	4.91	4.52	4.10	3.64	3.11
	1	8.53	6.23	5.29	4.77	4.44	4.20	3.89	3.55	3.18	2.75
	2.5	6.12	4.69	4.08	3.73	3.50	3.34	3.12	2.89	2.63	2.32
	5	4.49	3.63	3.24	3.01	2.85	2.74	2.59	2.42	2.24	2.01
	10	3.05	2.67	2.46	2.33	2.24	2.18	2.09	1.99	1.87	1.72
	20	1.79	1.78	1.74	1.70	1.67	1.64	1.61	1.56	1.51	1.43
17	0.1	15.72	10.66	8.73	7.68	7.02	6.56	5.96	5.32	4.63	3.85
	0.5	10.38	7.35	6.16	5.50	5.07	4.78	4.39	3.97	3.51	2.98
	1	8.40	6.11	5.18	4.67	4.34	4.10	3.79	3.45	3.08	2.65
	2.5	6.04	4.62	4.01	3.66	3.44	3.28	3.06	2.82	2.56	2.25
	5	4.45	3.59	3.20	2.96	2.81	2.70	2.55	2.38	2.19	1.96
	10	3.03	2.64	2.44	2.31	2.22	2.15	2.06	1.96	1.84	1.69
	20	1.78	1.77	1.72	1.68	1.65	1.63	1.59	1.55	1.49	1.42
18	0.1	15.38	10.39	8.49	7.46	6.81	6.35	5.76	5.13	4.45	3.67
	0.5	10.22	7.21	6.03	5.37	4.96	4.66	4.28	3.86	3.40	2.87
	1	8.28	6.01	5.09	4.58	4.25	4.01	3.71	3.37	3.00	2.57
	2.5	5.98	4.56	3.95	3.61	3.38	3.22	3.01	2.77	2.50	2.19
	5	4.41	3.55	3.16	2.93	2.77	2.66	2.51	2.34	2.15	1.92
	10	3.01	2.62	2.42	2.29	2.20	2.13	2.04	1.93	1.81	1.66
	20	1.77	1.76	1.71	1.67	1.64	1.62	1.58	1.53	1.48	1.40
19	0.1	15.08	10.16	8.28	7.26	6.61	6.18	5.59	4.97	4.29	3.52
	0.5	10.07	7.09	5.92	5.27	4.85	4.56	4.18	3.76	3.31	2.78
	1	8.18	5.93	5.01	4.50	4.17	3.94	3.63	3.30	2.92	2.49
	2.5	5.92	4.51	3.90	3.56	3.33	3.17	2.96	2.72	2.45	2.13
	5	4.38	3.52	3.13	2.90	2.74	2.63	2.48	2.31	2.11	1.88
	10	2.99	2.61	2.40	2.27	2.18	2.11	2.02	1.91	1.79	1.63
	20	1.76	1.75	1.70	1.66	1.63	1.61	1.57	1.52	1.46	1.39

(Continued)

TABLE A.6. Continued

df_2		df_1 1	2	3	4	5	6	8	12	24	∞
20	0.1%	14.82	9.95	8.10	7.10	6.46	6.02	5.44	4.82	4.15	3.38
	0.5%	9.94	6.99	5.82	5.17	4.76	4.47	4.09	3.68	3.22	2.69
	1 %	8.10	5.85	4.94	4.43	4.10	3.87	3.56	3.23	2.86	2.42
	2.5%	5.87	4.46	3.86	3.51	3.29	3.13	2.91	2.68	2.41	2.09
	5 %	4.35	3.49	3.10	2.87	2.71	2.60	2.45	2.28	2.08	1.84
	10 %	2.97	2.59	2.38	2.25	2.16	2.09	2.00	1.89	1.77	1.61
	20 %	1.76	1.75	1.70	1.65	1.62	1.60	1.56	1.51	1.45	1.37
21	0.1	14.59	9.77	7.94	6.95	6.32	5.88	5.31	4.70	4.03	3.26
	0.5	9.83	6.89	5.73	5.09	4.68	4.39	4.01	3.60	3.15	2.61
	1	8.02	5.78	4.87	4.37	4.04	3.81	3.51	3.17	2.80	2.36
	2.5	5.83	4.42	3.82	3.48	3.25	3.09	2.87	2.64	2.37	2.04
	5	4.32	3.47	3.07	2.84	2.68	2.57	2.42	2.25	2.05	1.81
	10	2.96	2.57	2.36	2.23	2.14	2.08	1.98	1.88	1.75	1.59
	20	1.75	1.74	1.69	1.65	1.61	1.59	1.55	1.50	1.44	1.36
22	0.1	14.38	9.61	7.80	6.81	6.19	5.76	5.19	4.58	3.92	3.15
	0.5	9.73	6.81	5.65	5.02	4.61	4.32	3.94	3.54	3.08	2.55
	1	7.94	5.72	4.82	4.31	3.99	3.76	3.45	3.12	2.75	2.31
	2.5	5.79	4.38	3.78	3.44	3.22	3.05	2.84	2.60	2.33	2.00
	5	4.30	3.44	3.05	2.82	2.66	2.55	2.40	2.23	2.03	1.78
	10	2.95	2.56	2.35	2.22	2.13	2.06	1.97	1.86	1.73	1.57
	20	1.75	1.73	1.68	1.64	1.61	1.58	1.54	1.49	1.43	1.35
23	0.1	14.19	9.47	7.67	6.69	6.08	5.65	5.09	4.48	3.82	3.05
	0.5	9.63	6.73	5.58	4.95	4.54	4.26	3.88	3.47	3.02	2.48
	1	7.88	5.66	4.76	4.26	3.94	3.71	3.41	3.07	2.70	2.26
	2.5	5.75	4.35	3.75	3.41	3.18	3.02	2.81	2.57	2.30	1.97
	5	4.28	3.42	3.03	2.80	2.64	2.53	2.38	2.20	2.00	1.76
	10	2.94	2.55	2.34	2.21	2.11	2.05	1.95	1.84	1.72	1.55
	20	1.74	1.73	1.68	1.63	1.60	1.57	1.53	1.49	1.42	1.34
24	0.1	14.03	9.34	7.55	6.59	5.98	5.55	4.99	4.39	3.74	2.97
	0.5	9.55	6.66	5.52	4.89	4.49	4.20	3.83	3.42	2.97	2.43
	1	7.82	5.61	4.72	4.22	3.90	3.67	3.36	3.03	2.66	2.21
	2.5	5.72	4.32	3.72	3.38	3.15	2.99	2.78	2.54	2.27	1.94
	5	4.26	3.40	3.01	2.78	2.62	2.51	2.36	2.18	1.98	1.73
	10	2.93	2.54	2.33	2.19	2.10	2.04	1.94	1.83	1.70	1.53
	20	1.74	1.72	1.67	1.63	1.59	1.57	1.53	1.48	1.42	1.33
25	0.1	13.88	9.22	7.45	6.49	5.88	5.46	4.91	4.31	3.66	2.89
	0.5	9.48	6.60	5.46	4.84	4.43	4.15	3.78	3.37	2.92	2.38
	1	7.77	5.57	4.68	4.18	3.86	3.63	3.32	2.99	2.62	2.17
	2.5	5.69	4.29	3.69	3.35	3.13	2.97	2.75	2.51	2.24	1.91
	5	4.24	3.38	2.99	2.76	2.60	2.49	2.34	2.16	1.96	1.71
	10	2.92	2.53	2.32	2.18	2.09	2.02	1.93	1.82	1.69	1.52
	20	1.73	1.72	1.66	1.62	1.59	1.56	1.52	1.47	1.41	1.32
26	0.1	13.74	9.12	7.36	6.41	5.80	5.38	4.83	4.24	3.59	2.82
	0.5	9.41	6.54	5.41	4.79	4.38	4.10	3.73	3.33	2.87	2.33
	1	7.72	5.53	4.64	4.14	3.82	3.59	3.29	2.96	2.58	2.13
	2.5	5.66	4.27	3.67	3.33	3.10	2.94	2.73	2.49	2.22	1.88
	5	4.22	3.37	2.98	2.74	2.59	2.47	2.32	2.15	1.95	1.69
	10	2.91	2.52	2.31	2.17	2.08	2.01	1.92	1.81	1.68	1.50
	20	1.73	1.71	1.66	1.62	1.58	1.56	1.52	1.47	1.40	1.31
27	0.1	13.61	9.02	7.27	6.33	5.73	5.31	4.76	4.17	3.52	2.75
	0.5	9.34	6.49	5.36	4.74	4.34	4.06	3.69	3.28	2.83	2.29
	1	7.68	5.49	4.60	4.11	3.78	3.56	3.26	2.93	2.55	2.10
	2.5	5.63	4.24	3.65	3.31	3.08	2.92	2.71	2.47	2.19	1.85
	5	4.21	3.35	2.96	2.73	2.57	2.46	2.30	2.13	1.93	1.67
	10	2.90	2.51	2.30	2.17	2.07	2.00	1.91	1.80	1.67	1.49
	20	1.73	1.71	1.66	1.61	1.58	1.55	1.51	1.46	1.40	1.30
28	0.1	13.50	8.93	7.19	6.25	5.66	5.24	4.69	4.11	3.46	2.70
	0.5	9.28	6.44	5.32	4.70	4.30	4.02	3.65	3.25	2.79	2.25
	1	7.64	5.45	4.57	4.07	3.75	3.53	3.23	2.90	2.52	2.06
	2.5	5.61	4.22	3.63	3.29	3.06	2.90	2.69	2.45	2.17	1.83
	5	4.20	3.34	2.95	2.71	2.56	2.44	2.29	2.12	1.91	1.65
	10	2.89	2.50	2.29	2.16	2.06	2.00	1.90	1.79	1.66	1.48
	20	1.72	1.71	1.65	1.61	1.57	1.55	1.51	1.46	1.39	1.30
29	0.1	13.39	8.85	7.12	6.19	5.59	5.18	4.64	4.05	3.41	2.64
	0.5	9.23	6.40	5.28	4.66	4.26	3.98	3.61	3.21	2.76	2.21
	1	7.60	5.42	4.54	4.04	3.73	3.50	3.20	2.87	2.49	2.03
	2.5	5.59	4.20	3.61	3.27	3.04	2.88	2.67	2.43	2.15	1.81
	5	4.18	3.33	2.93	2.70	2.54	2.43	2.28	2.10	1.90	1.64
	10	2.89	2.50	2.28	2.15	2.06	1.99	1.89	1.78	1.65	1.47
	20	1.72	1.70	1.65	1.60	1.57	1.54	1.50	1.45	1.39	1.29

(Continued)

TABLE A.6. Continued

df₂ \ df₁		1	2	3	4	5	6	8	12	24	∞
30	0.1%	13.29	8.77	7.05	6.12	5.53	5.12	4.58	4.00	3.36	2.59
	0.5%	9.18	6.35	5.24	4.62	4.23	3.95	3.58	3.18	2.73	2.18
	1 %	7.56	5.39	4.51	4.02	3.70	3.47	3.17	2.84	2.47	2.01
	2.5%	5.57	4.18	3.59	3.25	3.03	2.87	2.65	2.41	2.14	1.79
	5 %	4.17	3.32	2.92	2.69	2.53	2.42	2.27	2.09	1.89	1.62
	10 %	2.88	2.49	2.28	2.14	2.05	1.98	1.88	1.77	1.64	1.46
	20 %	1.72	1.70	1.64	1.60	1.57	1.54	1.50	1.45	1.38	1.28
40	0.1	12.61	8.25	6.60	5.70	5.13	4.73	4.21	3.64	3.01	2.23
	0.5	8.83	6.07	4.98	4.37	3.99	3.71	3.35	2.95	2.50	1.93
	1	7.31	5.18	4.31	3.83	3.51	3.29	2.99	2.66	2.29	1.80
	2.5	5.42	4.05	3.46	3.13	2.90	2.74	2.53	2.29	2.01	1.64
	5	4.08	3.23	2.84	2.61	2.45	2.34	2.18	2.00	1.79	1.51
	10	2.84	2.44	2.23	2.09	2.00	1.93	1.83	1.71	1.57	1.38
	20	1.70	1.68	1.62	1.57	1.54	1.51	1.47	1.41	1.34	1.24
60	0.1	11.97	7.76	6.17	5.31	4.76	4.37	3.87	3.31	2.69	1.90
	0.5	8.49	5.80	4.73	4.14	3.76	3.49	3.13	2.74	2.29	1.69
	1	7.08	4.98	4.13	3.65	3.34	3.12	2.82	2.50	2.12	1.60
	2.5	5.29	3.93	3.34	3.01	2.79	2.63	2.41	2.17	1.88	1.48
	5	4.00	3.15	2.76	2.52	2.37	2.25	2.10	1.92	1.70	1.39
	10	2.79	2.39	2.18	2.04	1.95	1.87	1.77	1.66	1.51	1.29
	20	1.68	1.65	1.59	1.55	1.51	1.48	1.44	1.38	1.31	1.18
120	0.1	11.38	7.31	5.79	4.95	4.42	4.04	3.55	3.02	2.40	1.56
	0.5	8.18	5.54	4.50	3.92	3.55	3.28	2.93	2.54	2.09	1.43
	1	6.85	4.79	3.95	3.48	3.17	2.96	2.66	2.34	1.95	1.38
	2.5	5.15	3.80	3.23	2.89	2.67	2.52	2.30	2.05	1.76	1.31
	5	3.92	3.07	2.68	2.45	2.29	2.17	2.02	1.83	1.61	1.25
	10	2.75	2.35	2.13	1.99	1.90	1.82	1.72	1.60	1.45	1.19
	20	1.66	1.63	1.57	1.52	1.48	1.45	1.41	1.35	1.27	1.12
∞	0.1	10.83	6.91	5.42	4.62	4.10	3.74	3.27	2.74	2.13	1.00
	0.5	7.88	5.30	4.28	3.72	3.35	3.09	2.74	2.36	1.90	1.00
	1	6.64	4.60	3.78	3.32	3.02	2.80	2.51	2.18	1.79	1.00
	2.5	5.02	3.69	3.12	2.79	2.57	2.41	2.19	1.94	1.64	1.00
	5	3.84	2.99	2.60	2.37	2.21	2.09	1.94	1.75	1.52	1.00
	10	2.71	2.30	2.08	1.94	1.85	1.77	1.67	1.55	1.38	1.00
	20	1.64	1.61	1.55	1.50	1.46	1.43	1.38	1.32	1.23	1.00

The value of F here is:

$$F = \frac{53.374/3}{79.608/42} = \frac{17.791}{1.895} = 9.39$$

To determine whether this value of F is large enough for the null hypothesis to be rejected, the value of F required for rejection is located in Table A.6. There are two degrees of freedom: df_1 would be 3 (i.e., the number of columns minus one) and df_2 would be 42 (i.e., the number of columns minus one times the number of rows minus one). The value of F required for rejection at the 0.05 alpha level when $df_1 = 3$ and $df_2 = 42$ is 2.84. Since the value computed—i.e., 9.39—exceeds this value, the null hypothesis would be rejected.

ANSWER: The second graders on the average tended to produce higher frequencies of some of the disfluency types than of others (F-test; alpha = 0.05).

REMARK: This example and the one that follows illustrate the simplest possible applications of analysis of variance. Other applications are described in a number of psychology and education statistical texts. Most can be computed with the Minitab Statistical Software described at the end of this appendix.

EXERCISE: Determine whether the third graders tended to produce higher fre-
(Number 19)   quencies of some of the four disfluency types than of others through
              the use of analysis of variance. (The value of F you compute should
              be approximately 7.77.)

5. One-Way Analysis of Variance (F-Test) for Independent Measures

QUESTION: Was there a tendency for the amount of part-word repetition produced
              by the children to vary as a function of grade level?
                  The first step in performing a one-way analysis of variance for
              independent measures (F) is selecting an *alpha* level, or maximum ac-
              ceptable probability for a *Type I* error (i.e., concluding there was a tend-
              ency for the amount of part-word repetition produced by the children
              to vary as a function of grade level when there was no such tendency).
              A 0.05 alpha level will be used for this test.
                  The next step is to compute the value of F. The following com-
              putations are made from the part-word repetition frequencies of the
              children at each grade level (see Table A.1).

Measure	2nd Grade	3rd Grade	4th Grade	5th Grade	6th Grade	
n_c	15	11	9	11	10	$N = 56$
T_c	12.28	13.70	9.84	6.82	4.11	$T = 46.75$
$\bar{X}_c$	0.819	1.245	1.093	0.620	0.411	
T_c^2/n_c	10.053	17.063	10.758	4.228	1.689	$\Sigma T_c^2/n_c = 43.791$
ΣX_c^2	17.100	30.695	14.947	6.238	2.700	$\Sigma\Sigma X^2 = 71.680$

Next, three sum square (SS) values are computed from these column
data analyses. The first is the sum of squares (SS) for columns (c) or
grade levels.

$$SS_c = \frac{\Sigma T_c^2}{n_c} - \frac{T^2}{N}$$

$$= 43.791 - \frac{(46.75)^2}{56}$$

$$= 43.791 - 39.028$$

$$= 4.763$$

The second is the total (T) sum of squares.

$$SS_T = \Sigma\Sigma X^2 - \frac{T^2}{N}$$

$$= 71.680 - \frac{(46.75)^2}{56}$$

$$= 71.680 - 39.028$$

$$= 32.652$$

The third is the within group (w), or residual, sum of squares, which is assumed to represent random measurement error.

$$SS_w = SS_T - SS_c = 32.652 - 4.763 = 27.889$$

The value of F can be computed by means of the following formula:

$$F = \frac{SS_c/c - 1}{SS_w/N - c}$$

where $c - 1$ is the degrees of freedom for SS_c and $N - c$ is the degrees of freedom for SS_w. The first is df_1 and the second df_2 (see p. 212). The value of F here is:

$$F = \frac{4.763/5 - 1}{27.889/56 - 5}$$

$$= \frac{1.191}{0.547}$$

$$= 2.18$$

To determine whether this value of F is large enough for the null hypothesis to be rejected, the value of F required for rejection is located in Table A.6. There are two degrees of freedom: df_1 would be 4 (i.e., the number of columns minus one), and df_2 would be 51 (i.e., the number of subjects minus the number of columns). The value of F required for rejection at the 0.05 alpha level, when $df_1 = 4$ and $df_2 = 51$, is 2.56. Since the value computed—i.e., 2.18—is smaller than this value, the null hypothesis would not be rejected.

ANSWER: There did not appear to be a tendency for the amount of part-word repetition produced by the children to vary as a function of grade level (F-test; alpha $= 0.05$).

EXERCISE: Determine whether there was a tendency for the amount of word repe-
(Number 20) tition produced by the children to vary as a function of grade level through the use of analysis of variance. (The value of F you compute should be approximately 2.32.)

CONFIDENCE INTERVAL ESTIMATION

A. Mean

QUESTION: Within what range is the mean interjection frequency of the *population* from which the children were selected (i.e., second- through sixth-grade nonstutterers) most likely to fall?

To answer this question, a 95 *percent confidence interval* will be computed. Theoretically, the limits of this interval define a range within which we can be 95 percent certain to find the mean interjection frequency for the *population* from which the sample was drawn. This 95 percent figure, however, should be regarded as only approximate, since certain assumptions underlying the computational procedure may not have been met (see Chapter 10).

The upper $(\bar{\mu})$ and lower $(\underline{\mu})$ limits of the confidence interval can be computed by means of the following formulas:

$$\bar{\mu} = \overline{X} + \frac{SD}{\sqrt{N-1}}(1.96)$$

$$\underline{\mu} = \overline{X} - \frac{SD}{\sqrt{N-1}}(1.96)$$

where

$\overline{X}$ = the mean frequency for the sample = 1.03 (see p. 296)
SD = the standard deviation for the sample = 1.39 (see p. 300)
N = the number of subjects = 56
1.96 = a constant for 95 percent confidence intervals

The *mean* value that would represent the *upper limit* of the confidence interval would be:

$$\bar{\mu} = 1.03 + \frac{1.39}{\sqrt{56-1}}(1.96)$$

$$= 1.03 + (0.187)(1.96)$$
$$= 1.40$$

The *mean* value that would represent the *lower limit* of the confidence interval would be:

$$\underline{\mu} = 1.03 - \frac{1.39}{\sqrt{56-1}}(1.96)$$

$$= 1.03 - (0.187)(1.96)$$

$$= 0.66$$

ANSWER: The mean interjection frequency of the population from which the children were selected is *approximately* 95 percent certain to fall between 0.66 and 1.40.

REMARK: The width of the confidence interval can be changed by substituting a different constant for 1.96. For a 99 percent confidence interval, for example, 2.58 would be used as the constant.

EXERCISE: Compute a 95 percent confidence interval for the mean part-word rep-
(Number 21) etition frequency of the population from which the children were se-

Selected Descriptive and Inferential Statistics

lected (see p. 296 and p. 300 for the sample mean and standard deviation). (The upper limit of the confidence interval you compute should be approximately 1.03, and the lower limit should be approximately 0.63.)

B. Median

QUESTION: Within what range is the median interjection frequency of the *population* from which the children were selected (i.e., second- through sixth-grade nonstutterers) most likely to fall?

To answer this question, a 95 *percent confidence interval* will be computed. Theoretically, the limits of this interval define a range within which we can be 95 percent certain of finding the median interjection frequency for the population from which the sample was drawn. This 95 percent figure, however, should be regarded as only approximate since certain assumptions underlying the computational procedure may not have been met (see Chapter 10).

The upper ($\bar{\xi}$) and lower ($\underline{\xi}$) limits of the confidence interval can be computed by means of the following formulas:

$$\bar{\xi} = \text{mdn} + \frac{1.25 \ SD}{\sqrt{N-1}}(1.96)$$

$$\underline{\xi} = \text{mdn} - \frac{1.25 \ SD}{\sqrt{N-1}}(1.96)$$

where

mdn = the median frequency for the sample = 0.51 (see p. 297)
SD = the standard deviation for the sample = 1.39 (see p. 300)
N = the number of subjects = 56
1.96 = a constant for 95 percent confidence intervals
1.25 = a constant

The median value that would represent the *upper boundary of* the confidence interval would be:

$$\bar{\xi} = 0.51 + \frac{(1.25)(1.39)}{\sqrt{56-1}}(1.96)$$

$$= 0.51 + (0.234)(1.96)$$
$$= 0.97$$

The median value that would represent the *lower boundary* of the confidence interval would be:

$$\underline{\xi} = 0.51 - \frac{(1.25)(1.39)}{\sqrt{56-1}}(1.96)$$

$$= 0.51 - (0.234)(1.96)$$
$$= 0.05$$

ANSWER: The median interjection frequency of the population from which the children were selected is *approximately* 95 percent certain to fall between 0.05 and 0.97.

REMARK: The width of the confidence interval can be changed by substituting a different constant for 1.96. For a 99 percent confidence interval, for example, 2.58 would be used as the constant.

EXERCISE: Compute a 95 percent confidence interval for the median part-word
(Number 22) repetition frequency of the population from which the children were selected (see p. 297 and p. 300 for the sample median and standard deviation). (The upper boundary of the confidence interval you compute should be approximately 1.07, and the lower boundary should be approximately 0.56.)

C. Difference between Means

QUESTION: Within what range is the *difference between mean* part-word repetition frequencies for third graders and sixth graders in the *populations* from which the children were selected (i.e., third-grade nonstutterers and sixth-grade nonstutterers) most likely to fall?

To answer this question, a 95 *percent confidence interval* will be computed. Theoretically, the limits of this interval define a range within which we can be 95 percent certain of finding the difference between mean part-word repetition frequencies for third graders and sixth graders in the populations from which the samples were drawn. This 95 percent figure, however, should only be regarded as approximate, since certain assumptions underlying the computational procedure may not have been met (see Chapter 10).

The upper $(\overline{\Delta})$ and lower $(\underline{\Delta})$ limits of the confidence interval can be computed by means of the following formulas:

$$\overline{\Delta} = \overline{D}_1 + (1.96)\sqrt{\frac{S_1^2}{n_1 - 1} + \frac{S_2^2}{n_2 - 1}}$$

$$\underline{\Delta} = \overline{D}_1 - (1.96)\sqrt{\frac{S_1^2}{n_1 - 1} + \frac{S_2^2}{n_2 - 1}}$$

where

$\overline{D}_1 = \overline{X}_1 - \overline{X}_2 = 1.245 - 0.411 = 0.834$
$n_1 =$ the number of third graders $= 11$
$n_2 =$ the number of sixth graders $= 10$
$S_1^2 =$ the variance of the third graders' part-word repetition frequencies

$$= \frac{\Sigma X_1^2}{n_1} - \overline{X}_1^2$$

$$= \frac{30.695}{11} - (1.245)^2$$

$$= 2.790 - 1.550 = 1.240$$

$S_2^2 =$ the variance of the sixth graders' part-word repetition frequencies

$$= \frac{\Sigma\ X_2^2}{n_2} - \overline{X}_2^2$$

$$= \frac{2.700}{10} - (0.411)^2$$

$$= 0.270 - 0.169 = 0.101$$

The mean difference that would represent the *upper boundary* of the confidence interval would be:

$$\overline{\Delta} = 0.834 + (1.96)\ \sqrt{\frac{1.240}{11 - 1} + \frac{0.101}{10 - 1}}$$

$$= 0.834 + (1.96)(0.368) = 1.56$$

The mean difference that would represent the *lower boundary* of the confidence interval would be:

$$\underline{\Delta} = 0.834 - (1.96)\ \sqrt{\frac{1.240}{11 - 1} + \frac{0.101}{10 - 1}}$$

$$= 0.834 - (1.96)(0.368) = 0.11$$

ANSWER: The difference between the means of the population from which the children were selected is *approximately* 95 percent certain to fall between 0.11 and 1.56.

REMARK: The width of the confidence interval can be changed by substituting a different constant for 1.96. For a 99 percent confidence interval, for example, 2.58 would be used as the constant.

EXERCISE: Compute a 95 percent confidence interval for the difference between (Number 23) mean part-word repetition frequencies for fourth graders and fifth graders in the populations from which the children were selected (see p. 295 for the values you will need). (The upper boundary of the confidence interval you compute should be approximately 1.01, and the lower boundary should be approximately −0.07.)

MINITAB STATISTICAL SOFTWARE COMMANDS

Data from Table A.1 has been utilized throughout this appendix for illustrating the computation of various statistics. To demonstrate how the Minitab Statistical Software can be used for this purpose, we will utilize the interjection, part-word repetition, and word repetition frequencies from it for the 26 second- and third-grade children (i.e., columns C1, C2, and C3).

Your first task after the program is ready to run is to input the data. Minitab stores data in a worksheet. The first command

READ C1 C2 C3

tells the computer to take the data from the lines that follow the READ command and put them into columns C1, C2, and C3 of the worksheet. After the data for the 26 children have been entered, the command

END

is issued. The display on your monitor screen will look something like that in Figure A.1. There may, however, be more lines in this figure than your screen can display at one time. If you want to print the data in the three columns, the appropriate command is

PRINT C1 C2 C3

FIGURE A.1   Monitor Display for MINITAB Worksheet

```
----------------------------------------------------
MTB  >     READ  C1   C2   C3
DATA >     0.50  1.16  0.50
DATA >     2.13  1.42  0.35
DATA >     1.40  0.00  0,00
DATA >     0.40  1.21  0.40
DATA >     0.31  0.94  0.63
DATA >     0.00  0.35  0.35
DATA >     0.00  0.00  1.28
DATA >     0.47  2.37  0.95
DATA >     0.30  1.80  1.50
DATA >     0.50  1.00  1.33
DATA >     8,53  0.34  2.39
DATA >     1.04  1.04  1.04
DATA >     1.46  0.29  0.44
DATA >     0.36  0.36  0.72
DATA >     1.87  0.00  0.75
DATA >     0.46  1.14  1.60
DATA >     3.78  1.13  2.64
DATA >     2.23  1.49  2.97
DATA >     0.33  0.99  0.99
DATA >     0.49  0.00  0.49
DATA >     1.07  1.43  1.07
DATA >     0.55  4.42  3.31
DATA >     0.84  0.28  0.28
DATA >     0.28  0.41  0.28
DATA >     3.40  1.51  1.89
DATA >     1.80  0.90  0.60
DATA >     END
MTB  >
----------------------------------------------------
```

Such a printout can be useful when checking for data entry errors.

After the columns of data are stored in the worksheet, various statistical analyses can be performed on them. By keyboarding the command

DESCRIBE C2

several descriptive statistics will be computed from the data in column C2 and displayed on the screen, including the mean, median, standard deviation, range, and interquartile range. If you wanted to compute the Pearson product-moment correlation coefficient (r) between disfluency frequencies for interjection (C1) and word repetition (C3) you would keyboard the following command

CORRELATION COEFFICIENT BETWEEN C1 AND C3

The value of *r* would be indicated on the screen. If you also wanted a scattergram to be plotted on it, you would keyboard

PLOT C1 VERSUS C3

Minitab can compute the other correlation coefficients mentioned in this appendix, but you have to use their computational formula rather than a single command (see Ryan, Joiner, and Ryan, 1985).

All of the significance tests described in this appendix can be computed with one or two commands. To determine whether the children had higher interjection than part-word repetition frequencies using the *Mann-Whitney U test,* you would keyboard

MANNWHITNEY C1 C2

and to determine this using the *t-test for related measures* the commands would be

LET C4 = C2 − C1
TTEST C4

The first tells the computer to subtract the numbers in column C1 from those in column C2 and store the differences in column C4. And the second tells it to do a *t*-test on the numbers in column C4. If the numbers in columns C1 and C2 were *independent* (e.g., the numbers in C1 were interjection frequencies for second- and third-grade children and those in C2 were interjection frequencies for fourth- and fifth-grade children), only a single command would be needed for a t-test between columns C1 and C2.

TWOSAMPLE-T C1 C2

Next, suppose you wanted to determine whether the frequencies for any of the three disfluency types were higher than the others (i.e., whether the difference between them was statistically significant) using the *Friedman two-way analysis of variance.* The command would be

FRIEDMAN C1 C2 C3

Strictly speaking, this would be a test of whether the frequencies in column C1 differ from those in columns C2 and C3. If, on the other hand, you wanted to determine whether the frequencies in column C3 differ from those in the others, the command would be

FRIEDMAN C3 C1 C2

The symbol used for the statistic here is S rather than X_r^2. You could also use a *one-way analysis of variance* to test the null hypothesis that these frequencies do not differ. The command would be

AOVONEWAY C1-C3

Strictly speaking, this is a test for indepedent measures.

There are commands in the manual (Ryan, Joiner, and Ryan, 1985) for computing the other significance tests mentioned in this appendix. There are also commands there for computing the three types of confidence intervals mentioned in it. Furthermore, there are commands in this manual for computing most of the multivariate statistics described in Chapters 9 and 10, including factor analysis, discriminant function analysis, and multiple correlation and regression.

Appendix B
3,500 Computer-Generated Random Digits

04433	80674	24520	18222	10610	05794	37515
60298	47829	72648	37414	75755	04717	29899
67884	59651	67533	68123	17730	95862	08034
89512	32155	51906	61662	64130	16688	37275
32653	01895	12506	88535	36553	23757	34209
95913	15405	13772	76638	48423	25018	99041
55864	21694	13122	44115	01601	50541	00147
35334	49810	91601	40617	72876	33967	73830
57729	32196	76487	11622	96297	24160	09903
86648	13697	63677	70119	94739	25875	38829
30574	47609	07967	32422	76791	39725	53711
81307	43694	83580	79974	45929	85113	72268
02410	54905	79007	54939	21410	86980	91772
18969	75274	52233	62319	08598	09066	95288
87863	82384	66860	62297	80198	19347	73234
68397	71708	15438	62311	72844	60203	46412
28529	54447	58729	10854	99058	18260	38765
44285	06372	15867	70418	57012	72122	36634
86299	83430	33571	23309	57040	29285	67870
84842	68668	90894	61658	15001	94055	36308
56970	83609	52098	04184	54967	72938	56834
83125	71257	60490	44369	66130	72936	69848
55503	52423	02464	26141	68779	66388	75242
47019	76273	33203	29608	54553	25971	69573
84828	32592	79526	29554	84580	37859	28504
68921	08141	79227	05748	51276	57143	31926
36458	96045	30424	98420	72925	40729	22337
95752	59445	36847	87729	81679	59126	59437
26768	47323	58454	56958	20575	76746	49878
42613	37056	43636	58085	06766	60227	96414
95457	30566	65482	25596	02678	54592	63607
95276	17894	63564	95958	39750	64379	46059
66954	52324	64776	92345	95110	59448	77249
17457	18481	14113	62462	02798	54977	48349
03704	36872	83214	59337	01695	60666	97410
21538	86497	33210	60337	27976	70661	08250
57178	67619	98310	70348	11317	71623	55510
31048	97558	94953	55866	96283	46620	52087
69799	55380	16498	80733	96422	58078	99643
90595	61867	59231	17772	67831	33317	00520
33570	04981	98939	78784	09977	29398	93896
15340	93460	57477	13898	48431	72936	78160
64079	42483	36512	56186	99098	48850	72527
63491	05546	67118	62063	74958	20946	28147
92003	63868	41034	28260	79708	00770	88643
52360	46658	66511	04172	73085	11795	52594
74622	12142	68355	65635	21828	39539	18988
04157	50079	61343	64315	70836	82857	35335
86003	60070	66241	32836	27573	11479	94114
41268	80187	20351	09636	84668	42486	71303

(Continued)
Commerce Commis-

48611	62866	33963	14045	79451	04934	45576
78812	03509	78673	73181	29973	18664	04555
19472	63971	37271	31445	49019	49405	46925
51266	11569	08697	91120	64156	40365	74297
55806	96275	26130	47949	14877	69594	83041
77527	81360	18180	97421	55541	90275	18213
77680	58788	33016	61173	93049	04694	43534
15404	96554	88265	34537	38526	67924	40474
14045	22917	60718	66487	46346	30949	03173
68376	43918	77653	04127	69930	43283	35766
93385	13421	67957	20384	58731	53396	59723
09858	52104	32014	53115	03727	98624	84616
93307	34116	49516	42148	57740	31198	70336
04794	01534	92058	03157	91758	80611	45357
86265	49096	97021	92582	61422	75890	86442
65943	79232	45702	67055	39024	57383	44424
90038	94209	04055	27393	61517	23002	96560
97283	95943	78363	36498	40662	94188	18202
21913	72958	75637	99936	58715	07943	23748
41161	37341	81838	19389	80336	46346	91895
23777	98392	31417	98547	92058	02277	50315
59973	08144	61070	73094	27059	69181	55623
82690	74099	77885	23813	10054	11900	44653
83854	24715	48866	65745	31131	47636	45137
61980	34997	41825	11623	07320	15003	56774
99915	45821	97702	87125	44488	77613	56823
48293	86847	43186	42951	37804	85129	28993
33225	31280	41232	34750	91097	60752	69783
06846	32828	24425	30249	78801	26977	92074
32671	45587	79620	84831	38156	74211	82752
82096	21913	75544	55228	89796	05694	91552
51666	10433	10945	55306	78562	89630	41230
54044	67942	24145	42294	27427	84875	37022
66738	60184	75679	38120	17640	36242	99357
55064	17427	89180	74018	44865	53197	74810
69599	60264	84549	78007	88450	06488	72274
64756	87759	92354	78694	63638	80939	98644
80817	74533	68407	55862	32476	19326	95558
39847	96884	84657	33697	39578	90197	80532
90401	41700	95510	61166	33757	23279	85523
78227	90110	81378	96659	37008	04050	04228
87240	52716	87697	79433	16336	52862	69149
08486	10951	26832	39763	02485	71688	90936
39338	32169	03713	93510	61244	73774	01245
21188	01850	69689	49426	49128	14660	14143
13287	82531	04388	64693	11934	35051	68576
53609	04001	19648	14053	49623	10840	31915
87900	36194	31567	53506	34304	39910	79630
81641	00496	36058	75899	46620	70024	88753
19512	50277	71508	20116	79520	06269	74173

Appendix C
Methodological Considerations for Quantifying Attributes of Speech, Language, and Hearing Using Psychological Scaling Methods

Once the scaling method has been selected, the next step is to prepare the stimuli for scaling. Since most of the stimuli scaled by speech-language pathologists and audiologists have been auditory—i.e., speech events or other acoustic signals recorded on audiotape—this discussion will emphasize the preparation of such stimuli for scaling. Most of the comments will be relevant, however, to the preparation of other types of stimuli for scaling, including videotaped ones.

A number of factors must be considered in preparing audiotaped stimuli for scaling, including: (1) method of assembling the tape (i.e., splicing versus dubbing), (2) ordering of the stimuli, (3) duration of the "judging interval" between stimuli, (4) selection, frequency of occurrence, and location of the standard stimuli, (5) definition and selection of stimuli, (6) equating stimuli for extraneous attributes, (7) numbering stimuli, (8) acquainting judges with the range of the target attribute present in the stimuli, and (9) determining the number of times each stimulus is to be presented. Comments relevant to each consideration are presented in the paragraphs that follow.

Method of Assembling. Two methods can be used to prepare audiotaped stimuli for scaling. The first is *splicing* together the segments of tape on which the stimuli were recorded. The second is *dubbing* the stimuli onto a master tape. The splicing method obviously cannot be used when a stimulus has to appear more than once on a master tape (as it would for pair comparisons and constant sums). The main limitation of the dubbing process is that some distortion of the signal is introduced by it. In many cases, this distortion would probably not be of sufficient magnitude to influence observers' ratings of the target attribute. While it would be unlikely to influence stuttering severity ratings, it may influence voice quality ratings.

Ordering of the Stimuli. The ordering of stimuli on the master tape should be random—i.e., determined by a table of random numbers (see Appendix B). If there is a possibility of order or sequence effects (see Chapter 6) influencing the ratings, these effects could be controlled for, at least partially, by preparing several randomizations of the stimuli. Since the possibility of order and sequence effects often cannot be ruled out, it is not desirable for all members of a panel to rate a set of stimuli in the same order.

Duration of the "Judging Interval" between Stimuli. This refers to the time interval following the presentation of a stimulus during which it is rated. It must be long enough to permit the judges to make their ratings with adequate levels of validity and reliability but not so long that it will unnecessarily extend the length of the judging session. An interval duration of approximately 15 seconds appears to be adequate for rating most attributes of audiotaped speech stimuli.

Selection, Frequency of Occurrence, and Location of the Standard Stimuli. Standard stimuli serve as anchor, or reference, points on a scale. They help to reduce intrarater and interrater variability. They usually are used with the method of direct magnitude-estimation. Standard stimuli also are used occasionally with the methods of equal-appearing intervals and successive intervals.

Several decisions must be made if standard stimuli are to be used: (1) which stimulus (for direct magnitude-estimation), or which stimuli (for equal-appearing intervals and successive intervals), to select, (2) how often to present the stimulus, or stimuli, and (3) at what points during the rating session to present the stimulus, or stimuli (i.e., at the beginning only, or at the beginning and periodically during the session). With direct magnitude-estimation, a stimulus is usually selected for the standard in which the amount of the attribute is at the approximate midpoint of the range (based on the judgment of the experimenter or that of a small panel of observers). Theoretically, the "location" of the standard in the range of possible values of the attribute should not influence the characteristics of the scale resulting from its use. As long as the scale is regarded as ordinal, this would probably be a safe assumption to make. However, if it is regarded as having interval or ratio properties, this assumption would be risky to make, since there is some evidence that suggests that the location of the standard used to construct a scale by the method of direct magnitude-estimation influences to some extent the spacings between points on that scale. For this reason, it would probably be most defensible to interpret direct magnitude-estimation scale values as if they had ordinal properties.

In scaling tape recorded stimuli with the method of direct magnitude-estimation, the standard stimulus usually appears two or three times (one after the other) at the beginning of the tape on which the stimuli are recorded. The standard may also appear on this tape after every third or fourth stimulus. Hence, the sequence of stimuli on a tape could be:

1. Standard Stimulus
2. Standard Stimulus

3. Standard Stimulus
4. Stimulus #1
5. Stimulus #2
6. Stimulus #3
7. Standard Stimulus
8. Stimulus #4
9. Stimulus #5
10. Stimulus #6
11. Standard Stimulus
    etc.

The more abstract or vague the target attribute, the more frequently the standard stimulus should be presented.

With the method of equal-appearing intervals and the method of successive intervals, if individual scale points are not defined, two stimuli are selected for the standard which represent the *extremes* of the range of possible values of the target attribute. It is crucial that the amounts of the target attribute present in these stimuli represent the extremes of the continuum. Otherwise, there may be an *end effect,* i.e., a piling up of ratings in one or both of the extreme intervals. Both stimuli that have a value of the target attribute *equal* to that in the standard and *exceeding* that in the standard will be assigned the most extreme ratings. (Such ratings on a seven-point scale would be 1 and 7.) Standard stimuli are often not used with these methods because of the difficulty in identifying stimuli that represent the extremes of the range of possible values of the target attribute. The extremes of the scale in such cases are usually defined verbally, e.g.,

    1 = *least* hypernasality and 7 = *most* hypernasality

or

    1 = *lowest* stuttering severity and 7 = *highest* stuttering severity

When standard stimuli are used with these scaling methods, they usually are presented several times at the beginning of the stimulus tape and after every third or fourth stimulus.

Definition and Selection of Stimuli. This is not a problem in many scaling experiments because the events, or stimuli, to be rated have "natural" boundaries. (Examples of events that can be treated as such are phonemes, syllables, and words.) This can present a problem, however, when the events to be rated do not have "natural" boundaries, e.g., conversational speech segments. To illustrate this point, suppose you wished to rate "before and after" therapy conversational speech segments for degree of nasality or degree of stuttering severity. How long a speech segment would be required to obtain ratings which are adequately reliable? Would 20-second segments be adequate? The answers to these questions would depend, in part, on the nature of the attribute being rated. Some attributes could be reliably rated from shorter segments than others. Nasality, for example, could probably be reliably rated from shorter segments than would be required for stuttering severity. Unfortunately, with the exception of a few attributes such as stuttering severity, there are no data in the literature that indicate the shortest segment lengths that can be expected to yield reliable ratings. The only possibly helpful observation from the literature is that in studies where the speech segments rated were 30 seconds in duration, ratings in almost all cases have been reported to be adequately reliable.

After a decision has been made concerning the duration of speech segments, it is then necessary to decide which segments of the available speech samples to rate. This obviously would be of concern only if the available samples were longer in duration than the segment length selected. There are several strategies that can be used for selecting such segments, including the following:

1. Segments are selected by the experimenter. The experimenter chooses segments that he or she feels are representative. One limitation of this strategy is that the experimenter, without being consciously aware of it, may select segments that instead of being representative would be likely to be rated in a manner consistent with his or her expectations or hypotheses. (The phenomenon of *experimenter bias* is discussed in several contexts in this book, which may be located by consulting the index.)
2. Segments are selected through the use of a random sampling procedure. The sample could be segmented, for example, into consecutive segments of the length to be rated. (A five-minute sample could be segmented into 10 consecutive, 30-second segments.) These segments would be numbered consecutively, and one or more would be selected by means of a table of random numbers. This sampling strategy is more likely than the first to provide representative samples for rating.

Equating Stimuli for Extraneous Attributes.   The stimuli the judges are asked to rate may possess a large number (perhaps, an infinite number) of attributes. The judges are usually instructed to attend to only one such attribute (i.e., the target attribute) when making their ratings. Two strategies have been used to *minimize* the impact of other attributes (i.e., extraneous attributes) on these ratings. The first is to instruct the judges to ignore these attributes when making their ratings, and the second is to equate the stimuli for them. Suppose you did not want judges to be influenced by disfluency level when they were rating speech segments for articulation defectiveness. If you used the first approach, you would tell them to ignore disfluency level when making their ratings. If you used the second approach, you would select speech segments in which no disfluency occurred. (If you were using a random sampling procedure for selecting such segments, you could exclude those containing instances of disfluency.)

Numbering Stimuli (or Stimulus Pairs).   Each stimulus (or stimulus pair) to be rated is usually given an identification number. If the stimuli are audio-tape-recorded speech segments, a carrier phrase and number is recorded on the stimulus tape preceding each segment, e.g., "sample number one." This carrier phrase-number combination performs two functions. First, it maximizes the odds that the judges will record their ratings at the appropriate places on the response sheet. Second, it alerts the judges immediately before the presentation of each stimulus, which maximizes the odds they will attend to it.

Acquainting Judges with the Range of the Target Attribute Present in the Stimuli.   With equal-appearing intervals, with successive intervals, and sometimes with direct magnitude-estimation, the judges are acquainted with the range of the target attribute present in the stimuli before beginning the rating task. This may be done by presenting 10 or 15 stimuli to them which represent the range of the attribute. It also may be done by presenting all the stimuli to the judges before they begin to rate them.

Determining the Number of Times Each Stimulus Is to Be Presented. It may sometimes be necessary to present a stimulus more than once before asking judges to rate it. If the duration of individual stimuli is relatively short, such as would be the case for isolated phonemes, judges may be unable to get a sufficiently good impression of the target attribute to rate isolated vowels for nasality. You might dub each vowel on the stimulus tape three times (with a few seconds between presentations) and have judges listen to the three presentations before assigning it a nasality rating.

Considerations in Writing Instructions to Judges

One of the most important tasks associated with designing a scaling experiment is writing the instructions of the judges. The instructions they are given influence both the validity and reliability of their ratings.

The instructions given the judges in scaling experiments usually provide them with three kinds of information: (1) a description of the attribute to be rated, (2) a description of the scaling task, and (3) descriptions of attributes to be ignored. Two representative sets of instructions which include these three kinds of information are reproduced here. The first is for the method of equal-appearing intervals; the second, for the method of direct magnitude-estimation. Both were used for rating the same attribute, i.e., intricacy of language usage (Sherman and Silverman, 1968).

I

You are asked to judge a series of samples of children's oral language which are presented in written form. You are to judge each sample in relation to a seven-point scale of "intricacy of language usage." Intricacy of language usage, for the purposes of this experiment, is defined as the intricacy of the arrangement of words for the purpose of conveying information. For example, consider the following four sets of words, which without reference to the specific meanings, might be judged to vary with respect to intricacy of language as defined here:

  (a) two good little boys
  (b) boys in your school
  (c) boys who are orphans
  (d) really very good boys

Although each of the above sets contains four words, it is obvious that they vary with respect to type of arrangement. .

Make your judgment on the basis of the whole sample. Avoid being influenced by grammatical correctness; for example, "we was" in place of the correct wording "we were." Obviously, the expressions "we was" and "we were" do not differ with respect to the intricacy of word arrangement. Also, do not give a rating based upon a judgment of the extent of vocabulary; for example, "big size" and "extensive area" are equivalent as far as the intricacy of arrangement is concerned, but they probably would not be considered equivalent if judged for the purpose of rating extent of vocabulary usage.

The scale is one of equal intervals—from 1 to 7—with 1 representing *least* intricacy of language usage and 7 representing *most* intricacy; 4 represents the midpoint between 1 and 7 with respect to intricacy, with the other numbers falling at equal distances along the scale. Do not attempt to place samples between any two of the seven points but only at these points.

Each language sample is preceded by a number. Your task will be to record your judgment on your response sheet to the right of the identifying number of the language sample.

On the following pages there are 50 samples to be rated on a seven-point scale. The experimenter obtained these samples by requesting the children to respond to a picture stimulus. He also encouraged the children to speak by asking them questions and by making comments, as needed. These questions and comments are not included in the material you are to judge. All of the samples are in response to the same picture.

Before you record any judgments, read quickly the first 25 samples to acquaint yourself with the experimental task and to acquaint yourself with the range of samples with respect to the intricacy of language usage which you are requested to judge.

After you have acquainted yourself with the task and the range, make a judgment on every sample. If you are somewhat doubtful, make a guess as to the most suitable scale position.

II

You are asked to judge a series of samples of children's oral language which are presented in written form. You are to judge each sample for *intricacy of language usage.* You are to estimate the relative intricacy of language usage of each language sample in relation to the intricacy of language usage of a standard sample which you will read before making your estimates. Your task will be to assign the number of points you believe represents the relative intricacy of language usage with reference to the standard sample.

Intricacy of language usage, for the purposes of this experiment, is defined as the intricacy of the arrangement of words for the purpose of conveying information. For example, consider the following four sets of words which, without reference to the specific meanings, might be judged to vary with respect to intricacy of language usage as here defined:

(a) two good little boys
(b) boys in our school
(c) boys who are orphans
(d) really good little boys

Although each of the above sets contains four words, it is obvious that they vary with respect to type of arrangement of words for the purpose of conveying information.

Make your judgment on the basis of the whole sample. Avoid being influenced by grammatical correctness; for example, "we was" in place of the correct wording "we were." Obviously, the expressions "we was" and "we were" do not differ with respect to the intricacy of word arrangement. Also, do not give a rating based upon a judgment of the extent of vocabulary; for example, "big size" and "extensive area" are equivalent as far as the intricacy of arrangement is concerned, but they probably would not be considered equivalent if judged for the purpose of rating extent of vocabulary.

The following sample is to be used as the *standard sample.*

"That's a grandpa lion and he is sitting down in a chair and he is thinking about something. And he's holding a pipe in his hand. And a little mouse is coming out of the mouse hole. Sneak up on the tiger. Cause he is gonna lay on the tiger's head. He would feel upon his head and he'd feel a mouse up on his head and try to catch him. Well, I would get out of there and crawl under the chair and go through there and run. Run away from him. I would run back under the chair and into my mousehole. He couldn't get under the chair."

You will assign *100 points* to this sample. The point assignments you make on the succeeding samples should represent, with reference to the standard, the relative intricacy of language usage of each sample. For example, if you believe that a sample is *twice* as intricate in language usage as the standard sample, you would assign *200 points* to it. On the other hand, if you believe that a sample is *half* as intricate in language usage as the standard, you would assign it *50 points.* You may, of course, use any point assignment you choose to represent your judgment of the intricacy of language usage. You need not limit yourself to even fractions and even multiples of the 100 points assigned to the standard. You might use, for example, 85, or 65, or 20, or even 57, or 112, or 120, or 215, or any other number you choose as long as it represents your judgment of the intricacy of language usage of the sample in relation to the standard sample.

On the following pages there are 50 samples to be judged in relation to the standard sample. The experimenter obtained these samples by requesting the children to respond to a picture stimulus. He also encouraged the children to speak by asking them questions and making comments, as needed. These questions and comments are not included in the material you are to judge. All of the samples are in response to the same picture.

Each experimental sample is preceded by a number. You are to record your judgments on your response sheet to the right of the identification numbers of the samples. Before you record any judgments, read quickly the first 25 samples to acquaint yourself with the experimental task. As you read think about the point assignments you would make if you were recording judgments. Now read the standard sample once again; record your judgments according to the instructions which have been given. Make a judgment on every sample. If you are somewhat doubtful about what number to assign, make a guess.

In the first set of instructions (for the method of equal-appearing intervals), the first paragraph gives a description of the attribute to be rated; the second, the attributes to be ignored; and the remaining paragraphs, a description of the scaling task. In the second set of instructions (for the method of direct magnitude-estimation), the second paragraph gives a description of the attribute to be rated; the third, the attributes to be ignored; and the remaining paragraphs, a description of the scaling task.

These sets of instructions can be modified fairly easily for rating other attributes of speech (or language). Also, the equal-appearing interval instructions can be used for the method of successive intervals, with minor modifications.

Instructions can be presented to judges in oral or written form. An oral mode of presentation can be either tape-recorded or "live." A written mode is usually typed (keyboarded) and duplicated (e.g., Xeroxed or photo-offset). These presentation modes are often combined. The experimenter reads the instructions aloud while the judges follow along on their copies. This combined mode may be the most satisfactory one (when it is possible to use it) since some judges would probably better comprehend "heard" than "read" instructions, and vice versa.

The judges usually record their ratings on a response sheet. A representative response sheet is reproduced in Figure C.1. This response sheet could be used for all the methods discussed, with the exception of constant sums. For the method of pair comparisons, a 1 or 2 would be recorded in the space to the right of each identification number to designate the stimulus in each pair which possessed the greater amount of the target attribute. For the method of rank order, the number recorded to the right of a stimulus identification number would designate the rank of that stimulus in an ordering. For the methods of equal-appearing intervals and successive intervals, this number would be a numeral that designates a point on scale (having a finite number of points). And for the method of direct magnitude-estimation, this number would be a magnitude estimate.

To make this response sheet usable for the method of constant sums, it would be necessary to have *two* response spaces to the right of each identification number, i.e.,

$$A \qquad B$$
$$1. \underline{\hspace{3em}} \quad \underline{\hspace{3em}}$$

The point value assigned to the first stimulus in a pair could be recorded in the *A* space and that assigned to the second member in the *B* space.

FIGURE C.1   Representative Response Sheet.

*Name*_____   *Date*_____

1____	26____
2____	27____
3____	28____
4____	29____
5____	30____
6____	31____
7____	32____
8____	33____
9____	34____
10____	35____
11____	36____
12____	37____
13____	38____
14____	39____
15____	40____
16____	41____
17____	42____
18____	43____
19____	44____
20____	45____
21____	46____
22____	47____
23____	48____
24____	49____
25____	50____

Considerations in the Selection of a Judging Panel

All scaling methods require a panel of judges, or raters. Several consider-ations concerning the selection of judges for a panel will be discussed in this section, including: (1) the number to be used, (2) their characteristics, and (3) the procedure by which they are to be selected.

Number of Judges to Be Used in the Panel.   If too few judges are used, the scale values for the stimuli may not be sufficiently reliable for the pur-poses of the experiment. If too many are used, the panel may be unnecessar-ily "costly." The added cost here includes: (1) judges' time in performing the rating task, (2) experimenter's time in administering the task, and (3) data analysis time and expense.

There is little in the literature to assist the experimenter in deciding how many judges to use, with the possible exception of information pertain-ing to the magnitude of reliability coefficients reported for scaling experi-ments in which different numbers of judges were used (e.g., Edwards, 1957, pp. 94–95). Such information has limited usefulness, since the number of judges required to attain a specific level of reliability would be expected to vary as a function of several factors, including: (1) the degree of ambiguity of the attribute being rated, (2) the complexity of the stimuli, and (3) the extent to which the judges are trained to share a common standard. However, in almost all studies reported in which speech segments were scaled by the methods of equal-appearing intervals, successive intervals, or direct magnitude-estimation and panels of approximately 50 judges were used, the investigators concluded that the resulting scale values were adequately reliable for their purposes. Panels of 50 judges, therefore, probably would be sufficiently large for scaling attributes of speech segments for most purposes.

With the approach described, the size of the judging panel is fixed before beginning the rating task, and the reliability of the scale values is permitted to vary. An alternative approach would be to fix the minimum level of reliability desired for the scale values before beginning the rating task and to permit the size of the judging panel to vary. That is, you would gradually increase the number of judges in the panel until the scale values computed from their ratings would possess a predetermined level of reliability. One such approach, based on the principle of sequential sampling, has been described by Silverman (1968a).

Definition of the Population from Which the Panel Is to Be Selected.

"Organismic" and related variables such as hearing acuity, visual acuity, intelligence, and previous exposure to the attribute being rated can systematically influence the ratings assigned by the members of a panel. A panel consisting of parents of children who stutter may tend to rate segments of disfluent speech as more abnormal than would a panel consisting of parents of children who do not stutter. Also, a panel of speech-language pathologists may tend to rate speech segments in which the speaker has a lateral lisp as more abnormal than would a panel consisting of laymen.

If it seems that a particular attribute might be rated differently by different subgroups of observers, it would be necessary for the experimenters to define the subgroup they wish to use for their panel. The characteristics of the members of this subgroup would be determined, at least in part, by the purpose to which the ratings were to be put. Suppose an investigator wished to determine whether the speech of severe stutterers would be regarded as less defective if they paced their speech with a miniature metronome than if they spoke in their usual manner. Since the ratings of speech-language pathologists might differ from those of laymen, and since the investigator would probably be interested primarily in how laymen would react to the "metronome" as opposed to the usual speech of such stutterers, the investigator would probably be wise to limit membership in the panel to persons who have not had training in speech-language pathology.

The more heterogeneous the members of a panel are with regard to organismic variables, the greater the probable dispersion of their ratings and the lower the probable *reliability* of the scale values computed from them (for a given size panel) will be. Also, the more heterogeneous the members of a panel are with regard to such variables, the less *valid* the scale values computed from their ratings are apt to be. If a panel consisted of two or more subgroups who would tend to rate a set of stimuli differently, scale values computed from the ratings of such a panel may not correspond to how the typical member of any subgroup would rate the stimuli. They may be merely "mathematical artifacts." (For a discussion of this point in two somewhat different contexts, see Silverman, 1974.)

Selection of the Panel.   The panel, strictly speaking, should consist of a random sample of persons from the defined population. Every member of this population should have an equal chance of being selected for the panel. Sometimes it is possible to have such a panel. For instance, suppose the population an investigator wished to sample for a panel consisted of speech-language pathologists who have been awarded the Certificate of Clinical Competence in Speech-Language Pathology by the American Speech-Language-Hearing Association. A reasonably complete list of such persons could be obtained from the most recent edition of the Association's Membership Directory. Each could be assigned a number, and a panel could be selected by means of a table of random numbers. Such a panel would be practical if the rating task could be mailed.

In some instances it is neither possible nor practical to sample randomly the defined population. All you can do in these instances is to try to select a panel of persons who appear to be representative of the defined population and to be cautious when generalizing from their ratings.

Modes of Stimulus Presentation

Once a scaling method has been selected, the stimuli have been prepared, the instructions have been written, and the panel has been selected, the stimuli can be presented to the panel for rating. The primary emphasis in this discussion will be on the presentation of audiotaped stimuli. Many of the comments, however, are relevant for the presentation of other types of stimuli.

A number of decisions have to be made on procedures for presenting audiotaped stimuli for scaling including the following: (1) individual versus group presentation, (2) headphones versus speakers, (3) loudness level of the stimuli, (4) physical environment, and (5) number of judging sessions.

Individual versus Group Presentation.   The issue here is whether the stimuli should be presented to one member of the panel at a time or to several (possibly even the entire panel). The main advantage of group presentation is efficiency. Ordinarily it takes less time to have a set of stimuli rated using a group presentation mode than using an individual one.

The individual presentation mode has several advantages that may outweigh the efficiency advantage of the group mode. First, it ordinarily allows more control to be exerted over the presentation of the stimuli. This permits you to maximize the odds that the stimuli presented to the members of a panel will be similar. They may not be similar if a group presentation mode is used. If, for example, tape recorded stimuli are presented to a group of judges over a loudspeaker, the judges may not "hear" the same stimuli because they are sitting at different distances from the speaker. With an individual presentation mode, judges could be seated the same distance from the speaker.

A second advantage of the individual over the group presentation mode is that it permits order and sequence effects (see Chapter 6) to be minimized. The stimuli can be presented to the members of a panel in different random sequences. This would ordinarily be quite difficult to do if a group presentation mode were used.

The third advantage of the individual over the group presentation mode is that it permits the use of the sequential approach for defining the size of a panel (Silverman, 1968a). The main advantage of this approach is that it ensures that the scale values derived from the judges' ratings will possess the required level of reliability and the panel will be no larger than necessary to achieve this end.

Headphones versus Speakers.   Two types of transducers can be used to present audiotape stimuli to judges: headphones and loudspeakers. The main advantage of loudspeakers is that they make it relatively easy to present a set of stimuli to more than one rater at a time. Their main disadvantage is that they permit the acoustic properties of the experimental room to interact with the stimuli. This can cause the properties of the stimuli to be distorted for at least some members of a panel. All members may not "hear" the same thing. Headphones (particularly those with a good acoustic seal) minimize the extent to which the stimuli the judges hear are distorted by the acoustical properties of the experimental room.

A second advantage of headphones over speakers is that they make the intensity level at which the stimuli are presented to the raters easier to control since the transducer-to-subject distance is constant. By the same token, headphones also make it relatively simple to compensate at least partially for differences in the hearing thresholds of judges.

Loudness Level of the Stimuli.   With audiotape recorded stimuli, it is necessary to define a loudness level for presenting the stimuli to the panel. This level usually is defined by the experimenter (implicitly or explicitly) as one the judges would regard as "comfortable." While such an approach would probably be satisfactory for rating some attributes (e.g., stuttering severity), it may not be satisfactory for others—i.e., those whose magnitudes might vary as a function of the loudness level or levels at which they were presented. For rating attributes that may be of the latter type, it would probably be a good idea to define the loudness level more precisely. One approach would be to determine each panel member's speech reception threshold (SRT) and present the stimuli a given number of decibels above this threshold.

Physical Environment. The environment in which the stimuli are rated can influence the level of reliability of the ratings. As previously indicated, the acoustical properties of the experimental room can interact with those of audiotape recorded stimuli. Such an interaction would tend to increase the dispersion of the ratings and hence reduce their reliability.

The temperature and humidity levels within the experimental room also can influence the reliability of the ratings. If the judges are uncomfortable while rating the stimuli, they may divert some of the attention they should be devoting to the stimuli to their feelings of discomfort. This could reduce the reliability of their ratings.

Number of Judging Sessions. The rating task may be administered at a single session or divided into several sessions. While it is usually most efficient to have all the stimuli rated at a single session, this may not be possible or desirable. If the rating task is relatively long (i.e., longer than one hour), it almost always is desirable to divide the task into several sessions. It would also be desirable to divide the task into several sessions if the task were relatively short but so demanding that raters would likely become fatigued before completing it. Fatigue, of course, can reduce the reliability of the judges' ratings.

Analyses of Judges' Ratings

Once the judges have rated the stimuli, the next task is to analyze their ratings to yield: (1) a scale value for each of the stimuli, (2) an estimate of the reliability of these scale values, and (3) an index of the degree of agreement among the judges in their ratings of individual stimuli. Computational procedures for these three types of analyses are presented in the references cited for the six scaling methods in the section in Chapter 8 dealing with psychological scaling methods as measuring instruments. Here a general description of each type of analysis will be presented. We will also discuss two related topics: (1) the desirability of eliminating the ratings of judges who did not appear to be following instructions, and (2) the use of multiple regression analysis for inferring the attributes of the stimuli that influenced judges' ratings.

Computation of Scale Values. A stimulus's scale value is a number that designates the amount (relative or absolute) of the attribute rated that it possesses. This number indicates the location of the stimulus on the continuum, or scale, of possible values of this attribute. If a stimulus, for example, had a scale value of 4.0 on a seven-point, equal-appearing interval scale of stuttering severity where 1 designated least possible severity and 7 designated most possible severity, its location on this continuum, or scale, would be at the midpoint.

For the methods of equal-appearing intervals and direct magnitude-estimation, either the mean or median of the ratings assigned to a stimulus can be used as its scale value. Which of these is used may not make too much difference even though mean and median scale values for a stimulus will differ somewhat in magnitude, since both appear to order a set of stimuli in approximately the same manner (Silverman, 1967a).

For the methods of pair comparisons, constant sums, rank order, and successive intervals, the computational procedures for deriving scale values are fairly complex. Computer programs are available for computing scale values from sets of ratings yielded by these methods.

Estimating Reliability of Scale Values.   Before a set of scale values can be interpreted, it is necessary to establish whether they are sufficiently reliable for the purpose they were intended for. If they are not sufficiently reliable for this purpose, they cannot be used to answer the question or questions they were intended to answer. Both intrasubject and intersubject differences and relationships can be obscured.

Suppose you wished to determine whether dysarthrics were less hypernasal after being fitted with some sort of palatal prosthesis. You could have "before and after" treatment speech segments from such persons rated for degree of nasality. If the ratings were not adequately reliable, you could end up concluding the treatment made no difference when, in fact, it did.

What would be the minimum acceptable level of reliability for most purposes? Unless a difference were quite large or a relationship quite strong, you would stand a good chance of failing to detect it if the reliability of your scale values were less than 0.85. A reliability coefficient of 0.90 would probably be adequate except in instances where you were attempting to detect relatively small differences or relatively weak relationships. In such instances, a reliability coefficient of at least 0.95 probably would be necessary. This level probably could be achieved by using a fairly large judging panel—i.e., one with more than 50 judges.

Several approaches have been used for estimating the reliability level of a set of scale values. One such approach that can be used with any scaling method is *test-retest*. With this approach, the panel either rates the entire set of stimuli twice (usually on different days) or a randomly selected sample of the set of stimuli twice (e.g., at the beginning and at the end of the rating session). Two sets of scale values are computed from these ratings and correlated.

Suppose you wished to use the test-retest approach and the number of stimuli you were having rated were 75. You could select from these a sample of 25 by means of a table of random numbers and have them rated twice in different random orders—once at the beginning and once at the end of the rating session. The observers, then, would rate a total of 100 stimuli. Sets of scale values for the 25 stimuli could be computed from the first and second ratings, and these two sets of scale values could be correlated, possibly using a Pearson product-moment correlation coefficient (see Chapter 9). The magnitude of this coefficient would indicate whether the ratings were likely to be adequately reliable.

Another approach that can be used with any scaling method for estimating reliability is the *split-half* method. With this approach, each member of a panel is randomly assigned to one of two groups. Two sets of scale values are computed—one from the ratings of the judges in each group. These sets of scale values are correlated, usually with a Pearson product-moment correlation coefficient. The resulting correlation coefficient can be interpreted as a reliability estimate for a panel *one half* the size of the panel used. This would tend to be a conservative estimate for the entire panel. A more accurate estimate for the entire panel would be obtained by inserting the value of the Pearson product-moment correlation coefficient that was computed into the Spearman-Brown formula (Guilford, 1954, p. 391).

The main disadvantage of the split-half approach is that it is necessary to compute three sets of scale values—two of which are used solely for estimating reliability.

A third approach to estimating the reliability of scale values that can be used with the methods of equal-appearing intervals and direct magnitude-estimation utilizes the *intraclass correlation coefficient for average ratings* (Ebel, 1951). With this approach, the ratings assigned to the stimuli are subjected to an analysis of variance (see Chapter 10). An intraclass correlation coefficient is computed from the resulting mean square values, i.e.,

$$r_{\text{intraclass}} = 1 - \frac{MS_{AS}}{MS_A}$$

One interpretation of this coefficient (which was paraphrased from Winer, 1962) is that if the experiment were to be repeated with another random sample of the same number of judges, but with the same stimuli, the correlation between the *mean* ratings obtained from the two sets of data on the same stimuli would be approximately the value obtained for this coefficient. Because of the close correspondence between mean and median scale values, this coefficient can also be used to estimate the reliability of *median* ratings (Silverman, 1968b).

The intraclass correlation coefficient discussed here provides a reliability estimate for the average of the ratings of a *group* of judges. Sometimes it may be necessary to estimate the reliability of the ratings of the *individual* judges in a panel. Ebel (1951) provides formulas for two intraclass correlation coefficients which can be used for this purpose. One provides an estimate of the reliability of single ratings that is adjusted for systematic differences in judges' frames of reference (i.e., internal standards). It is approximately equal to the average intercorrelation between ratings given by all possible pairs of judges (Winer, 1962). This coefficient provides an estimate of how closely judges' ratings order a set of stimuli in the same manner. Suppose three judges rated five speech segments for degree of nasality by the method of direct magnitude-estimation and assigned the ratings given in Table C.1.

While the absolute ratings assigned by these judges are quite different, the five segments have been ordered by them in the same manner. For this reason, the magnitude of the intraclass correlation coefficient computed with this formula would be quite high, indicating good interjudge agreement.

Ebel's other formula provides an estimate of the reliability of the *absolute* ratings assigned by individual judges. It indicates how closely the absolute ratings assigned by individual judges agree. This formula could be used for such a purpose as estimating how well speech-language pathologists agree in their assignment of stutterers to one of the eight points on the Iowa Scale for Rating Severity of Stuttering (Darley and Spriestersbach, 1978). If it were applied to the data used to illustrate the other intraclass correlation coefficient for the ratings of individual judges, the formula would yield a coefficient that was considerably lower because of the differences in the absolute magnitudes of the judges' ratings. The magnitude of this coefficient will almost always be lower than that of the other.

One other approach that has been used for estimating the reliability of scale values utilizes the *mean Q value*. This strategy has only been used in conjunction with the method of equal-appearing intervals. The mean Q value is the mean semi-interquartile range (see Chapter 9) of the ratings assigned to each of a set of stimuli. A semi-interquartile range is computed for the ratings assigned to each stimulus in a set, and the mean of these ranges is computed.

The mean Q value is a measure of average interjudge agreement. The smaller the mean Q value, the closer the agreement of the judges in their

TABLE C.1   Direct magnitude-estimation ratings of five speech segments by three judges for degree of nasality.

Segment	Judge #1	Judge #2	Judge #3
A	150	150	95
B	375	250	165
C	333	200	125
D	400	300	175
E	270	185	115

ratings. And the closer the agreement of the judges in their ratings, the higher the reliability (or stability) of the scale values.

Information on the distribution of mean Q values for stimuli rated on a seven-point, equal-appearing interval scale has been reported (Silverman, 1967b). The relative magnitude of an obtained mean Q value can be estimated by locating it in this distribution.

Degree of Agreement among Judges in Their Ratings of Individual Stimuli.

Judges do not usually assign identical ratings to stimuli. There is ordinarily some variability in their ratings. It is sometimes useful to be able to describe the degree of agreement among the judges in their ratings of specific stimuli. Such information is useful, for example, in the construction of master scales. Suppose you wished to construct an equal-appearing interval master scale of nasality. You could have a large number of speech segments from persons with cleft palates rated on a seven-point, equal-appearing interval scale of degree of nasality. You would compute from the ratings assigned to each stimulus both a scale value and a measure of dispersion, or spread (e.g., the semi-interquartile range). Next, you would identify segments that had scale values of 1.0, 2.0, 3.0, 4.0, 5.0, 6.0, and 7.0. From the segments having scale values at each of these points, you would select the one on which the dispersion of their ratings was the smallest. These seven segments ordered on a tape would constitute a seven-point master scale of nasality.

Several measures of dispersion have been used to describe the degree of agreement among the judges in their ratings of individual stimuli, including: (1) the range, (2) the interquartile range, (3) the semi-interquartile range, and (4) the standard deviation. These measures are described in Chapter 9.

Desirability of Eliminating Judges Who Did Not Appear to Follow Instructions.

There are a few judges on almost every panel whose ratings are so different from those of the others that it appears likely they failed to follow instructions. Should the ratings of such judges be thrown out? Unfortunately, this isn't an easy question to answer. It is usually quite difficult to discriminate between judges who did not follow instructions and judges who did follow instruction but reacted to the stimuli differently than the other panel members. Suppose, for example, that a judge who was instructed to rate a set of stimuli by the method of equal-appearing intervals assigned 1s, 4s, and 7s to the stimuli. While it is likely that he or she failed to follow instructions, it is possible that all the stimuli fell at one of these points on his or her internally generated scale.

If the ratings of only a small proportion of the members of a panel are questionable, the scale values would probably not be influenced very much by including them. There would be no need in such a case to throw them out. If, on the other hand, a relatively high percentage of the members of a panel assigned ratings in a manner that suggested they were not following instructions, it would be important to determine whether this was the case. If it were established that they were not following instructions, it would be justifiable to throw out their ratings.

Use of Multiple Regression for Inferring Characteristics of the Stimuli That Influenced Judges' Ratings.   A speech-language pathologist or audiologist may on occasion wish to answer a question such as the following:

1. What aspects of a stutterer's communicative behavior are apt to influence observers' judgments of his or her stuttering severity?
2. What aspects of the communicative behavior of an esophageal speaker are apt to influence observers' judgments of the "acceptability" of his or her speech?

Obviously many aspects of communicative behavior could influence observer judgments such as these. A procedure will be outlined in this section that can be helpful in identifying relevant aspects. This procedure utilizes multiple regression analysis (see Chapter 9). Representative studies from the speech-language pathology literature in which it has been used include those of Jordan (1960) and Shriner and Sherman (1967).

The procedure can be summarized briefly as follows:

1. A set of stimuli is rated by one of the scaling methods for the attribute the investigator wishes to study. This attribute for the first question would be stuttering severity and for the second question would be acceptability of speech. A scale value is computed from these ratings for each of the stimuli in the set. (These scale values serve as the *dependent variable* in the multiple regression analysis.)

2. Aspects of the stimuli that the investigator feels may have influenced the observers' ratings are measured. One such aspect relevant to the first question would be stuttering frequency; to the second question, speaking rate. (These measures serve as the *independent variables* in the multiple regression analysis.)

3. A coefficient of multiple correlation (see Chapter 9) is computed between the dependent variable (i.e., the scale values) and the composite of the independent variables (i.e., the measures of the aspects of the stimuli the investigator felt may have influenced the observers' ratings). A multiple regression equation (see Chapter 9) is also computed. It is used for predicting the dependent variable from the independent variables.

4. Independent variables that do not appear to be related to the dependent variable are eliminated. Such variables are unlikely to have influenced the observers' ratings. The basic strategy here is to identify the independent variable that is least related to the observers' ratings and eliminate it. The coefficient of multiple correlation then is recomputed without this variable. If this coefficient is not significantly lower than the original one, the independent variable that is least related to the observers' ratings is identified and eliminated from among the remaining ones. The coefficient of multiple correlation is then recomputed. If it is not significantly (in a statistical sense) lower than the original one, the identification and elimination process is continued until the point is reached where a statistically significant difference exists between a multiple correlation coefficient computed on a reduced set of independent variables and the original multiple correlation coefficient. The independent variables remaining at this point are *hypothesized* to have influenced the observers' ratings. They are not, of course, the only independent variables that could have influenced the observers' ratings. There may have been other aspects of the stimuli which, if measured, would have been found to correlate with the observers' ratings.

Appendix D
Representative Regulations Governing the Use of Human Subjects

NUREMBERG CODE (1946)*

Note: The Nuremberg Code, which was one of the first attempts to regulate human experimentation, consists of ten points that delimit permissible experimentation on human subjects. It was motivated by abuses in such experimentation that occurred in Nazi Germany during World War II.

1. The voluntary consent of the human subject is absolutely essential. This means that the person involved should have legal capacity to give consent; should be so situated as to be able to exercise free power of choice, without the intervention of any element of force, fraud, deceit, duress, overreaching, or other ulterior form of constraint or coercion, and should have sufficient knowledge and comprehension of the elements of the subject matter involved as to enable him to make an understanding and enlightened decision. This latter element requires that before the acceptance of an affirmative decision by the experimental subject there should be made known to him the nature, duration, and purpose of the experiment; the method and means by which it is to be conducted, all inconveniences and hazards reasonably to be expected; and the effects upon his health or person which may possibly come from his participation in the experiment.

The duty and responsibility for ascertaining the quality of the consent rests upon each individual who initiates, directs or engages in the experiment. It is a personal duty and responsibility which may not be delegated to another with impunity.

2. The experiment should be such as to yield fruitful results for the good of society, unprocurable by other methods or means of study, and not random and unnecessary in nature.

3. The experiment should be so designed and based on the results of animal experimentation and a knowledge of the natural history of the disease or other problem under study that the anticipated results will justify the performance of the experiment.

4. The experiment should be so conducted as to avoid all unnecessary physical and mental suffering and injury.

5. No experiment should be conducted where there is an *a priori* reason

*Reprinted from "Permissible medical experiments" in *Trials of War Criminals before the Nuremberg Military Tribunals under Control Council Law No. 10: Nuremberg 1946 to April 1949*. Washington, D.C.: U.S. Government Printing Office (no date).

to believe that death or disabling injury will occur; except, perhaps, in those experiments where the experimental physicians also serve as subjects.

6. The degree of risk to be taken should never exceed that determined by the humanitarian importance of the problem to be solved by the experiment.

7. Proper preparations should be made and adequate facilities provided to protect the experimental subject against even remote possibilities of injury, disability, or death.

8. The experiment should be conducted only by scientifically qualified persons. The highest degree of skill and care should be required through all stages of the experiment of those who conduct or engage in the experiment.

9. During the course of the experiment the human subject should be at liberty to bring the experiment to an end if he has reached the physical or mental state where continuation of the experiment seems to him to be impossible.

10. During the course of the experiment the scientist in charge must be prepared to terminate the experiment at any stage, if he has probable cause to believe, in the exercise of the good faith, superior skill and careful judgment required of him that a continuation of the experiment is likely to result in injury, disability, or death of the experimental subject.

DECLARATION OF HELSINKI (1964)*

Note: This document has replaced the Nuremberg Code to some extent. The recommendations contained in it for conducting experiments using human subjects have been adopted by the World Medical Association. It represents one of the first attempts by the international scientific community to regulate human experimentation. Though its emphasis is medical, most of the recommendations are applicable to research in speech-language pathology and audiology. You may wish to substitute the word "clinician" for "doctor" while reading it. A somewhat expanded version of this code was adopted by the World Medical Association in 1975.

Introduction

It is the mission of the doctor to safeguard the health of the people. His knowledge and conscience are dedicated to the fulfillment of this mission. . . .

Because it is essential that the results of laboratory experiments be applied to human beings to further scientific knowledge and to help suffering humanity, the World Medical Association has prepared the following recommendations as a guide to each doctor in clinical research. It must be stressed

*Reprinted with permission of *The World Medical Journal.*

that the standards as drafted are only a guide to physicians all over the world. Doctors are not relieved from criminal, civil and ethical responsibilities under the laws of their own countries.

In the field of clinical research a fundamental distinction must be recognized between clinical research in which the aim is essentially therapeutic for a patient, and the clinical research, the essential object of which is purely scientific and without therapeutic value to the person subjected to the research.

I. *Basic Principles*

1. Clinical research must conform to the moral and scientific principles that justify medical research and should be based on laboratory and animal experiments or other scientifically established facts.

2. Clinical research should be conducted only by scientifically qualified persons and under the supervision of a qualified medical man.

3. Clinical research cannot legitimately be carried out unless the importance of the objective is in proportion to the inherent risk to the subject.

4. Every clinical research project should be preceded by careful assessment of inherent risks in comparison to foreseeable benefits to the subject or to others.

5. Special caution should be exercised by the doctor in performing clinical research in which the personality of the subject is liable to be altered by drugs or experimental procedure.

II. *Clinical Research Combined with Professional Care*

1. In the treatment of the sick person, the doctor must be free to use a new therapeutic measure, if in his judgment it offers hope of saving life, reestablishing health, or alleviating suffering.

   If at all possible, consistent with patient psychology, the doctor should obtain the patient's freely given consent after the patient has been given a full explanation. In case of legal incapacity, consent should also be procured from the legal guardian; in the case of physical incapacity the permission of the legal guardian replaces that of the patient.

2. The doctor can combine clinical research with professional care, the objective being the acquisition of new medical knowledge, only to the extent that clinical research is justified by its therapeutic value for the patient.

III. *Non-Therapeutic Clinical Research*

1. In the purely scientific application of clinical research carried out on a human being, it is the duty of the doctor to remain the protector of the life and health of that person on whom clinical research is being carried out.

2. The nature, the purpose and the risk of clinical research must be explained to the subject by the doctor.

3a. Clinical research on a human being cannot be undertaken without his free consent after he has been informed; if he is legally incompetent, the consent of the legal guardian should be procured.

3b. The subject of clinical research should be in such a mental, physical and legal state as to be able to exercise fully his power of choice.

3c. Consent should, as a rule, be obtained in writing; However, the responsibility for clinical research always remains with the research worker; it never falls on the subject even after consent is obtained.

4a. The investigator must respect the right of each individual to safeguard his personal integrity, especially if the subject is in a dependent relationship to the investigator.

4b. At any time during the course of clinical research the subject or his guardian should be free to withdraw permission for research to be continued.

   The investigator or the investigating team should discontinue the research if in his or their judgment, it may, if continued, be harmful to the individual.

Glossary

Many of the terms relevant to statistics and research design that were used in this book are briefly defined here. For definitions of other terms or for more complete definitions of those defined, consult the index. For a glossary of symbols used in Appendix A, see p. 294. Words set in CAPITAL LETTERS are defined elsewhere in the Glossary.

Alpha Level. See LEVEL OF CONFIDENCE.

Answerable Question. A question that can be answered by observations which can be made and that implicitly or explicitly (preferably the latter) specifies the observation or observations necessary to answer it.

Applied Research. RESEARCH that implicitly or explicitly is intended to increase our understanding of how to prevent the development of, or modify behaviors contributing to, communicative disorders.

Attributes of Events. Measurable or verbally describable properties of EVENTS.

"Before and After" Design. Research design in which measures are made before and after the administration of a TREATMENT (e.g., a therapy program).

Bivariate Distribution. A DISTRIBUTION in which observations are assigned to categories on the basis of two of their ATTRIBUTES.

Causality. Assumption of the scientific method that every event has a cause.

Chance. See RANDOM FLUCTUATION.

Clinician-Investigator. A speech-language pathologist or audiologist who functions as both a clinician and a clinical investigator.

Confidence Interval. An INFERENTIAL STATISTIC for estimating POPULATION values of DESCRIPTIVE STATISTICS and differences between such statistics.

Constant Sums. A PSYCHOLOGICAL SCALING METHOD.

Correlation Coefficient. An INDEX OF ASSOCIATION.

Criterion Measure. A measure of an ATTRIBUTE of an EVENT.

Cubic Relationship. A NONLINEAR RELATIONSHIP between VARIABLES (see Figure 6.6).

Curvilinear Relationship. A NONLINEAR RELATIONSHIP between VARIABLES (see Figure 6.5).

Data. Symbolic representations (numerical or verbal description) of ATTRIBUTES of EVENTS. See QUALITATIVE and QUANTITATIVE DATA.

Degrees of Freedom. This value for a set of DATA designates the DISTRIBUTION in a table that contains the critical value of the statistic for testing the NULL HYPOTHESIS.

Dependent Measures. Sets of measures made on the same subjects or on matched groups of subjects.

Dependent Variable. A VARIABLE whose value one seeks to determine.

Descriptive Statistics. Indices that describe an ATTRIBUTE of a set of measures. See MEASURES OF ASSOCIATION, CENTRAL TENDENCY, and VARIABILITY.

df. Abbreviation for DEGREES OF FREEDOM.

Direct Magnitude-Estimation. A PSYCHOLOGICAL SCALING METHOD.

Distribution. A set of categories to which measures are assigned. See BIVARIATE, MULTIVARIATE, and UNIVARIATE DISTRIBUTIONS.

End Effect. A piling up of ratings in one or both of the extreme intervals when the method of EQUAL-APPEARING INTERVALS is used.

Equal-Appearing Intervals. A PSYCHOLOGICAL SCALING METHOD.

Event. A phenomenon that occurs in a certain place during a particular interval of time.

Experimental Condition. A set of circumstances under which observations are made.

Experimenter Bias. The impact of an experimenter's expectations and beliefs on his or her observations.

Extensional Definition. Pointing to or exhibiting in some way the actual objects, phenomena, and so on which the term you wish to define refers to.

Face Validity. Refers to a test or observational procedure intuitively appearing to be valid for the purpose intended.

Generality. The extent to which the persons or events observed are representative of those in the POPULATION to which a question refers.

Hypothesis. A tentative theory adopted to explain certain observations.

Independent Measures. Sets of measures made on different groups of persons.

Independent Variable. A VARIABLE whose values are known.

Index of Association. See MEASURE OF ASSOCIATION.

Index of Central Tendency. See MEASURE OF CENTRAL TENDENCY.

Index of Variability. See MEASURE OF VARIABILITY.

Inferential Statistics. Indices that allow one to answer several kinds of questions about a set of data that go beyond analyses that were made of it. See SIGNIFICANCE TESTS and CONFIDENCE INTERVALS.

Interval Scale. A measurement SCALE in which NUMERALS designate points on a continuum which have equal amounts of the ATTRIBUTE being MEASURED between them.

Laboratory Setting. An artificial controlled environment in which observations are made.

Level of Confidence. States how small the PROBABILITY of a NULL HYPOTHESIS being true has to be before it is rejected. See SIGNIFICANCE TESTS.

Linear Relationship. When two VARIABLES are linearly related, an increase (or decrease) in the magnitude of one is associated with a proportional increase (or decrease) in the magnitude of the other. The points in a SCATTERGRAM for two VARIABLES that are linearly related lie on a straight line.

Logarithmic Scale. A measurement SCALE in which NUMERALS designate points on a continuum which have unequal, but known, mathematically defined amounts of the ATTRIBUTE being MEASURED between them.

Mean. An INDEX OF CENTRAL TENDENCY which is the arithmetic average of a set of measures.

Measurement. The assignment of NUMERALS to ATTRIBUTES of EVENTS according to rules.

Measurement Error. Various forms of RANDOM and SYSTEMATIC ERROR which influence the RELIABILITY of observations.

Measures of Association. Indices used to describe the strength and direction of the relationships between sets of measures.

Measures of Central Tendency. Indices that designate the "average," "typical," or most frequently occurring NUMERAL in a set of numerals. See MEAN, MEDIAN, and MODE.

Measures of Variability. Indices that designate the spread, dispersion, homogeneity, or variability of a set of NUMERALS.

Median.   An INDEX OF CENTRAL TENDENCY; it is that measure which occurs at the mid-point of a set of measures when they are ordered from lowest to highest (or from highest to lowest).

Mode.   An INDEX OF CENTRAL TENDENCY; it is the most frequently occurring measure in a set of measures.

Multivariate Distribution.   A DISTRIBUTION in which observations are assigned to categories on the basis of two or more of their attributes.

N.   Abbreviation for number of subjects.

Negative Relationship.   A relationship between two VARIABLES in which individuals who tend to score highly on one tend to have relatively low scores on the other, and vice versa (see Figure 6.4).

Nominal Scale.   A measurement SCALE in which NUMERALS merely designate, or label, categories.

Nonlinear Relationship.   When two VARIABLES are not linearly related, an increase (or decrease) in the magnitude of one is not associated with a proportional increase (or decrease) in the magnitude of the other. The points in a SCATTERGRAM for the two VARIABLES would not lie on a straight line.

Nonrandom Sample.   A SAMPLE that was not generated by a RANDOM SAMPLING METHOD.

Normal Distribution.   A symmetrical, bell-shaped curve in which certain relationships hold regarding its height at specified distances from its center (see Figure 9.1).

Null Hypothesis.   The hypothesis tested by a SIGNIFICANCE TEST; it states that observed differences or relationships are due to CHANCE, or RANDOM FLUCTUATION.

Numerals.   Number symbols; their meanings are determined by the rules used to assign them.

One-Tailed Test.   A SIGNIFICANCE TEST intended to detect a difference between measures (e.g., means) in one direction only.

Order Effect.   A phenomenon that systematically improves or impairs a subject's performance on a series of tasks (e.g., fatigue).

Ordinal Scale.   A measurement SCALE in which NUMERALS designate locations in a rank order.

Organismic Variables. Properties, or ATTRIBUTES, of the individual. Examples are sex, chronological age, and educational level.

Paired Comparison.   A PSYCHOLOGICAL SCALING METHOD.

Placebo Effect.   Changes produced by placebos, i.e., therapeutic procedures that are objectively without specific activity for the condition being treated.

Population.   The group of persons to whom a question refers.

Positive Relationship.   A relationship between two VARIABLES in which individuals who tend to score highly on one also tend to score highly on the other, and vice versa.

Probability.   The likelihood of the occurrence of an event.

Psychological Scaling Methods.   Techniques for MEASURING, or quantifying, ATTRIBUTES of EVENTS through the use of observer judgments.

Pure Research.   Research that implicitly or explicitly is intended to increase our understanding of the etiology of communicative disorders.

Qualitative Data (or Concepts).   Verbal descriptions of ATTRIBUTES of EVENTS.

Quantitative Data (or Concepts).   Numerical descriptions of ATTRIBUTES of EVENTS.

Random Error.   A form of error present to some degree in all MEASUREMENT processes that does not bias the data resulting from such processes.

Random Fluctuation. Unpredictable variation in measures of ATTRIBUTES of EVENTS.

Random Sample. A SAMPLE selected by a random sampling process, e.g., a table of random numbers.

Ratio Scale. A measurement SCALE in which NUMERALS designate points on a continuum which both have equal amounts of an ATTRIBUTE between them and are related to an absolute 0.

Reliability. This refers to the repeatability of the observations used to answer a question.

Replication. Repetition of a study or observational procedure used to answer a question or questions.

Representativeness. Refers to the extent to which the ATTRIBUTES of the persons or EVENTS in a SAMPLE are similar to those in the POPULATION from which the sample was selected.

Research. This refers to the processes underlying the asking and answering of questions. See APPLIED RESEARCH and PURE RESEARCH.

Research Hypothesis. The hypothesis an investigator seeks to test.

Sample. Part of a POPULATION.

Scale. A succession or progression of steps or degrees, or a graduated series of categories.

Scale Value. The point, or value, on a SCALE to which an event (e.g., speech segment) is assigned. Scale values are computed for ratings generated by PSYCHOLOGICAL SCALING METHODS.

Scaling Methods. See PSYCHOLOGICAL SCALING METHODS.

Scattergram. A two-dimensional graphical display used for assessing the relationship between two variables (see Figures 6.2 through 6.7).

Scientific Method. A set of rules for asking and answering questions.

Sequence Effect. Occurs when a subject's performance on a task is enhanced or impaired by his having performed a particular task prior to it.

Significance Tests. INFERENTIAL STATISTICS used to estimate the PROBABILITY that observed differences and relationships between DESCRIPTIVE STATISTICS resulted from RANDOM FLUCTUATION.

Statistical Inference. Statistical techniques that provide information needed to generalize beyond a set of DATA or SAMPLE of subjects. See CONFIDENCE INTERVALS and SIGNIFICANCE TESTS.

Statistically Significant Result. A finding is regarded as statistically significant if the NULL HYPOTHESIS is rejected.

Statistics. Numerical procedures for analyzing, organizing, and summarizing QUANTITATIVE DATA. See DESCRIPTIVE STATISTICS and INFERENTIAL STATISTICS.

Subject Bias. Results from subjects responding to experimental conditions in the manner in which they feel the experimenter either would like them to respond or expects them to respond.

Successive Intervals. A PSYCHOLOGICAL SCALING METHOD.

Systematic Error. A form of error that can be present in a MEASUREMENT process which can bias the DATA resulting from that process.

Systematic Observation. A process that permits individual ATTRIBUTES of EVENTS to be described with adequate levels of RELIABILITY and VALIDITY.

Treatment. An experimental condition under which subjects are observed.

Two-Tailed Test. A SIGNIFICANCE TEST intended to detect a difference between measures (e.g., means) in either direction.

Type I Error. Rejection of the NULL HYPOTHESIS when it should not have been rejected, i.e., when the observed difference or relationship really was the result of RANDOM FLUCTUATION.

Type II Error.   Failure to reject the NULL HYPOTHESIS when it should have been rejected.

Univariate Distribution.   A DISTRIBUTION in which observations are assigned to categories on the basis of one of their ATTRIBUTES.

Validity.   The appropriateness of observations for answering a question they are used to answer.

Variable.   A quantity that can assume more than one value. See DEPENDENT VARIABLE and INDEPENDENT VARIABLE.

References

AGNEW, N. M., & PYKE, S. W. (1975). *The Science Game*. Englewood Cliffs, N.J.: Prentice-Hall.

ALBRIGHT, R. G. (1988). *A Basic Guide to Online Information Systems for Health Care Professionals*. Arlington, Va.: Information Resources Press.

ANGLE, E. (1907). *Malocclusion of the Teeth* (7th Ed.). Philadelphia: S. S. White Dental Manufacturing Company.

ATTANASIO, J. S. (1986). Therapy and research: Response to Siegel and Spradlin (1985). *Journal of Speech and Hearing Disorders, 51,* 378.

BAER, D. M., WOLF, M. M., & RISLEY, T. R. (1968). Some current dimensions in applied behavior analysis. *Journal of Applied Behavior Analysis, 1,* 91–97.

BARBER, T. X. (1976). *Pitfalls in Human Research*. New York: Pergamon Press.

BARLOW, D. H., & HAYES, S. C. (1979). Alternating treatments design: One strategy for comparing the effects of two treatments on a single subject. *Journal of Applied Behavior Analysis, 12* (2), 199–210.

BARLOW, D. H., & HERSEN, M. (1973). Single-case experimental designs: Uses in applied clinical research. *Archives of General Psychiatry, 29,* 319–325.

BARLOW, D. H., & HERSEN, M. (1984). *Single Case Experimental Designs: Strategies for Studying Behavior Change* (2nd Ed.). New York: Pergamon Press.

BEASLEY, D. S., & MANNING, J. I. (1973). Experimenter bias and speech pathologists' evaluation of children's language skills. *Journal of Communication Disorders, 6,* 93–101.

BENCH, R. J. (1989). Science and theory in communication disorders: A response to Siegel and Ingham (1987). *Journal of Speech and Hearing Disorders, 54,* 296–298.

BENNETT, M. J., & WEATHERBY, L. A. (1982). Newborn acoustic reflexes to noise and pure-tone signals. *Journal of Speech and Hearing Research, 25,* 383–387.

BERKMAN, R. I. (1990). *Find It Fast*. New York: Harper & Row.

BERRY, R. C., & SILVERMAN, F. H. (1972). Equality of intervals on the Lewis-Sherman scale of stuttering severity. *Journal of Speech and Hearing Research, 15,* 185–188.

BERRY, W. R., DARLEY, F. L., ARONSON, A. E., & GOLDSTEIN, N. P. (1974). Dysarthria in Wilson's disease. *Journal of Speech and Hearing Research, 17,* 160–183.

BEST, J. W., & KAHN, J. V. (1989). *Research in Education* (6th Ed.). Englewood Cliffs, N.J.: Prentice-Hall.

BIRNBAUER, J. S., PETERSON, C. R., & SOLNICK, J. V. (1974). Design and interpretation of studies of single subjects. *American Journal of Mental Deficiency, 79,* 191–203.

BLOODSTEIN, O. (1987). *A Handbook on Stuttering*. Chicago: National Easter Seal Society for Crippled Children and Adults.

BLOODSTEIN, O. (1988). Science in communication disorders: Letter to the editor. *Journal of Speech and Hearing Disorders, 53,* 347–348.

BLOOM, C. M., & SILVERMAN, F. H. (1973). Do all stutterers adapt? *Journal of Speech and Hearing Research, 16,* 518–521.

BORDEN, G. J., & HARRIS, K. S. (1980). *Speech Science Primer*. Baltimore: Williams & Wilkins.

BORGMAN, C. L., MOGHDAM, D., & CORBETT, P. K. (1984). *Effective Online Searching.* New York: Marcel Dekker.

BRIDGMAN, P. W. (1927). *The Logic of Modern Physics.* New York: The Macmillan Company.

BRIGGS, J., & PEAT, F. D. (1989). *Turbulent Mirrors: An Illustrated Guide to Chaos Theory and the Science of Wholeness.* New York: Harper & Row.

BROMLEY, D.B. (1986). *The Case-study Method in Psychology and Related Disciplines.* New York: John Wiley & Sons.

BROOKSHIRE, R. H. (1983). Subject description and generality of results in experiments with aphasic adults. *Journal of Speech and Healing Disorders,* 48, 342–346.

BUCKLEY, W. (Ed.) (1968). *Modern Systems Research for the Behavioral Scientist.* Chicago: Aldine Publishing Company.

BUSH, S. G. (1974). Should the history of science be rated X? *Science,* 183, 1164–1172.

CAMPBELL, D. T. (1963). From description to experimentation: Interpreting trends as quasi-experiments. In C. W. Harris (Ed.), *Problems in Measuring Change.* Madison: University of Wisconsin Press, 212–242.

CAMPBELL, D. T., & STANLEY, J. C. (1966). *Experimental and Quasi-Experimental Designs for Research.* Chicago: Rand McNally.

CAMPBELL, S. K. (1974). *Flaws and Fallacies in Statistical Thinking.* Englewood Cliffs, N. J. Prentice-Hall.

CATLETT, C. (1989). Constructing a competitive proposal. *Asha,* 31 (2), 70–72.

CHADWICK, B. A., BAHR, H. M., & ALBRECHT, S. L. (1984). *Social Science Research Methods.* Englewood Cliffs, N.J.: Prentice-Hall.

CHRISTENSEN, M., & HANSON, M. (1981). An investigation of the efficacy of oral myofunctional therapy as a precursor to articulation therapy for pre-first grade children. *Journal of Speech and Hearing Disorders,* 47, 160–167.

CLARK, J. G., & STEMPLE, J. C. (1982). Assessment of three modes of alaryngeal speech with a synthetic sentence identification (SSI) task in varying message-to-completion ratios. *Journal of Speech and Hearing Research,* 25, 333–338.

CODE, C., & BALL, M. (Eds.) (1984). *Instrumentation in Speech-Language Pathology.* San Diego: College-Hill.

CONNELL, P. J., & THOMPSON, C. K. (1986). Flexibility of single-subject experimental designs. Part III: Using flexibility to design or modify experiments. *Journal of Speech and Hearing Disorders,* 51, 204–214.

COOK, T. D., & CAMPBELL, D. T. (1979). *Quasi-experimentation.* Boston: Houghton Mifflin.

COSTELLO, J. M. (1979). Clinicians and researchers: A necessary dichotomy? *Journal of the National Student Speech and Hearing Association,* 7, 6–26.

CUDAHY, E. (1988). *Introduction to Instrumentation in Speech and Hearing.* Baltimore: Williams and Wilkins.

CULATTA, R. A. (1984). Why articles don't get published in Asha. *Asha,* 26 (3), 25–27.

CURETON, E. E., & D'AGOSTINO, R. B. (1983). *Factor Analysis: An Applied Approach.* Hillsdale, N.J.: L. Erlbaum Associates.

CURTIS, J. F., & SCHULTZ, M. C. (1986). *Basic Laboratory Instrumentation for Speech and Hearing.* Boston: Little, Brown.

CUVO, A. J. (1979). Multiple-baseline design in instructional research: Pitfalls of measurement and procedural advantages. *American Journal of Mental Deficiency,* 84, 219–228.

DANILOFF, J. K., NOLL, J. D., FRISTOE, M., & LLOYD, L. L. (1982). Gestural recognition in patients with aphasia. *Journal of Speech and Hearing Disorders,* 47, 43–49.

DARLEY, F. L., & SPRIESTERSBACH, D. C. (1978). *Diagnostic Methods in Speech Pathology* (2nd Ed.). New York: Harper and Row, Publishers.

DAVIDSON, P. O., & COSTELLO, C. G. N. (1969). $N = 1$: *Experimental Studies of Single Cases*. New York: Van Nostrand-Reinhold.

DAVISON, M. L. (1983). *Multidimensional Scaling*. New York: Wiley.

DECKER, T. N. (1989). *Instrumentation: An Introduction for Students in Speech and Hearing Sciences*. White Plains, N.Y.: Longman.

DOWELL, R. C. et al. (1982). A 12-consonant confusion study of a multiple-channel cochlear implant patient. *Journal of Speech and Hearing Research, 25,* 509–516.

DOYLE, P. C. (1990). A SINDSCAL analysis of perceptual features for consonants produced by esophageal and tracheoesophageal talkers. *Journal of Speech and Hearing Disorders, 55,* 756–760.

DUFFY, J. R., WATT, J., & DUFFY, R. J. (1981). Path analysis: A strategy for investigating multivariate causal relationships in communication disorders. *Journal of Speech and Hearing Research, 24,* 474–490.

DUKES, W. F. (1965). $N = 1$. *Psychological Bulletin, 64,* 74–79.

EBEL, R. (1951). Estimation of the reliability of ratings. *Psychometrika, 16,* 407–424.

EDGAR, E., & BILLINGSLEY, F. (1974). Believability when $N = 1$. *Psychological Record, 24,* 147–160.

EDGINGTON, E. S. (1967). Statistical inference from $N = 1$ experiments. *Journal of Psychology, 65,* 195–199.

EDGINGTON, E. S. (1972). $N = 1$ experiments: Hypothesis testing. *Canadian Psychology, 13,* 121–135.

EDGINGTON, E. S. (1984). Statistics and single case analysis. In M. Hersen, R. M. Eisler, & P. M. Miller (Eds.), *Progress in Behavior Modification* (Volume 16). Orlando: Academic Press.

EDWARDS, A. L. (1957). *Techniques of Attitude Scale Construction*. New York: Appleton-Century-Crofts.

EDWARDS, A. L., & CRONBACH, L. J. (1966). Experimental design for research in psychotherapy. In Arnold P. Goldstein and Stanford J. Dean (Eds.), *The Investigation of Psychotherapy: Commentaries and Readings*. New York: John Wiley and Sons, Inc., 71–79.

EINSTEIN, A., & INFELD, L. (1938). *The Evolution of Physics*. New York: Simon and Schuster.

ELBERT, M., SHELTON, R. L., & ARNDT, W. B. (1967). A task for evaluation of articulation change: I. Development of methodology. *Journal of Speech and Hearing Research, 10,* 281–288.

ELLIOTT, C. R. (1951). *Bibliography of stuttering*. Evanston, Ill.: The Book Box.

ELLIOTT, L. L., HAMMER, M. A., & SCHOLL, M. E. (1989). Fine-grained auditory discrimination in normal children and children with language-learning problems. *Journal of Speech and Hearing Research, 32,* 112–119.

FEIGL, H. (1953). The scientific outlook: Naturalism and humanism. In Herbert Feigl and May Brodbeck (Eds.), *Readings in the Philosophy of Science*. New York: Appleton-Century-Crofts, 8–18.

FERGUSON, G. A. (1989). *Statistical Analysis in Psychology and Education* (6th Ed.). New York: McGraw-Hill.

FIMIAN, M. J., LIEBERMAN, R. J., & FASTENAU, P. S. (1991). Development and validation of an instrument to measure occupational stress in speech-language pathology. *Journal of Speech and Hearing Research, 34,* 439–446.

Final regulations amending basic HHS policy for the protection of human research subjects (1981). *Federal Register, 46,* 8366–8392.

FINN, P., & GLOW, M. (1990). Clinical implications from Meyers (1989) on preschool stutterers and their conversational partners: Too much ado about null. *Journal of Speech and Hearing Disorders*, 55, 172-173.

FITZ-GIBBON, C. T. (1984). Meta-analysis: An explication. *British Educational Research Journal*, 10, 135-144.

FITZ-GIBBON, C. T. (1986). In defence of randomized controlled trials, with suggestions about the possible use of meta-analysis. *British Journal of Disorders of Communication*, 21, 117-124.

FORSCHER, B. K., & WERTZ, R. T. (1970). Organizing the scientific paper. *Asha*, 12, 494-497.

FREUND, P. (Ed.) (1970). *Experimentation with Human Subjects*. New York: George Braziller.

FRIED, C. (1974). *Medical Experimentation: Personal Integrity and Social Policy*. New York: American Elsevier.

GARDNER, M. J., & ALTMAN, D. G. (1990). Confidence—and clinical importance—in research findings. *British Journal of Psychiatry*, 156, 472-474.

GELATT, J. P. (1989). Obtaining grant funding: Ten steps to success. *Asha*, 31 (2), 67-69.

GELFAND, S. A., PIPER, N., & SILMAN, S. (1983). Effects of hearing levels at the activator and other frequencies upon the expected levels of the acoustic reflex threshold. *Journal of Speech and Hearing Disorders*, 48, 11-17.

GENTILE, J. R., RODEN, A. H., & KLEIN, R. D. (1972). An analysis of variance model for the intrasubject replication design. *Journal of Applied Behavior Analysis*, 5, 193-198.

GLASS, G. V., McGAW, B., & SMITH, M. L. (1981). *Meta-analysis in Social Research*. Beverly Hills, Calif.: Sage Publications.

GLASS, G. V., WILSON, V. L., & GOTTMAN, J. M. (1975). *Design and Analysis of Time-series Experiments*. Boulder: Colorado Associated University Press.

GOLDSTEIN, R. (1972). Presidential address: 1971 national convention. *Asha*, 14, 58-62.

GOLENPAUL, D. (Ed.) (1973). *Information Please Almanac, Atlas, and Yearbook 1974*. New York: Simon and Schuster.

GOODWIN, P. E. (1982). Ratings of professional journals by ASHA members. *Asha*, 24, 185-189.

GORSUCH, R. L. (1983). *Factor Analysis* (2nd Ed.). Hillsdale, N.J.: L. Erlbaum Associates.

GOSLING, C. G., KNIGHT, N. H., & McKENNEY, L. S. (1989). *Search PsycINFO*. Washington, D.C.: American Psychological Association.

GOTTMAN, J. M. (1973). N-of-one and N-of-two research in psychotherapy. *Psychological Bulletin*, 80, 93-105.

GOTTMAN, J. M. (1981). *Time-Series Analysis*. Cambridge: Cambridge University Press.

GOTTMAN, J. M., & GLASS, G. V. (1978). Analysis of interrupted time-series experiments. In Thomas R. Kratochwill (Ed.), *Single Subject Research—Strategies for Evaluating Change*. New York: Academic Press, 197-236.

GREEN, P. E. (1989). *Multidimensional Scaling: Concepts and Applications*. Boston: Allyn & Bacon.

GREENWALD, A. (1975). Consequences of prejudice against the null hypothesis. *Psychological Bulletin*, 82, 1-20.

GREENWALD, M. K., RYAN, M. K., & MULVIHILL, J. E. (Eds.) (1982). *Human Subject Research: A Handbook for Institutional Review Boards*. New York: Planum Press.

Guidelines for nonsexist language in journals of ASHA (1979). *Asha*, 21, 973-978.

GUILFORD, J. P. (1954). *Psychometric Methods*. New York: McGraw-Hill.

GUILFORD, J. P. (1978). *Fundamental Statistics in Psychology and Education* (6th Ed.). New York: McGraw-Hill.

HALL, M. (1988). *Getting Funded: A Complete Guide to Proposal Writing.* Portland, Oreg.: Continuing Education Publications.

HAMRE, C. E. (1972). Research and clinical practice: A unifying model. *Asha,* 14, 542–545.

HAYS, W. L. (1973). *Statistics for the Social Sciences.* New York: Holt, Reinhart and Winston.

HEAD, H. (1926). *Aphasia and Kindred Disorders of Speech.* New York: Cambridge University Press.

HEAD, H. (1963). *Aphasia and Kindred Disorders of Speech,* Vol. 1. New York: Hafner.

HEDGES, L. V., & OLKIN, I. (1985). *Statistical Methods for Meta-analysis.* New York: Academic Press.

HELM-ESTABROOKS, N., FITZPATRICK, P. M., & BARRESI, B. (1982). Visual action therapy for global aphasia. *Journal of Speech and Hearing Disorders,* 47, 385–389.

HEMPEL, C. G. (1952). *Fundamentals of Concept Formation in Empirical Science.* Chicago: University of Chicago Press.

HENERSON, M. E., MORRIS, L. L., & FITZ-GIBBON, C. T. (1987). *How to Measure Attitudes.* Beverly Hills, Calif: Sage Publications.

HENNEKENS, C. H., BURING, J. E., & HEBERT, P. R. (1987). Implications of overviews of randomized trials. *Statistics in Medicine,* 6 (3), 397–409.

HINDS, P. S., SCANDRETT-HIBDEN, S., & MCAULAY, L. S. (1990). Further assessment of a method to estimate reliability and validity of qualitative research findings. *Journal of Advanced Nursing,* 15 (4), 430–435.

HIRSHOREN, A., HURLEY, O. L., & KAVALE, K. (1979). Psychometric characteristics of the WISC-R Performance Scale with deaf children. *Journal of Speech and Hearing Disorders,* 44, 73–79.

HOLLAND, A. L. (1982). Observing functional communication of aphasics. *Journal of Speech and Hearing Disorders,* 47, 50–56.

HOLLAND, A. L., GREENHOUSE, J. B., FROMM, D., & SWINGELL, C. S. (1989). Predictors of language restitution following stroke: A multivariate analysis. *Journal of Speech and Hearing Research,* 32, 332–338.

HOLTZMAN, W. H. (1963). Statistical models for the study of change in the single case. In C. W. Harris (Ed.), *Problems in Measuring Change.* Madison: University of Wisconsin Press, 199–211.

HORNER, R. D., & BAER, D. M. (1978). Multiple-probe technique: A variation of the multiple baseline. *Journal of Applied Behavior Analysis,* 11 (1), 189–196.

How to be sure you don't get funded (1989). *Asha,* 31 (2), 76.

HOWARD, D. (1986). Beyond randomised controlled trials: The case for effective case studies of the effects of treatment in aphasia. *British Journal of Disorders of Communication,* 21, 89–102.

HSU, L. M. (1989). Random sampling, randomization, and equivalence of contrasted groups in psychotherapy outcome research. *Journal of Consulting and Clinical Psychology,* 57, 131–137.

HUNTER, J. E. (1982). *Cumulating Research Findings Across Studies.* Beverly Hills, Calif.: Sage Publications.

HUNTER, J. E., & SCHMIDT, F. L. (1990). *Meta-analysis: Correcting Error and Bias in Research Findings.* Beverly Hills, Calif.: Sage Publications.

ILER, K. L., DANHAUER, J. L., & MULAC, A. (1982). Peer perceptions of geriatrics wearing hearing aids. *Journal of Speech and Hearing Disorders,* 47, 433–438.

INGHAM, R. J., & SIEGEL, G. M. (1989). On statements and overstatements: A response to Bench (1989). *Journal of Speech and Hearing Disorders,* 54, 298–299.

IWAN, S. J., & SIEGEL, G. M. (1982). The effect of feedback on referential communication of preschool children. *Journal of Speech and Hearing Research*, 25, 224–229.

JERGER, J. (1960). Bekesy audiometry in analysis of auditory disorders. *Journal of Speech and Hearing Research*, 3, 275–287.

JERGER, J. (1962). Scientific writing can be readable. *Asha*, 4, 101–104.

JERGER, J. (1963a). Viewpoint. *Journal of Speech and Hearing Research*, 6, 203–206.

JERGER, J. (1963b). Who is qualified to do research? *Journal of Speech and Hearing Research*, 6, 301.

JERGER, J. (1964a). More on "Who is qualified to do research." *Journal of Speech and Hearing Research*, 7, 4–6.

JERGER, J. (1964b). Subject-oriented research. *Journal of Speech and Hearing Research*, 7, 207–208.

JERGER, J., & SPEAKS, C. (1967). Annual review of JSHR research, 1966. *Journal of Speech and Hearing Disorders*, 32, 197–211.

JOHNSON, W. (1946). *People in Quandaries*. New York: Harper and Row.

JOHNSON, W. and ASSOCIATES (1959). *The Onset of Stuttering*. Minneapolis: University of Minnesota Press.

JOHNSON, W., DARLEY, F. L., & SPRIESTERSBACH, D. C. (1963). *Diagnostic Methods in Speech Pathology*. New York: Harper and Row.

JORDAN, E. P. (1960). Articulation test measures and listener ratings of articulation defectiveness. *Journal of Speech and Hearing Research*, 3, 303–319.

Journals in Communication Sciences and Disorders (1991). Rockville, Md.: American Speech-Language-Hearing Association.

KATT, D., & SPRAGUE, H. (1981). Determining the pure-tone frequencies to be used in identification audiometry. *Journal of Speech and Hearing Disorders*, 46, 433–436.

KAZDIN, A. E. (1981). External validity and single case experimentation: Issues and limitations. *Analysis and Intervention in Developmental Disabilities*, 1, 133–143.

KAZDIN, A. E. (1982a). Single-case experimental designs in clinical research and practice. In A. E. Kazdin & A. H. Tuma (Eds.), *Single-case Research Designs*. San Francisco: Jossey-Bass, pp. 33–47.

KAZDIN, A. E. (1982b). *Single-Case Research Designs: Methods for Clinical and Applied Settings*. London: Oxford University Press.

KEARNS, K. P. (1986). Flexibility of single-subject experimental designs. Part II: Design selection and arrangement of experimental phases. *Journal of Speech and Hearing Disorders*, 51, 204–214.

KELLY, C. A., & DALE, P. S. (1989). Cognitive skills associated with the onset of multi-word utterances. *Journal of Speech and Hearing Research*, 32, 645–656.

KELLY, D. J., & MCREYNOLDS, L. V. (1987). The role of research in the clinic. Paper presented at the 1987 annual meeting of the American Speech-Language-Hearing Association, New Orleans.

KEMPSTER, G. B., KISTLER, D. J., & HILLENBRAND, J. (1991). Multidimensional scaling analysis of dysphonia for two speaker groups. *Journal of Speech and Hearing Research*, 34, 534–543.

KENDALL, P. C. (1981). Assessing generalization and the single subject strategies. *Behavior Modification*, 5 (3), 307–319.

KEPPEL, G. (1982). *Design and Analysis: A Researcher's Handbook* (2nd Ed.). Englewood Cliffs, N.J.: Prentice-Hall.

KIMBALL, A. W. (1957). Errors of the third kind in statistical consulting. *Journal of the American Statistical Association*, 52, 133–142.

KLITCH, R. J., & MAY, G. M. (1982). Spectrographic study of vowels in stutterers' fluent speech. *Journal of Speech and Hearing Research*, 25, 364–370.

KORZYBSKI, A. (1958). *Science and Sanity: An Introduction to Non-Aristotelian Systems and General Semantics.* Lakeville, Conn.: Institute of General Semantics.

KRAEMER, H. C., & THIEMANN, S. (1989). A strategy to use soft data effectively in randomized controlled clinical trials. *Journal of Consulting and Clinical Psychology,* 57, 148–154.

KRATOCHWILL, T. R. (Ed.) (1978). *Single Subject Research.* New York: Academic Press.

KRATOCHWILL, T. R., & BRODY, G. H. (1978). Single subject designs—A perspective on the controversy over employing statistical inference and implications for research and training in behavior modification. *Behavior Modification,* 2 (3), 291–307.

KRATOCHWILL, T. R., & LEVIN, J. R. (1980). On the applicability of various data analysis procedures to the simultaneous and alternating treatment designs in behavior therapy research. *Behavioral Assessment,* 2, 353–360.

KUBASKA, C. A., & KEATING, P. A. (1981). Word duration in early child speech. *Journal of Speech and Hearing Research,* 24, 615–621.

KUHN, T. S. (1962). *The Structure of Scientific Revolutions.* Chicago: University of Chicago Press.

LADIMER, I. (1970). Protection and compensation for injury in human studies. In Paul A. Freund (Ed.), *Experimentation with Human Subjects.* New York: George Braziller.

LADOUCEUR, R., COTE, C., LEBLOND, G., & BOUCHARD, L. (1982). Evaluation of regulated-breathing method and awareness training in the treatment of stuttering. *Journal of Speech and Hearing Disorders,* 47, 422–426.

LAIRD, N. M., & MOSTELLER, F. (1990). Some statistical methods for combining experimental results. *International Journal of Technology Assessment in Health Care,* 6 (1), 5–30.

LAMBERT, S. (1984). *Presentation Graphics on the Apple Macintosh.* Bellevue, Wash.: Microsoft Press.

LASKY, E., & Klopp, K. (1982). Parent-child interactions in normal and language-disordered children. *Journal of Speech and Hearing Disorders,* 47, 7–18.

LEITENBERG, H. (1973). The use of single case methodology in psychotherapy research. *Journal of Abnormal Psychology,* 82, 87–101.

LEVIN, J. R., MARASCUILO, L. A., & HUBERT, L. J. (1978). N = 1: Nonparametric randomization tests. In Thomas R. Kratochwill (Ed.), *Single Subject Research—Strategies for Evaluating Change.* New York: Academic Press, 167–196.

LEWIS, D., & SHERMAN, D. (1951). Measuring the severity of stuttering. *Journal of Speech and Hearing Disorders,* 16, 320–326.

LEWIS, K. E. (1991). The structure of disfluency behavior in the speech of adult stutterers. *Journal of Speech and Hearing Research,* 34, 492–500.

LIEBER, R. L. (1990). Statistical significance and statistical power in hypothesis testing. *Journal of Orthopedic Research,* 8 (2), 304–309.

LILLY, D. J., SHERMAN, D., COMPTON, A. J., FISHER, C. G., & CARNEY, P. J. (1968). Annual review of JSHR research, 1967. *Journal of Speech and Hearing Disorders,* 33, 303–317.

LINDQUIST, E. F. (1953). *Design and Analysis of Experiments in Psychology and Education.* Boston: Houghton Mifflin.

LINVILLE, S. E., SKARIN, B. D., & FORNATTO, E. (1989). The interrelationship of measures related to vocal function, speech rate, and laryngeal appearance in elderly women. *Journal of Speech and Hearing Research,* 32, 323–330.

LLOYD, L. L. (1980). Unaided nonspeech communication for severely handicapped individuals: An extensive bibliography. *Education and Training of the Mentally Retarded,* 15, 15–34.

LORE, J. I., & GUTTER, F. J. (1968). The embryogeny of an NIH research grant. *Asha,* 10, 7–9.

LUICK, A. H., KIRK, S. A., AGRANOWITZ, A., & BUSBY, R. (1982). Profiles of children with severe oral language disorders. *Journal of Speech and Hearing Disorders,* 47, 88–92.

MALLARD, A. R., HICKS, D. M., & RIGGS, D. E. (1982). A comparison of stutterers and nonstutterers in a task of controlled voice onset. *Journal of Speech and Hearing Research,* 25, 287–290.

MATT, G. E. (1989). Decision rules for effect sizes in meta-analysis: A review and reanalysis of psychotherapy outcome studies. *Psychological Bulletin,* 105, 106–115.

MCCALL, G. J., & SIMMONS, J. L. (1969). *Issues in Participant Observation: A Text and Reader.* Reading, Mass.: Addison-Wesley.

MCCULLOUGH, J. P. (1984). Single case investigative research and its relevance for the nonoperant clinician. *Psychotherapy,* 21, 382–388.

MCDONALD, R. P. (1985). *Factor Analysis and Related Methods.* Hillsdale, N.J.: L. Erlbaum Associates.

MCPHERSON, D. L., & THATCHER, J. W. (1977). *Instrumentation in the Hearing Sciences.* New York: Grune and Stratton.

MCREYNOLDS, L. V., & KEARNS, K. P. (1983). *Single-subject Experimental Designs in Communicative Disorders.* Baltimore: University Park Press.

MCREYNOLDS, L. V., & THOMPSON, C. K. (1986). Flexibility of single-subject experimental designs. Part I: Review of the basics of single-subject designs. *Journal of Speech and Hearing Disorders,* 51, 194–203.

MEITUS, I. J., RINGEL, R. L., HOUSE, A. S., & HOTCHKISS, J. C. (1973). Clinical bias in evaluating speech proficiency. *British Journal of Disorders of Communication,* 8, 146–151.

MERRIAM, S. B. (1988). *Case Study Research in Education: A Qualitative Approach.* San Francisco: Jossey-Bass.

MESLIN, E. M. (1990). Protecting human subjects from harm through improved risk judgments. *IRB: A Review of Human Subjects Research,* 12 (1), 7–10.

METZ, D. E., & FOLKINS, J. W. (1985). Protection of human subjects in speech and hearing research. *Asha,* 27 (3), 25–29.

METZ, D. E., SCHIEVATTI, N., SAMAR, V. J., & SITLER, R. W. (1990). Acoustic dimensions of hearing-impaired speakers' intelligibility: Segmental and suprasegmental characteristics. *Journal of Speech and Hearing Research,* 33, 476–487.

MEYERS, S. C. (1990). Tempest in a *t* test: A reply to Finn and Glow. *Journal of Speech and Hearing Disorders,* 55, 173–174.

MICHAEL, J. (1974). Statistical inference for individual organism research: Mixed blessing or curse? *Journal of Applied Behavior Analysis,* 7, 647–653.

MILES, J. (1987). *Design for Desktop Publishing.* San Francisco: Chronicle Books.

MOORE, M. V. (1969). Pathological writing. *Asha,* 11, 535–538.

MOWER, D. E. (1969). Evaluating speech therapy through precision recording. *Journal of Speech and Hearing Disorders,* 34, 329–344.

MOWER, D. E., WAHL, P., & DOOLAN, S. J. (1978). Effects of lisping on audience evaluation of male speakers. *Journal of Speech and Hearing Disorders,* 43, 140–148.

MURRAY, G. D. (1989). Confidence intervals. *Nuclear Medicine Communications,* 10 (6), 387–388.

MURRY, T. (1978). Speaking fundamental frequency characteristics associated with voice pathologies. *Journal of Speech and Hearing Disorders,* 43, 374–379.

NELSON, D. A., & PAVLOV, R. (1989). Auditory time constants for off-frequency forward masking in normal-hearing and hearing-impaired listeners. *Journal of Speech and Hearing Research,* 32, 298–306.

OHLSSON, A., BRINK, O., & LÖFQVIST, A. (1989). A voice accumulator—Validation and application. *Journal of Speech and Hearing Research,* 32, 451–457.

OLSWANG, L. B. (1990). Treatment efficacy research: A path to quality assurance. *Asha,* 32 (1), 45–47.

ORNE, M. T. (1969). Demand characteristics and the concept of quasi-controls. In Robert Rosenthal and Ralph L. Rosnow (Eds.), *Artifacts in Behavioral Research.* New York: Academic Press, 143–179.

OSGOOD, C. E., SUCI, G. J., & TANNENBAUM, P. H. (1957). *The Measurement of Meaning.* Urbana: University of Illinois Press.

PANUSH, R. (1989). The limits of science in communication disorders: A reply to Siegel. *Journal of Speech and Hearing Disorders,* 54, 301–302.

PAP, A. (1949). *Elements of Analytic Philosophy.* New York: The Macmillan Company.

PAP, A. (1953). Does science have metaphysical presuppositions? In Herbert Feigl and May Brodbeck (Eds.), *Readings in the Philosophy of Science.* New York: Appleton-Century-Crofts, 21–33.

PARSONSON, B. S., & BAER, D. M. (1978). The analysis and presentation of graphic data. In Thomas R. Kratochwill (Ed.), *Single Subject Research—Strategies for Evaluating Change.* New York: Academic Press, 101–166.

PAULOSKI, B. R., FISHER, H. B., KEMPSTER, G. B., & BLOM, E. D. (1989). Statistical differentiation of tracheoesophageal speech produced under four prosthetic/occlusion speaking conditions. *Journal of Speech and Hearing Research,* 32, 591–599.

PENNER, M. J., & BILGER, R. C. (1989). Adaptation and the masking of tinnitus. *Journal of Speech and Hearing Research,* 32, 339–346.

PERKINS, W. H. (1986). Functions and malfunctions of theories in therapies. *Asha,* 28 (2), 31–33.

PERKINS, W. H., & CURLEE, R. F. (1969). Causality in speech pathology. *Journal of Speech and Hearing Disorders,* 34, 231–238.

PEZZEI, C., & ORATIO, A. R. (1991). A multivariate analysis of the job satisfaction of public school speech-language pathologists. *Language, Speech, and Hearing Services in Schools,* 22, 139–146.

PFAFFENBERGER, B. (1990). *Democratizing Information: Online Databases and the Rise of End-User Searching.* Boston: G. K. Hall.

PlusNet2 Medline System: End-user Introduction (1990). New York: CD Plus.

POLANYI, M. (1967). *The Tacit Dimension.* Garden City, N.Y.: Doubleday Anchor Books.

PORCH, B. (1971). Multidimensional scoring in aphasia testing. *Journal of Speech and Hearing Research,* 14, 776–792.

PORTNOY, R. A., & ARONSON, A. E. (1982). Diadochokinetic syllable rate and regularity in normal and in spastic and ataxic dysarthric subjects. *Journal of Speech and Hearing Disorders,* 47, 324–328.

POWERS, M. H. (1955). The dichotomy in our profession. *Journal of Speech and Hearing Disorders,* 20, 4–10.

PRATHER, E. M. (1960). Scaling defectiveness of articulation by direct magnitude-estimation. *Journal of Speech and Hearing Research,* 3, 380–392.

Preparing a Research Grant Application to the National Institutes of Health (1989). Bethesda, Md.: National Institutes of Health.

PRING, T. R. (1986). Evaluating the effects of speech therapy for aphasics: Developing the single case methodology. *British Journal of Disorders of Communication,* 21, 103–115.

PRUTTING, C. A., MENTIS, M., & NELSON, P. (1989). Critique of Siegel: The limits of

"The Limits of Science in Communication Disorders." *Journal of Speech and Hearing Disorders*, 54, 299–300.

The Publication Process: A Guide for Authors (1991). Rockville, Md.: American Speech-Language-Hearing Association.

Publications Manual for the American Psychological Association (3rd Ed.) (1983). Washington, D.C.: American Psychological Association.

PURTILO, R., & CASSEL, C. K. (1981). *Ethical Dimensions in the Health Professions.* Philadelphia: W. B. Saunders.

RABUSH, D. R., LLOYD, L. L., & GERDES, M. (1982, 1983). Aided nonspeech communication: An extensive bibliography (Parts I, II, and III). *Communication Outlook*, 3 (4) and 4 (1, 2).

RADIL-WEISS, T. (1983). Men in extreme conditions: Some medical and psychological aspects of the Auschwitz Concentration Camp. *Psychiatry*, 46, 259–268.

REINER, B. J., & LUDLOW, C. L. (1979a). *MEDLINE Users Manual and Thesaurus for Specialists in Communicative Disorders*, Vol. I (Users Manual NIH 79-1997). Bethesda, Md.: U. S. Department of Health Services, Public Health Service, National Institutes of Health.

REINER, B. J., & LUDLOW, C. L. (1979b). *MEDLINE Users Manual and Thesaurus for Specialists in Communicative Disorders*, Vol. II (Thesaurus NIH 79-1998). Bethesda, Md.: U. S. Department of Health Services, Public Health Service, National Institutes of Health.

REINER, B. J., & LUDLOW, C. L. (1981). Using MEDLINE for literature retrieval in the communicative disorders. *Asha*, 23, 655–662.

REVUSKY, S. H. (1967). Some statistical treatments compatible with individual organism methodology. *Journal of Experimental Analysis of Behavior*, 10, 319–330.

RICKELS, K., SCHWEIZER, E., & CASE, W. G. (1988). The uncontrolled case report: A double-edged sword. *Journal of Nervous and Mental Diseases*, 176 (1), 50–52.

RINGEL, R. L. (1972). The clinician and the researcher: An artificial dichotomy. *Asha*, 14, 351–353.

RINGEL, R. L., TACHTMAN, L. E., & PRUTTING, C. A. (1984). The science in human communication sciences. *Asha*, 26 (12), 33–36.

RIZZO, J. M., & STEPHENS, M. I. (1981). Performance of children with normal and impaired oral language production on a set of auditory comprehension. *Journal of Speech and Hearing Disorders*, 46, 150–159.

ROCHON, J. (1990). A statistical model for the "N-of-1" study. *Journal of Clinical Epidemiology*, 43, 499–508.

ROSENTHAL, D., & FRANK, J. D. (1956). Psychotherapy and the placebo effect. *Psychological Bulletin*, 53, 294–302.

ROSENTHAL, R. (1963). On the social psychology of the psychological experiment: The experimenter's hypothesis as unintended determinant of experimental results. *American Scientist*, 51, 268–283.

ROSENTHAL, R. (1966). *Experimental Bias in Behavioral Research.* New York: Appleton-Century-Crofts.

ROSENTHAL, R. (1969). Interpersonal expectations: Effects of the experimenter's hypothesis. In Robert Rosenthal and Ralph L. Rosnow (Eds.), *Artifact in Behavioral Research.* New York: Academic Press, Inc., 182–277.

ROSENTHAL, R. (1976). *Experimenter Effects in Behavioral Research.* New York: Halsted Press.

ROSENTHAL, R. (1978). Combining results of independent studies. *Psychological Bulletin*, 85, 185–193.

ROSENTHAL, R., & ROSNOW, R. (1969). *Artifacts in Behavioral Research.* New York: Academic Press.

ROTH, C. R., ARONSON, A. E., & DAVIS, L. J., JR. (1989). Clinical studies in psychogenic stuttering of adult onset. *Journal of Speech and Hearing Disorders*, 54, 634–646.

RUSCH, F. R., & KAZDIN, A. E. (1981). Toward a methodology of withdrawal designs for the assessment of response maintenance. *Journal of Applied Behavior Analysis*, 14 (2), 131–140.

RYAN, B. F., JOINER, B. L., & RYAN, T. A., JR. (1985). *MINITAB Handbook* (2nd Ed., Revised Printing). Boston: PWS-KENT Publishing Company.

SARNO, M. T., & SANDS, E. (1967). A selected bibliography of acquired verbal impairment secondary to brain damage. *Rehabilitation Monographs*, 34.

SCHIFFMAN, S. S., REYNOLDS, M. L., & YOUNG, F. W. (1981). *Introduction to Multidimensional Scaling*. New York: Academic Press.

SCHOBER-PETERSON, D., & JOHNSON, C. J. (1989). Conversational topics of 4-year-olds. *Journal of Speech and Hearing Research*, 32, 857–870.

SCHUELL, H., JENKINS, J., & JIMENEZ-PABON, E. (1964). *Aphasia in Adults*. New York: Harper and Row.

SCHULTZ, M. C., ROBERTS, W. H., & YAIRI, E. (1972). The clinician and the researcher: Comments. *Asha*, 14, 539–541.

SEYMOUR, H. N., & SEYMOUR, C. M. (1981). Black English and Standard American English contrasts in consonantal development of four- and five-year-old children. *Journal of Speech and Hearing Disorders*, 46, 274–280.

SHAPIRO, A. K. (1964). Factors contributing to the placebo effect: Implications for psychotherapy. *American Journal of Psychotherapy*, 18 (Supplement 1), 73–88.

SHELTON, R. L., PAESANI, A., MCCLELLAND, K. D., & BRADFIELD, S. S. (1975). Panendoscope feedback in the study of voluntary velopharyngeal movements. *Journal of Speech and Hearing Disorders*, 40, 232–244.

SHERMAN, D., & SILVERMAN, F. H. (1968). Three psychological methods applied to language development. *Journal of Speech and Hearing Research*, 11, 837–841.

SHIPLEY, K. G. (Ed.) (1982). *A Style Manual for Writers in Communicative Disorders*. Tucson: Communication Skill Builders.

SHRIBERG, L. D., & KWIATKOWSKI, J. (1982). Phonological disorders III: A procedure for assessing severity of involvement. *Journal of Speech and Hearing Disorders*, 47, 256–270.

SHRINER, T. H., HOLLOWAY, M. S., & DANILOFF, R. G. (1969). The relationship between articulation defects and syntax in speech defective children. *Journal of Speech and Hearing Research*, 12, 319–325.

SHRINER, T. H., & SHERMAN, D. (1976). An equation for assessing language development. *Journal of Speech and Hearing Research*, 10, 41–48.

SIDMAN, M. (1960). *Tactics of Scientific Research*. New York: Basic Books.

SIEGEL, G. M. (1988). Science and communication disorders: A reply to Bloodstein. *Journal of Speech and Hearing Disorders*, 53, 348–349.

SIEGEL, G. M., & INGHAM, R. J. (1987). Theory and science in communication disorders. *Journal of Speech and Hearing Disorders*, 52, 99–104.

SIEGEL, G. M., & SPRADLIN, J. E. (1985). Therapy and research. *Journal of Speech and Hearing Disorders*, 50, 226–230.

SIEGEL, S. (1956). *Nonparametric Statistics for the Behavioral Sciences*. New York: McGraw-Hill.

SIEGEL, S. (1988). *Nonparametric Statistics for the Behavioral Sciences* (2nd Ed.). New York: McGraw-Hill.

SILVERMAN, E. M. (1972). Generality of disfluency data collected from preschoolers. *Journal of Speech and Hearing Research*, 5, 84–92.

SILVERMAN, F. H. (1967a). Correspondence between mean and median scale values for sets of stimuli scaled by the method of equal-appearing intervals. *Perceptual and Motor Skills*, 25, 727–728.

SILVERMAN, F. H. (1967b). Interpretation of mean Q values for sets of stimuli rated on a seven-point equal-appearing interval scale. *Perceptual and Motor Skills, 24,* 842 (1967).

SILVERMAN, F. H. (1968a). An approach to determining the number of judges needed for scaling experiments. *Perceptual and Motor Skills, 17,* 1333–1334.

SILVERMAN, F. H. (1968b). Intraclass correlation coefficient as an index of reliability of median scale values for sets of stimuli rated by equal-appearing intervals. *Perceptual and Motor Skills, 26,* 878.

SILVERMAN, F. H. (1977a). A bibliography of literature relevant to nonspeech communication modes for the speechless. *Ohio Journal of Speech and Hearing, 12,* 83–102.

SILVERMAN, F. H. (1977b). Criteria for assessing therapy outcome in speech pathology and audiology. *Journal of Speech and Hearing Research, 20,* 5–20.

SILVERMAN, F. H. (1978). Bibliography of literature pertaining to stuttering in elementary school children. *Journal of Fluency Disorders, 3,* 87–102.

SILVERMAN, F. H. (1983). *Legal Aspects of Speech-Language Pathology and Audiology.* Englewood Cliffs, N.J.: Prentice-Hall.

SILVERMAN, F. H. (1984). Speech-Language Pathology and Audiology: An Introduction. Columbus, Ohio: Merrill.

SILVERMAN, F. H. (1987). *Microcomputers in Speech-Language Pathology and Audiology.* Englewood Cliffs, N.J.: Prentice-Hall.

SILVERMAN, F. H. (1988). The "Monster" Study. *Journal of Fluency Disorders, 13,* 225–231.

SILVERMAN, F. H. (1989). *Communication for the Speechless* (2nd Ed.). Englewood Cliffs, N.J.: Prentice-Hall.

SILVERMAN, F. H. (1992). *Legal-Ethical Considerations, Restrictions, and Obligations for Clinicians Who Treat Communicative Disorders* (2nd Ed). Springfield, IL: Charles Thomas.

SILVERMAN, F. H., & JOHNSTON, R. G. (1975). Direct interval-estimation: A ratio scaling method. *Perceptual and Motor Skills, 41,* 464–466.

SILVERMAN, F. H., SILVERMAN, E.-M., & MEAGHER, M. (1979). Bibliography of literature pertaining to the onset, development, and treatment of stuttering during the preschool years. *Journal of Fluency Disorders, 4,* 171–203.

SILVERMAN, F. H., & TROTTER, W. D. (1973a). Bibliography: Literature related to the use of instrumental aids in stuttering therapy. *Perceptual and Motor Skills, 36,* 247–251.

SILVERMAN, F. H., & TROTTER, W. D. (1973b). Impact of pacing speech with a miniature electronic metronome upon the manner in which a stutterer is perceived. *Behavior Therapy, 4,* 414–419.

SILVERMAN, F. H., & WILLIAMS, D. E. (1973). Use of revision by elementary-school stutterers and nonstutterers during oral reading. *Journal of Speech and Hearing Research, 16,* 584–585.

SIMES, J. (1990). Meta-analysis: Its importance in cost-effectiveness studies. *Medical Journal of Australia, 153* (Supplement), 13–16.

SMITH, K. J., & ANDERSON, J. L. (1982). Relationship of perceived effectiveness to verbal interaction/content variables in supervisory conferences in speech-language pathology. *Journal of Speech and Hearing Research, 25,* 252–261.

SMITH, R. C., REID, W. M., & LUCHSINGER, A. E. (1980). *Smith's Guide to the Literature of the Life Sciences.* Minneapolis: Burgess Publishing Company.

SNIDER, J. G., & OSGOOD, C. E. (Eds.) (1968). *Semantic Differential Technique: A Sourcebook.* Chicago: Aldine Publishing Company.

SOMMERS, R. K. (1991). Approaches to the prediction of language abilities in a sample of children who have developmental delays. *Journal of Speech and Hearing Research*, 34, 317–324.

SPARKS, R. D. (1989). Matching ideas and funds. *Asha*, 31, (2), 77, 99.

STANLEY, B. (1985). Toward "applicable" single-case research. *Bulletin of the British Psychological Society*, 38, 33–36.

STEELE, J. A., BINNIE, C. A., & COOPER, W. A. (1978). Combining auditory and visual stimuli in the adaptive testing of speech discrimination. *Journal of Speech and Hearing Disorders*, 43, 115–122.

STEVENS, S. S. (1951). Mathematics, measurement, and psychophysics. In S. S. Stevens (Ed.), *Handbook of Experimental Psychology*. New York: John Wiley and Sons, 1–49.

STOUT, M. B. (1962). *Basic Electrical Measurements* (2nd Ed.). Englewood Cliffs, N.J.: Prentice-Hall.

STRAIN, P. S., & SHORES, R. E. (1979). Additional comments on multiple baseline designs in instructional research. *American Journal of Mental Deficiency*, 84, 229–234.

STUTT-L for researchers, clinicians (1990). *Asha*, 32 (2), 12.

SUMMERS, R. R. (1987). Research and training programs of the National Institute of Neurological and Communicative Disorders and Stroke. In Herbert J. Oyer (Ed.), *Administration of Programs in Speech-Language Pathology and Audiology*. Englewood Cliffs, N.J.: Prentice-Hall.

TALBOTT, R. E. (1969). Bacteriology of earphone contamination. *Journal of Speech and Hearing Research*, 12, 326–329.

The Task Force on Research (1989). *Asha*, 31 (9), 41–44.

TAWNEY, J. W., & GAST, D. L. (1984). *Single Subject Research in Special Education*. Columbus, Ohio: Charles C. Merrill.

THOMPSON, R. A. (1990). Behavioral research involving children: A developmental perspective on risk. *IRB: A Review of Human Subjects Research*, 12 (2), 1–6.

TOMES, L., & SHELTON, R. L. (1989). Children's categorization of consonants by manner and place characteristics. *Journal of Speech and Hearing Research*, 32, 432–438.

TOWNSEND, T. H., & OLSON, C. C. (1982). Performance of new hearing aids using the ANSI S3.22-1976 standard. *Journal of Speech and Hearing Disorders*, 47, 376–382.

TROTTER, W. D., & KOOLS, J. A. (1955). Listener adaptation to the severity of stuttering. *Journal of Speech and Hearing Disorders*, 29, 385–387.

TYLER, R. S., MOORE, B. C. J., & KUK, F. K. (1989). Performance of some of the better cochlear-implant patients. *Journal of Speech and Hearing Research*, 32, 887–911.

VAN RIPER, C. (1958). Experiments in stuttering therapy. In Jon Eisenson (Ed.), *Stuttering: A Symposium*. New York: Harper and Row, 273–390.

VAN RIPER, C. (1982). *The Nature of Stuttering* (2nd Ed.). Englewood Cliffs, N.J.: Prentice-Hall.

VILLARRUEL, F., MATHY-LAIKKO, P., RATCLIFF, A., & YODER, D. (1987). *Alternative and Augmentative Communication Bibliography*. Madison: Trace Research & Development Center, University of Wisconsin.

WACHTER, K. W., & STRAF, M. E. (Eds.) (1990). *The Future of Meta-analysis*. New York: Russell Sage Foundation.

WATSON, P. J., & WORKMAN, E. A. (1981). The non-concurrent multiple baseline across-individuals design: An extension of the traditional multiple baseline design. *Journal of Behavior Therapy and Experimental Psychiatry*, 12 (3), 257–259.

WEBB, E. J., CAMPBELL, D. T., SCHWARTZ, R. D., & SCHREST, L. (1966). *Unobtrusive Measures: Nonreactive Research in the Social Sciences*. Chicago: Rand McNally.

WEISMER, G., & ELBERT, M. (1982). Temporal characteristics of "functionally" misarticulated /s/ in 4- to 6-year-old children. *Journal of Speech and Hearing Research, 25,* 275–287.

WEISS-LAMBROU, R. (1989). *The Health Professionals Guide to Writing for Publication.* Springfield, Ill.: Charles C. Thomas.

WESTON, A. D., SHRIBERG, L. D., & MILLER, J. F. (1989). Analysis of language-speech samples with Salt and Pepper. *Journal of Speech and Hearing Research, 32,* 755–766.

WHITAKER, V. B., DILL, C. A., & WHITAKER, R., JR. (1990). Experimenter behavior: Influences on research outcomes? *Insight,* 15 (4), 18–19.

WILLIAMS, D. E. (1968). Stuttering therapy: An overview. Hugo H. Gregory (Ed.), *Learning Theory and Stuttering Therapy.* Evanston, Ill.: Northwestern University Press, 52–66.

WILLIAMS, R., INGHAM, R. J., & ROSENTHAL, J. (1981). A further analysis for developmental apraxia of speech in children with defective articulation. *Journal of Speech and Hearing Research, 24,* 496–505.

WILSON, P. H., HENRY, J., BOWEN, M., & HARALAMBOUS, G. (1991). Tinnitus Reaction Questionnaire: Psychometric properties of a measure of distress associated with tinnitus. *Journal of Speech and Hearing Research, 34,* 197–201.

WINER, B. J. (1962). *Statistical Principles in Experimental Design.* New York: McGraw-Hill Book Company.

WINER, B. J. (1991). *Statistical Principles in Experimental Design* (3rd Ed.). New York: McGraw-Hill.

WOLERY, M., & HARRIS, S. R. (1982). Interpreting results of single-subject research designs. *Physical Therapy,* 62 (4), 445–452.

WOLF, F. M. (1986). *Meta-Analysis: Quantitative Methods for Research Synthesis.* Beverly Hills, Calif.: Sage Publications.

YAIRI, E. (1974). A sudden onset of high-pitched voice associated with unilateral vocal fold paralysis: A case report. *Journal of Speech and Hearing Disorders, 39,* 373–375.

YIN, R. K. (1984). *Case Study Research: Design and Methods.* Beverly Hills, Calif.: Sage Publications.

YOUNG, M. A. (1961). Predicting ratings of severity of stuttering. *Journal of Speech and Hearing Disorders,* Monograph Supplement 7, 31–54.

ZINKUS, P. W., & GOTTLIEB, M. I. (1983). Patterns of auditory processing and articulation deficits in academically deficient juvenile delinquents. *Journal of Speech and Hearing Disorders, 48,* 36–40.

Author Index

Subject Index

Instrumentation magnetic tape recorders, 131, 132
Instrumentation schemes for physical measurement, 126–40
International Association for Logopedics and Phoniatrics, 235, 248
International Fluency Association, 248
International Society for Augmentative and Alternative Communication, 235, 248
INTERNET, 238
Interval scale (see Measurement)
Investigation, 76
Isomorphism (see Map-territory relationships)

Journal for Computer Users in Speech and Hearing, 250
Journal of the Acoustical Society of America, 249
Journal of Auditory Research, 249
Journal of Child Language, 249
Journal of Communication Disorders, 248, 249
Journal of Fluency Disorders, 43, 249
Journal of Learning Disabilities, 249
Journal of Psycholinguistic Research, 18, 62, 249
Journal of Speech and Hearing Disorders, 5, 18, 64, 105, 168, 222, 247, 248, 249
Journal of Speech and Hearing Research, 5, 6, 7, 8, 9, 151, 152, 194, 208, 222, 244, 247, 248, 249
Journal of Verbal Learning and Verbal Behavior, 249
Journals in Communication Sciences and Disorders, 235

Language, Speech, and Hearing Services in Schools, 5, 9, 18, 62, 222, 235, 247, 249
Language and Speech, 249
Laryngoscope, 249
Legal considerations in clinical research (see Ethical/legal considerations in clinical research)
Letters to the editor, 222, 235–36
Level of confidence, 203, 209, 210, 212, 213, 228
Lewis-Sherman Scale of Stuttering Severity, 116–17
Likert methodology, 146–47
Line graphs, 193
Linear relationship, 97, 98, 100, 101, 133, 189
Linguistics and Language Behavior Abstracts, 56, 59, 235, 248
Literature searching (see Searching literature)
Loading effects, 139
Logarithmic scale (see Measurement)
Longitudinal diary studies, 87
Longitudinal research, 61, 76

Map-territory relationships, 104–108, 239
Mean (see Statistics)
Measurement, 108–21, 258 (see also Psychological scaling methods)
 definition, 111–12
 errors:
  gross, 138, 141
  random, 79, 80, 123, 140, 141, 142, 222–29, 260
  readout devices and, 138–40
  systematic, 124, 138–40, 141, 229, 232
 interval scale, 109, 111, 116–17, 141, 154, 155, 158, 174, 175, 178, 179, 180, 182, 186, 189, 190, 193, 194, 195, 206, 215
 logarithmic scale, 110, 111, 119–21, 141, 194, 195
 nominal scale, 109, 111, 112–13, 141, 175, 178, 184, 186, 195, 196, 206

ordinal scale, 109, 111, 113–16, 141, 153, 158, 174, 179, 180, 183, 184, 186, 189, 190, 193, 194, 195, 206, 208, 215
 physical, 122–23
 ratio scale, 109–10, 111, 117–20, 141, 156, 158, 174, 175, 179, 180, 182, 186, 189, 190, 193, 194, 195, 206, 215
 role of observer, 122–26
 schemes that utilize electronic instrumentation, 125, 126–40
  data reduction and analysis, 135–38
  diagram, 127
 schemes that utilize tests and structured tasks, 140–42
Median (see Statistics)
MEDLINE, 42, 43, 44, 235, 248
Meta-analysis (see Statistics)
Meters, 129–30, 135
Minitab software, 170, 294, 333–36
Mode (see Statistics)
Modification and shaping stage, 127, 128 (see also Instrumentation schemes for physical measurement)
Multidimensional scaling (see Statistics)
Multiple regression and correlation (see Statistics)
Multiple baseline designs, 92
Multitreatment designs, 91–92
Multivariate distributions, 172
Mutually exclusive categories, 93, 112

National Institute of Health, 289
National Science Foundation, 289
Natural experiment, 76
Negative relationship, 98–99, 133, 183, 184, 188
Negligence tort, 272
Newman-Keuls post hoc tests, 208
Nominal scales (see Measurement)
Nonlinear relationships, 191–92 (see also Cubic relationship; Curvilinear relationship)
Normal distribution (see Distributions)
Null hypothesis, 202–205, 208, 209, 211, 212, 213, 214, 224, 225, 228, 255, 256, 263 (see also Appendix A; Statistics)
Nuremberg Code, 359–60
Nuremberg trials, 272
Numerals, 111–12 (see also Measurement)

Objects, 111–12 (see also Events)
Observation with systematic classification, 160–61
Observational errors, 140, 142 (see also Measurement)
Office for Protection from Research Risks, 279
Office of Education, 289
Online information retrieval systems (see Searching literature)
One-tailed tests, 210–12
Operational definition, 28
Order effect, 79, 81–82, 84, 340
Order of merit (see Rank order)
Ordinal scale (see Measurement)
Organismic variables, 27, 264
Oscillographic recorders, 130, 134, 135, 136, 137, 138
Oscilloscopes, 131, 132, 134, 135, 136, 137, 138

Pair comparisons (*see* Psychological scaling methods)
Path analysis, 27
Perceptual and Motor Skills, 248
Permutations, 112, 113, 156
Photoelectric cells, 128
Pie graphs, 195–96
Placebo effect, 27, 265–66
Pneumotactographs, 128
Population, 67, 68, 200
Positive relationship, 93–94, 98, 133, 183, 184, 187, 188
Post hoc analyses, 87
Power of significance tests, 206 (*see also* Statistics)
Preamplifiers, 127, 134
Precedence relation, 114, 115
Prediction (*see* Scientific method; Prognosis)
Pretest-posttest design, 76, 260, 263
Probability, 27–28, 201–202, 209, 223 (*see also* Statistics)
Prognosis, 28
Psychological Abstracts, 41, 42, 44, 56, 248
Psychological scaling methods, 122, 125–26, 138, 149–64, 340–58 (*see also* Measurement)
 analyses of judges' ratings, 352–58
  degree of agreement among judges, 356
  multiple regression application, 357–58
  reliability of scale values, 353–56, 348–49
  scale values, 352–53
 considerations in the choice of, 157–60
  age and intellect of judges, 159
  computational ease, 159
  duration of individual stimuli, 160
  judges' reactions to task, 160
  maximum length of judging session, 159
  maximum number of judges available, 159
  minimum level of measurement required, 158
  necessity that ratings be comparable, 160
  number of stimuli to be rated, 158–59
  statistical sophistication of audience, 160
 constant sums, 151, 156, 158, 159, 160
 direct magnitude-estimation, 118–19, 151, 156–57, 158, 159, 160
 equal-appearing intervals, 151, 153, 158, 159, 160
  end effect, 342
 as measuring instruments, 151–57
 modes of stimulus presentation, 350–52
  headphones vs. speakers, 351
  individual vs. group presentation, 350–51
  loudness level, 351–52
  number of judging sessions, 352
  physical environment, 352
 need for, 149–51
 paired comparisons, 151, 153, 158, 159, 160
 preparation of stimuli for scaling, 340–44
  acquainting judges with stimuli, 344
  definition and selection of stimuli, 342–43
  duration of interval between stimuli, 341
  equating stimuli for extraneous attributes, 343–44
  method of assembling, 340
  numbering stimuli, 344
  number of times to present each stimulus, 344
  ordering of stimuli, 340–41
  standard stimuli, 341–42
 rank order, 125, 151, 153–54, 158, 159, 160
 representative attributes
  quantified by means of, 152
 selection of judging panel, 348–50

 definition of population from which selected, 349–50
 number of judges, 348–49
 successive intervals, 151, 155–56, 158, 159, 160
 writing instructions for judges, 344–48
  direct magnitude-estimation, 345–47
  equal-appearing intervals, 345
PsycINFO, 43
PsycLIT, 42, 43, 44
Public law 94–142, 12

Qualitative data (*see* Data)
Quantitative data (*see* Data)
Quasi-experimental designs, 89
Questionnaires, 147–49
Questions:
 answering, 3–4
 answers, tentative nature of, 13
 asking questions that are relevant and answerable, 12–13, 60–74
 clinical effectiveness and, 2–3
 examples of how research can provide data for answering, 6–8
 generating, 62–72
 identifying problem area from which to generate, 63–66
 identifying relevant questions from problem area, 66–72
 "importance" criterion, 60–61, 64
 need for selection being relevant, 62–63
 need for systematic observation in, 3–5
 research as a process of asking and answering, 1, 22–39
 structuring questions to make them answerable, 72–74

Radio transmitter, 134
Random assignment of subjects, 277
Random digits, 337–39, 340
Random error (*see* Measurement)
Random fluctuation, 203–204, 212, 263 (*see also* Null hypothesis)
Random sampling, 67, 200, 214, 220, 225–26
Randomized controlled trials, 76
Rank order, 113–16, 187 (*see also* Measurement; Psychological scaling methods)
Ratio scale (*see* Measurement)
RCT (*see* Randomized controlled trials)
Readout devices, 127, 129–40 (*see also* Instrumentation scheme for physical measurement)
Reflexive property, 113, 114
Related measures, 206, 208
Reliability, 4, 21, 22, 29–30, 67, 77, 78, 79, 84, 88, 102, 107, 110, 174, 199, 202, 223, 224–25, 226, 228–29, 232, 240, 255, 348
Replication, 28–29, 68, 76, 90
Reprint request form, 238
Research:
 applied, 1, 5
 clinical effectiveness and, 2–3
 consumer role, 10
 definition, 1
 need for, 1–8
 pure, 1, 5
 relevance for clinical decision making, 5–8
Research hypothesis, 203, 256

Research programs (clinical), achieving administrative support, 285–86
    funding, 288–90
    preparing a research proposal, 286–88
    use of consultants, 62, 66, 291–92
Retrospective design, 77
Reversal design (*see* "A-B-A-B" design)
Review papers, 69

Sample, 200
Sample size, 228
Sampling error, 68
Scales, 151 (*see also* Measurement; Psychological scaling methods)
Scandinavian Audiology, 249
Scattergrams, 96–101, 189, 193
Scientific justification, 62–63, 240
Scientific method, 22–39
    as a game, 23
    as a set of rules for asking and answering questions, 22–24, 38–39
    characteristics, 28–35
        coherence or systematic structure, 31–33, 39
        comprehensiveness or scope of knowledge, 33–35, 39
        definiteness and precision, 30–31, 38–39
        intersubjective testability, 28–29, 38, 240
        reliability, 29–30, 38
    historical perspective, 22–23, 37–38
    objectives, 24–28
        description, 24–25
        explanation, 25–27, 35–36
        prediction, 27–28, 35–36
    underlying assumptions, 35–37
        principle of causality, 35–36
        principle of the finitude of relevant factors, 36–37
        principle of uniformity, 36
Searching literature, 41–59, 68–69, 71
    abstracts journals, 56–59
    bibliographies, 42
    computer-based retrieval
        systems, 42–56
        doing, 45–56
        planning, 44–45
        deciding when to use, 44
Search strategies, 45, 47–51 (*see also* Boolean logic connectors)
    AND and OR, 48, 50, 51
    AND NOT, 48, 49
    BUT NOT, 48, 49
    compound AND and AND NOT, 48, 50, 51
    inclusive OR, 45, 48
    exclusive OR, 45, 48, 49
    multiple AND, 48, 50
    NOT, 48, 49
    single AND, 45, 47, 54
    single keyword, 45, 47
Semantic differential, 142–46, 267
Sequence effect, 79, 81–82, 84, 340
Sheffe post hoc tests, 208
Significance tests (*see* Statistics)
Single subject designs, 75–84, 86–93, 101–102
    advantages and disadvantages of, 83–84
    definition, 77
    generalization to population, 79, 83, 84
    inferential statistics for, 202
    variations in, 86–93

versus group designs, 77–83
Societa Italiana di Foniatria e Logopedia, 248
Sonograph, 137
Split-half reliability, 354
Sponsored Programs Information Network, 290
Static-group comparison design, 77
Statistics, 79, 82–83, 134, 165–220, 293–336
    analysis of variance, 205, 207, 208, 209, 322–29
    association measures, 182–93
    binomial test, 207
    central tendency measures, 173–78
    chi square test, 205, 207, 305–307
    confidence intervals, 201, 207, 212–15, 220, 329–33
    contingency coefficient, 183–87, 213, 301–302
    correlation coefficients, 182–93, 201, 209, 216
    descriptive, 165–66, 170–93, 213–15, 258
    discriminant function analysis, 28, 207, 215, 217–19
    factor analysis, 207, 215–17
    Fisher exact test, 207
    Friedman two-way analysis of variance, 205, 207, 313–15
    geometric mean, 178
    harmonic mean, 178
    inferential, 67, 170, 199–220, 258
        representative studies using, 207
    interquartile range, 179–80, 300
    intraclass correlation coefficient, 193, 354–55
    Kendall coefficient of concordance, 193
    Kruskal-Wallis analysis of variance, 205, 207, 315–16
    Mann-Whitney U test, 205, 207, 310–13
    McNemar test for the significance of change, 208
    mean, 94, 173–77, 181, 201, 209, 214, 296–97
    median, 94, 176–77, 180, 201, 209, 213, 214, 297–98
    meta-analysis, 207, 215, 219–20
    mode, 177–78, 201, 298–99
    multidimensional scaling, 207, 215, 219
    multiple correlation, 192
    multiple regression analysis, 28, 207, 357–58
    multivariate, 37
    Newman-Keuls post hoc tests, 208
    partial correlation, 192
    Pearson product-moment correlation coefficient, 187, 189–91, 216, 304–305
    phi coefficient, 187, 189, 302–303
    range, 178–79, 299–300
    semi-interquartile range, 179–80, 300, 355–56
    Sheffe post hoc tests, 208
    significance tests, 177, 200–13
    sign test, 205, 208, 307–10
    Spearman rank-order coefficient, 187–89, 303–304
    standard deviation, 180–82, 201, 300–301
    table of significance tests, 205–208
    t-test, 205, 207, 208, 316–22
    Tukey post hoc tests, 208
    variability measures, 178–82
    Wilcoxon signed-ranks matched-pairs test, 207
Strain gages, 127–28, 131
Strip chart recorders, 130–31, 134, 135, 137, 138
Structured interviews, 147–49
Structures tasks, 140–42 (*see also* Measurement)
STUTT-L, 238
Subject bias, 124–25, 220
Subpopulations, 225–26
Successive categories (*see* Successive intervals)

Successive intervals (*see* Psychological scaling methods)
Symmetrical property, 113, 114
Systematic error (*see* Measurement)
Systematic observation, 3–5
  filters and, 3–4

Tables, use of, 168
Tacit knowing, 70
Taft Corporate Giving Directory, 290
t-distribution, 209, 210
Test-retest reliability, 353–54
Tests, 140–42 (*see also* Measurement)
Therapist variables, 27, 265
Therapy outcome research, 13–17, 36, 84, 88–92, 125, 158, 165–67, 199, 204–205, 208, 213–14, 226, 229, 232, 342 (*see also* Ethical/legal consideration in clinical research; Research programs)
  assessing for relapse, 267, 271
  choice of presumption, 254–56
  choosing a criterion measure, 259
  controlling placebo effect contamination, 265–66
  establishing a baseline, 259–60
  establishing a measurement interval, 260–62
  identifying organismic variables, 264
  identifying therapist variables, 265
  measuring attitudes, 143, 267
  questions to consider, 256–58
  reducing effects of experimenter bias, 263–64
  research design considerations, 258–71
Time-series designs, 77, 88–89, 260–62
Transducers, 127
Transmitting stage, 127, 129 (*see also* Instrumentation scheme for physical measurement)

Transitive property, 113, 114, 115
Tukey post hoc tests, 208
Two-tailed tests, 210–212
Type I analysis-of-variance design, 95–96 (*see also* Statistics)
Type I error, 204–205, 211, 220
Type II error, 204–206, 211, 220, 224, 225, 228, 260, 263
Typical subject design (*see* Group design)

United Cerebral Palsy, 289
Univariate distributions, 171–72
U.S. Department of Health and Human Services regulations, 278
U.S. Public Health Service, 290

Validity, 4, 21, 22, 67, 72, 102, 105, 107, 110, 150, 223–24, 226–28, 240
Voltmeter, 139
Volta Review, 249
V U meter, 135

Wilcoxon signed-ranks matched-pairs test (*see* Statistics)
Watch analogy, 33
Withdrawal design (*see* "A-B-A" design; "A-B-A-B" design)

X-Y recorder, 133, 134, 135, 137, 138

Z-fold packs, 130